Philips Technical Lib

Principles of Diagnostic X-Ray Apparatus

Edited by
D.R. Hill

To Pat Boyle
with compliments

Dennis R. Hill.
1979

M

Published 1975 by
THE MACMILLAN PRESS LTD
London and Basingstoke
Associated companies in Delhi Dublin
Hong Kong Johannesburg Lagos Melbourne
New York Singapore and Tokyo

Reprinted 1977

ISBN 0 333 17731 2

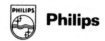

Trademarks of N.V. Philips' Gloeilampenfabrieken

Reproduced and printed by photolithography and bound in
Great Britain at The Pitman Press, Bath

Preface

This technical publication has been written primarily for students of diagnostic radiography, X-ray engineering and medical electronics. It will also serve as an introduction to the principles of X-ray apparatus and its associated medical electronic equipment for those embarking upon a career in radiology.

The authors are actively involved with the design, service, installation and application of the equipment discussed and have written as a team to ensure a comprehensive treatment of the subject on an up-to-date basis.

Acknowledgements

The authors wish to thank Norman Bush for the production of many line-drawings, Malcolm Pyke for the graphic artwork and presentation and Ann Horner for the laborious task of typing the complete manuscript.

The authors are indebted to various organisations for permission to publish illustrations of specialised equipment, in particular Sierex Ltd., London for figure 3 in chapter 18 and figures 1,4,5,7,11 & 12 in chapter 19, and Medicamundi, Holland for figures 1 and 3 in chapter 1.

The writing of the book was encouraged and supported by the Directors of Philips Medical Systems Ltd., London to whom thanks are also due.

Contents

Chapter 1

A History of X-Rays

1.1 The Discovery of a New Kind of Ray

Less than 100 years ago an event took place in Germany which was to have a dramatic effect on science and particularly in the field of medicine. On the evening of the 8th November, 1895, a physicist named Wilhelm Konrad Roentgen discovered a radiation which passes through matter.

Roentgen's "new kind of ray" he called X-rays, X for the unknown. With these new rays he made a photograph of his wife's hand showing the bones and wedding ring. The exposure time required was some 30 minutes.

At the first public lecture by Roentgen, on January 25th 1896, Professor Albert von Kolliker proposed that "these new rays not be called X-rays" as Roentgen continued to name them throughout his life, "but should be named Roentgen rays in honour of the discoverer". Both forms of nomenclature persist today. However, the accepted international unit of X-ray quantity became the Roentgen in 1925.

1.2 Cathode Rays

In 1837 Michael Faraday carried out research studies on the luminous effects produced by passing an electric current through various gases. In 1838 he produced a discharge of electricity through space in a partially evacuated glass tube. Such glass tubes were produced by Heinrich Geissler.

The observations of Faraday led Wilhelm Hittorf, in 1869, to describe "cathode rays" and the passage of electricity in a vacuum tube. Plucker had

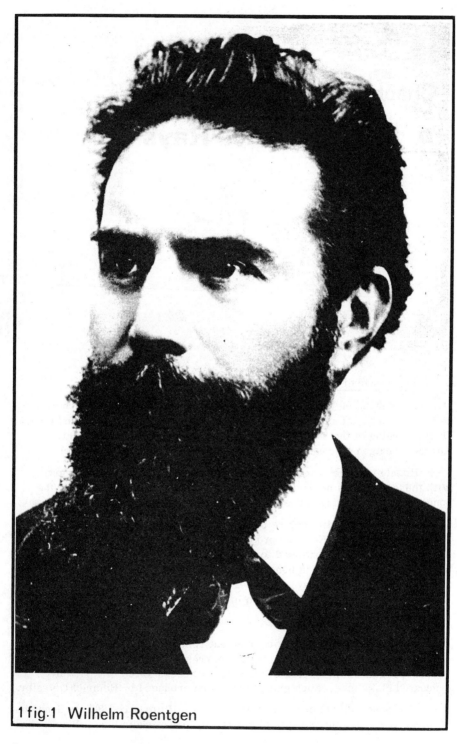

1 fig.1 Wilhelm Roentgen

already noticed that objects placed between the negative electrode (cathode) and the glass wall would cast shadows on the glass wall. Plucker and Hittorf therefore announced that "cathode rays move straight from the negative electrode," a statement which was soon to be qualified.

Shortly afterwards, William Crookes of England became interested in making glass tubes, from which nearly all the air had been pumped, for experiments he was conducting. By 1877 he was able to produce a very low gas pressure in a glass tube, thereafter called a Crookes' tube. Two years later Crookes had greatly clarified the phenomenon of cathode rays, particularly by his discovery that the rays were deflected by electric and magnetic fields. See 1 Fig. 2.

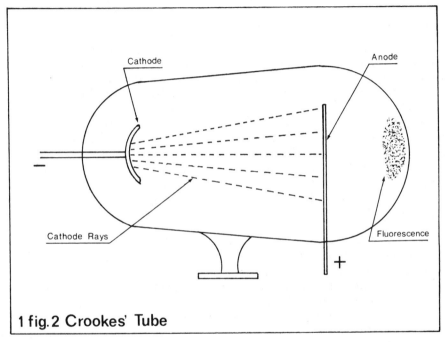

Cathode

Anode

Cathode Rays

Fluorescence

+

1 fig. 2 Crookes' Tube

Crookes continued to experiment and came to the conclusion that "cathode rays are a stream of particles carrying negative electricity . . . . . and can be deflected by an electromagnetic field or focussed by a convex electrode". He also showed that "the particles heat up bodies upon which they fall". Crookes must have been producing X-rays at the same time but they went unnoticed until Roentgen, using the same type of tube, made his discovery at the end of the 19th century.

In 1892 Heinrich Hertz conducted experiments from which he concluded that the stream of cathode rays could pass through the glass wall of a vacuum tube. Hertz therefore believed that the cathode rays were a form of electromagnetic waves. He was not happy to refer to them as a stream of particles.

3

It is about this time that Roentgen became interested in the subject. He was at the German University of Wuerzburg when he made his important discovery. Fortunately, he had a deep interest in photography. Thus on November 8th 1895, Roentgen noticed some objects fluorescing in the vicinity of a Crookes' tube which he was supplying with a current from an induction coil connected to a battery. Upon closer examination he found that the photographic plates were affected by this radiation,while the radiation was found to be stopped by extra glass shielding. The objects which fluoresced, he noted, were those coated with a particular chemical.

It was obvious that the cathode rays in the tube were the origin of the new phenomenon, so Roentgen made his first report of the discovery on December 28th.

1.3   The Early Production of the New Kind of Rays

Within a month of Roentgen's discovery, X-rays were being deliberately generated and studied all over the world by those who had a Crookes' tube. The daily newspapers seized on the news and by the end of the month many interested readers were able to produce excellent X-ray photographs of their own. "The Times" ignored the discovery throughout January and "The Morning Post" was lukewarm, having interviewed an official of the Science Museum in London, who said that he did not see very much in it. The Medical Journals were unimpressed until one interested reader, Campbell-Swinton, convinced them by producing X-ray photographs, around January 7th, among the first to be taken in England. In March he announced a service in his laboratory in London for X-ray photography of patients sent by doctors.

1.4   The First Claim to the Discovery of X-rays

Crookes' tubes were in use all over the world. Dr. Monell of New York, reported that in 1896 Crookes' tubes were available at the reduced price of $7 to $15. So much activity was generated as a result of Roentgen's announcement that it is impossible to sort out all the claims for a "first". Strangely enough, however, the pages of history have to be turned back six years for one of these claims. A.W. Goodspeed of Philadelphia, although accidentally, made an X-ray photograph on February 22nd 1890.

Goodspeed demonstrated the effect to his colleague, Jennings, by photographing spark discharges in a Crookes' tube. He displayed his picture after Roentgen's announcement. However, he stated in 1896 "we claim no merit for the discovery for no discovery was made. All we ask is that you remember that six years ago the first picture in the world by cathodic rays was taken". By 1890 Crookes' tubes had been in use for over 20 years, so X-rays could have been discovered any time between 1870 and 1890. Roentgen's fame is due to the fact that he was aware of a discovery. By 1895 he had been, to use his own words, "interested for a long time in the problem of the cathode rays from a vacuum tube as studied by Hertz and Lenard". However, Helmholtz, who died one year before the discovery of X-rays, had predicted that a radiation would one day be found of such a

4

short wavelength that it would readily pass through matter.

1.5   X-rays, Cathode Rays, and the Physicist

Historical events recounted so far have left important questions unanswered. What are cathode rays? Are they streams of particles as postulated by Crookes, or radio waves as proposed by Hertz? What are X-rays and how do they differ from cathode rays? These problems faced the physicists in 1895.

Roentgen's interest was not in the gas discharge phenomenon, nor was it to continue after his discovery of X-rays. He was primarily concerned with the physics of solids. It was only the challenge of the problem, apparently, that caused him to deviate temporarily from his main interests. In 1893 the subject was confused and only empirically based. Ten years later it was laid open to mathematical treatment based on the concept of a charged particle called an electron.

In 1893, thirty-four years after Plucker's discovery of cathode rays and after much investigation, there was still no agreement concerning their nature. Controversy centred on the nature of cathode rays and X-rays for many years following Roentgen's discovery.

1.6   The Nature of Cathode Rays

It was known that cathode rays were deflected by magnetic fields, produced thermal and mechanical effects on materials in their path and induced phosphorescence in certain materials.

However, two rival theories remained open: the ether-wave theory of Goldstein and the corpuscular theory of Crookes.

Thomson favoured the corpuscular theory and, from his point of view, the position became confused when Lenard confirmed the observations of Hertz, made in 1892. These showed that to all appearances cathode rays could pass through thin foils and produce effects a few centimetres away in the air outside the discharge tube. At first sight the experiments of Lenard and Hertz provided the greatest obstacle to the acceptance of the corpuscular theory.

Roentgen, on the other hand, had been aroused by the work of Hertz and his pupil Lenard, and was consequently a cautious advocate of the ether-wave theory. This caused him to be initially more concerned with effects observable outside the tube rather than with those taking place in the rarefied gas inside. There is no evidence that he provided himself with a thin-windowed tube, but he must have done, for he soon discovered that some rays outside the tube passed more easily through bodies than cathode rays and they did not appear to be deflected by a magnet.

Roentgen had certainly discovered a new effect outside the tube as important, fundamentally, as Lenard's observation that cathode rays could pass through thin foil.

1.7 The Nature of X-rays

Roentgen, working on a wave theory, questioned whether the new rays (X-rays) should be ascribed to vibrations in ether. Schuster was inclined to postulate that they were of a very short wavelength and that the radiation being produced, was most likely, not homogeneous.

Thomson showed that longitudinal waves might exist in a medium containing moving ions, i.e. charged atomic residues. He also commented that "transverse waves would not be refracted" and thus agreed with Schuster. Thomson was able to report on February 15th 1896 that the discharging effect of X-rays was not the same as that of ultra-violet light which had previously been observed. He wrote ".... this, again, is in favour (of the theory) that these rays turn air into an electrolyte". Consequently the ionisation of air by X-rays was established. This principle will be met in the description of ionisation chambers for the measurement of X-ray intensity and radiographic exposure control.

1.8 The Difference Between Cathode Rays and X-rays

Thomson and his pupil Rutherford (later to become the father of nuclear physics) reported on September 17th that "when a current is passing through a gas exposed to X-rays, the current destroys and the rays produce the structure which gives conductivity to the gas".

Schuster's first reaction on the nature of cathode rays was that they were corpuscular and he suggested that X-rays were produced "by an impact" on the wall of the tube. However, Lenard, eight months later was still opposed to the corpuscular theory, and the identification of the cathode rays as a stream of electrons was not proposed for another year.

In his first paper on X-rays, Roentgen indicated that the transparency of different substances is determined by their density. Thomson commented that this appeared to favour Prout's theory of 1815 of chemicals being compounds of atoms, as investigations indicated that each atom shared in stopping the Roentgen rays. Later, when the electron had been identified as forming the cathode rays, mainly by his own work, Thomson was able to give the first satisfactory explanation of the scattering of X-rays on their passage through matter.

Throughout 1896, at the age of 76 years, Stokes advocated the corpuscular theory of cathode rays. Thomson considered the question of phosphorescence of the glass as either being produced by impact of charged particles or by the reversal of the velocity of negatively charged particles. Stokes resolved the matter on November 9th and can rightly claim to be the originator of the classical theory of X-ray production by braking, called bremsstrahlung. The discovery in 1898 of the electron was required to give weight to the bremsstrahlung theory and this honour goes to Thomson.

So cathode rays were identified as a stream of particles called electrons. However, the actual nature of the X-ray was in doubt until 1912 when it was shown that X-rays were electromagnetic radiation similar to light or radio waves, but of a shorter wavelength. This was followed by Lawrence Bragg's work in 1913 which resulted in the absolute measurement of X-ray wavelength.

1.9 Application of the New Ray

To satisfy public interest, demonstration of X-ray phenomena soon became popular. As early as May 1896, a special exhibition was staged in New York using the technique of observing the X-ray image on a screen; the technique of fluoroscopy was thus born. The demonstration that a hand held in front of a screen produced a skeletal outline caused the Pall Mall Gazette, published in London in 1895, to comment "One consequence of it appears that you can see other peoples bones with the naked eye. On the revolting indecency of this there is no need to dwell and it will call for legislative restriction of the severest kind".

X-ray apparatus found its way into hospitals as early as 1896; mainly by the efforts of "queer practitioners of medicine" as they were often considered. In 1897 a patent applicant referred to himself as a radiographer and this appears to be the earliest recorded use of such a term. Many people started to construct apparatus to support the X-ray tube and eventually the patient. Until then he had been comfortably supported on an upright chair alongside a fancy inlaid table (See 1 Fig. 3).

The first British patent on an X-ray subject appeared on 24th September 1896 and was concerned with the aspect of maintaining the required gas pressure in the X-ray "bulb", as it was often called. A great deal of activity centred around attempts to improve the X-ray bulb. The Crookes' tube, which Roentgen used, had an electrode known as the cathode. See 1 Fig. 2.

The tube was pear-shaped and two electrodes were placed at opposite ends. After the tube had been made the air was pumped out. As soon as the gas pressure was low enough and a voltage had been applied between the cathode and the second electrode, called the anode, a current was found to pass through the residual gas and a luminous effect was observed. A further reduction in gas pressure led to the production of X-rays in the glass wall. Positive ions, formed in the gas, bombarded the cathode to liberate negatively charged electrons which travelled directly to the positive anode. The bombardment of the anode by electrons also produced X-radiation. The tube Roentgen used had to be continuously evacuated and it took days to reach the low pressure required.

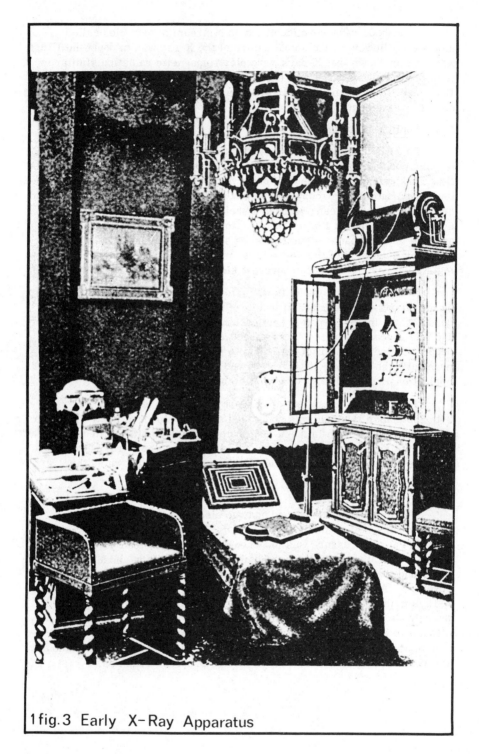

1 fig. 3 Early X-Ray Apparatus

The X-ray tube often bore a label which read "foot" or "upper leg" or some other locality of the human body. A selection of tubes was often kept and the one found to be most suitable used for the particular part of the anatomy to be examined.

In 1897, Dr. Max Levy (an engineer in Berlin) was granted a patent which specified that the X-ray sensitised plate could be made more sensitive by coating the emulsion on both sides of the support, which in those days was a glass plate. He also suggested that plates could be piled on top of each other, if made thin enough for transmission of the X-rays, to achieve a similar increase in speed. It was not until later that Pupin of Columbia University discovered that fluorescent screens could be placed in close proximity to the emulsion in order to increase the speed. Around 1918, the glass plate was replaced by celluloid based film. Today the improvement might appear insignificant but this simple invention ushered in many of the advantages and techniques which were to follow.

1.10 The Early X-ray Tube

Roentgen's experimental tube contained only an anode and a cathode. The advantage of a concave aluminium cathode in focussing the cathode rays to produce greater detail in the X-ray image was soon discovered. In 1896 an additional heavy metal electrode, called the anticathode, was introduced to increase the X-ray output. The X-rays were then produced by the anticathode rather than the glass and anode which previously had tended to melt. The anode itself was retained purely to steady the discharge. As the X-ray tube evolved the anticathode became known as the anode and the electrode formerly of that name ceased to be a separate feature of the tube. This was brought about by an invention by William Coolidge discussed in Section 1.14.

Roentgen, in his second paper, stated "as far as my experience goes up till now, platinum is best suited to generate the most intense X-rays possible". In the same paper, Roentgen described his experiments on this ability of X-rays to pass through thin foil anodes by using a pin-hole camera observation technique. So early on we see serious thought being given to improving the X-ray bulb. Modern terminology uses the word bulb only for the glass section itself.

It was found that platinum anodes soon deposited a metal film on the glass wall of the bulb and therefore tubes with anodes of tungsten and uranium were made before the end of 1896. As the X-rays were emitted from all parts of the tube struck by the cathode particles, the shadows cast by the rays from the tube first used by Roentgen were indistinct. Moreover, if the current was at all large the cathode rays rapidly fused the glass walls on which they fell. Thus in 1896 Swinton improved the design by placing a target obliquely in the path of the cathode beam.

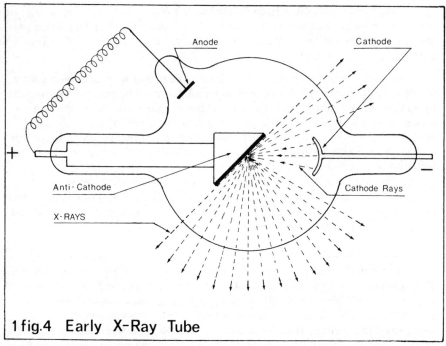

1 fig.4   Early X-Ray Tube

1.11 Improvements in the Apparatus Associated with X-rays

Among the many inventions of Thomas Edison was that of the electric
light bulb in 1881. It was while working on the electric lamp that he
discovered electricity would flow from the fine wire filament to a plate
fixed inside. This became known as the Edison effect.

Inspired by the first incandescent bulbs brought to Europe in 1881 by
Edison, C.H.F. Mueller of Hamburg immediately foresaw their vast
potential and, it is said, in 1882 was Germany's only light bulb maker. In
1896 he began to fashion X-ray bulbs too and in 1901, the year Roentgen was
awarded the Nobel prize, the London Roentgen Society recognised the
superiority of Mueller's X-ray tube by awarding him its Gold Medal
(See 1 Fig. 5). Almost forty-eight years after he had started his own
business he retired. However, the eight years left to him were not pleasant
ones. Like many X-ray pioneers, he became a victim of the radiation that
took toll of so many lives before its inherent danger was fully recognised.

As early as 1899 Dr. George Pfahler, of Philadelphia, believed that he
had probably saved his own life by placing an aluminium screen between
himself and the X-ray tube. This was not intended to protect him from the
rays but to provide protection from the electrical circuits which it concealed.
Dr. Russell Reynolds in England evidently suspected the connection between
his X-ray apparatus and dermatitis of his hands; he therefore enclosed the
tube in a box coated with a lead-base paint. The epilating effect of
X-radiation had been demonstrated by J. Daniel of Vanderbilt University as

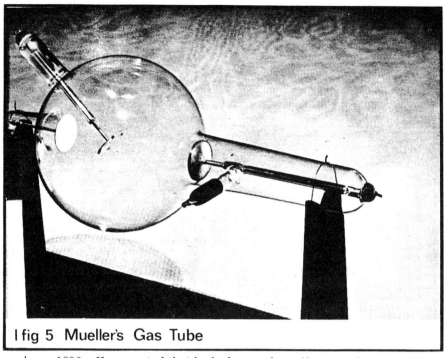

| fig 5   Mueller's Gas Tube

early as 1896. He reported that he had caused a colleague's hair to fall out by X-raying the skull.

Despite these early warning signs, it became common practice to test the hardness (gaseous state) of the tube by placing a hand in the beam and adjusting the current and various other factors, until a good image could be produced.

1.12   Early Attempts to Shorten the Exposure Time

A reminder of the exposure times common in the early days will serve to emphasise the need in those days to improve the sensitivity of the plates and X-ray output of the tube. Probably one of the first military applications of X-rays was during the Spanish-American War of 1898, for locating and removal of bullets and the examination of underlying bones. Dr. W.C. Borden, of the United States Army listed exposure times required with apparatus in use at the front, under fire of the enemy. These were as follows :

Hip joint, head, pelvis	. . . . .	20 minutes
Shoulder and chest	. . . . .	10 minutes
Knee	. . . . .	9 minutes
Forearm and hand	. . . . .	2 minutes

11

The exposures in use today can be listed in the same way but by replacing the unit of minutes by hundredths of a second.

The fact that the X-ray tube was inefficient soon became apparent. Even today it is less than 1% efficient, as 99% of the energy applied to it is converted to useless heat rather than useful radiation. It should also be noted that very little of the X-radiation produced forms part of the collimated beam. However, the output was soon greatly increased by the efforts of those early pioneers. To accommodate the heat, the anode block was made larger and so the tiny square foil anode, which even in those days often bore the mark of having been melted by the cathode rays, began to be replaced by heavy copper blocks with tungsten insets.

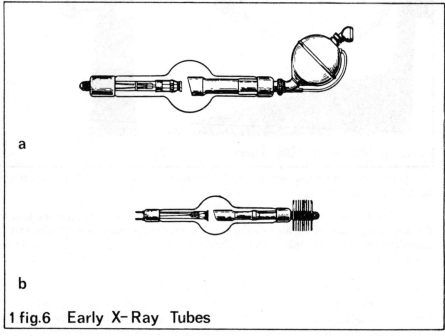

a

b

1 fig.6 Early X-Ray Tubes

Cooling of the anode was then achieved in a variety of ways. At the turn of the century tubes were being devised with water-cooled anodes. Attached to the X-ray tube was a secondary bulb which acted as a water reservoir and condenser for the steam produced (See 1 Fig. 6a). Later, detachable cooling fins were fitted over the anode neck and these were exchanged for cool ones with the aid of special tongs provided (See 1 Fig. 6b). As we have seen already, the need for protection from unnecessary radiation was realised very early on. By the 1930's X-ray dermatitis was commonly referred to as Radiologists' Dermatitis. The therapeutic effect of X-rays was also observed. Therapy with the new rays was tried in 1896 for a skin condition and even for a tumour. In November 1899 a paper was read to the Roentgen Society on the use of radiation in the treatment of skin diseases. Consequently, by 1907, a range of X-ray tubes, specially made for therapy was already available.

1.13 Further Developments of the X-ray Tube

In the very beginning the tubes were continuously evacuated by being connected to an air pump. When it was found possible to maintain the required vacuum they were sealed off. In fairly soft tubes, that is tubes with higher gas pressure, it was possible to see the cathode beam as a faint blue stream. In harder tubes the only visible effect of the discharge was the vivid green fluorescence, excited by the rays in the hemisphere of glass in front of the anticathode. The colour of the fluorescence, which depended on the nature of the glass,changed slightly with the hardness of the tube, becoming greyer and less brilliant as the gas pressure diminished. In those days an expert radiographer could gauge the gas pressure of his tube with some accuracy by observing the fluorescence. Campbell-Swinton studied the phenomenon of the tube becoming harder in use and produced evidence in 1908, that molecules of the gas were driven into the walls of the tube by the discharge. The absorption of too much gas resulted in less ionisation and less X-ray production. So absorbent substances, such as asbestos and glass wool, were enclosed in a side tube communicating with the bulb. These substances liberated occluded gas when heated.

A further possibility of increasing the X-ray tube output, limited by the anode heat, was the suggestion of rotating the anode to present a cooler target area during the exposure time. The task was formidable when one bears in mind that the anode was inside a vacuum. However, in "Revue Scientifique Industrielle de l''annee 1898-99" we find mention of the book "Les Rayons Cathodiques et Rayons X" by J.L. Breton containing a description of an X-ray tube with a revolving anode. A quarter of a century was to elapse before this idea could be realised practically.

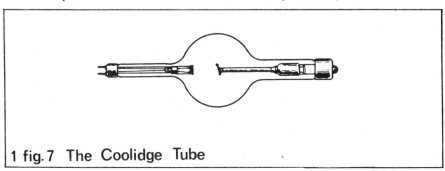

1 fig. 7 The Coolidge Tube

Edison's first lamp contained a carbon filament (thread) but was improved by making the filament of fine glowing wire instead. Platinum, osmium, tantalum and tungsten filaments were all used in turn. As early as 1883 Geddes discovered the effect of electrons being emitted from a hot metal. In 1913 Lanmuir showed by experiments that a hot tungsten cathode in a high vacuum emits electrons continuously at a rate determined only by the temperature. He found that the current increased with a heated filament in an evacuated tube. Against this background Dr. William Coolidge was led to evolve an X-ray tube with a hot cathode in 1913. This tube contained an electrically heated filament which was surrounded by a molybdenum cylinder or bowl to focus the cathode ray stream i.e. electron stream (See 1 Fig. 7). Coolidge met Roentgen in Leipzig in 1895; a meeting which may have spurred him on to his invention. Crookes died in 1919 and, no doubt, was able to witness the progress made up till 1913.

1.14 Gas Tubes Versus the Coolidge Tube

Gas tubes were used for many more years because radiographers at first claimed that Coolidge tubes gave less defined radiographs and that gas tubes, at low pressure, gave twice the X-ray output of a Coolidge tube. However, the hot filament tube was found to be more stable and the gas tube was used less and less.

Roentgen, himself, showed that the penetrating power of an X-ray beam increased once it had been filtered through metal. Therefore, the X-ray beam must be heterogeneous, the more easily absorbed component being filtered out first. It was this characteristic, influenced by the type of high voltage system employed, which gave the radiographer cause to compare the output from the gas tubes and the hot filament tubes. Roentgen contributed little further to our knowledge of X-rays beyond 1897 and died on February 10th 1923, in his 78th year. Roentgen must have been impressed by the progress made in the design of the X-ray tube.

Methods of preventing the liberation of X-rays except at the desired aperture, engaged the developers' attention and X-ray tubes were housed in ray-proof materials. Thus, for the Coolidge type tubes, lead and lead-glass tube holders were devised. The next step was the screening of tubes with radiopaque materials around the source of the rays. Lead cylinders with suitable windows were employed. The first tube of this type, was demonstrated by Dr. Heilbron in London in December 1923 before the British Institute of Radiology.

This was the first X-ray tube manufactured by Philips. The brothers Anton and Gerard Philips, with the aid of their father, Frederik Philips, had established their firm on May 5th 1891 for the manufacture of light bulbs. During the 1914-1918 war new X-ray tubes were unobtainable in Europe and consequently the practice of repairing tubes (quite common in those early days) was established at the Philips factory in Eindhoven, Holland.

1.15 Historical Refinements in X-ray Tube Design

Apart from knowledge of vacuum work, glass-to-metal seals, getters (to serve to bind gas residues) and measuring apparatus, only high voltage experience was needed to construct an X-ray tube and apparatus. So was born the Philips X-ray and Medical Equipment activity which led to the production of the first ray-proof tube, the Metalix. The filament was circular and the focal size was regulated by a circular diaphragm in the cathode beam. In the first Metalix a conical focus was used to improve the loading, a cone being cut out of the anode in the area of cathode bombardment (See 1 Fig. 8). It can be seen that if the beam was collimated at a small angle to the face of the anode this resulted in a loss of output.

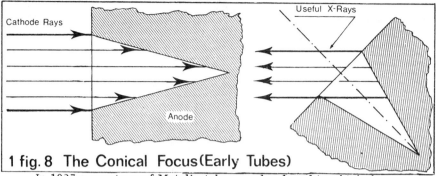

1 fig. 8 The Conical Focus (Early Tubes)

In 1927 a new type of Metalix tube was developed in which the centre part, surrounding the electrodes, was made of metal. The rays emerged through a window in the metal centre part at an angle of about 20 degrees with the target surface. The conical focus could not be employed due to the anode angle and so use was made of a new principle known as the "line" focus evolved by Goetze.

The major advantage was the increased definition of the radiographs produced with this tube as the "apparent" focus was smaller than that on the previous type, yet the intensity of radiation substantially the same. The explanation of this is given in Chapter 8.

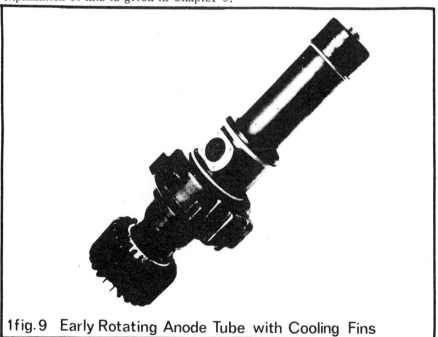

1fig. 9 Early Rotating Anode Tube with Cooling Fins

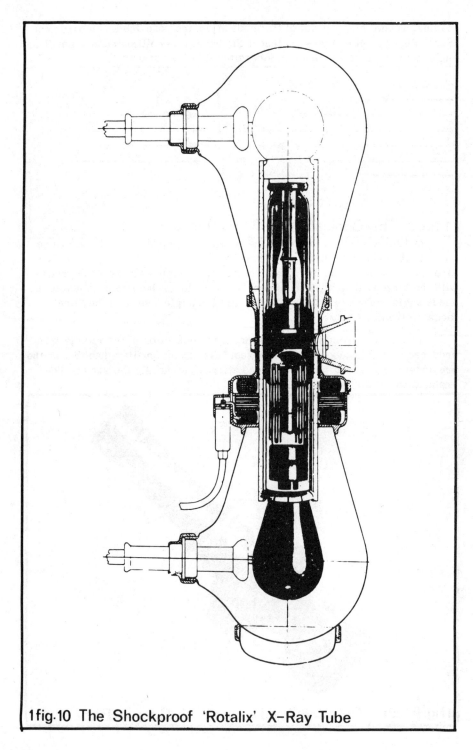

1fig.10 The Shockproof 'Rotalix' X-Ray Tube

In an effort to increase the X-ray output from the tube following Breton's suggestion of 1898, a tube with a rotating anode was devised. This was demonstrated by E. Pohl in 1928.

In 1929 the first rotating anode tube made by Philips , aptly named the Rotalix, was launched (See 1 Fig. 9). The rotating anode of this tube was a long copper cylinder with a tungsten face. It was not until later that the tungsten disc anode appeared.

In 1930 the first double-focus Rotalix tube was introduced. The smaller focus could be used for finer definition and the larger focus when a higher loading was required. Protection from electrical hazards was also provided by metal shields. An example is shown in 1 Fig. 10.

The focus size of the X-ray tube partly determines the degree of definition produced in the radiographic image. Consequently over the years attempts were made to obtain higher and higher X-ray output from smaller and smaller target area. A practical tube was manufactured which had an effective focal size of 0.3 mm^2 and tube shields filled with oil for insulation were also available before the second World War. This enabled the manufacturer to make shields smaller in size.

In 1926 a Dr. Barry examined radiographically the mummy of Tutankhamen, the 18th Dynasty Pharaoh who reigned from 1339 BC, and established that death had occurred at the age of 18 years. Many discoveries have been made with the aid of Roentgen's rays, not least of those being the function or malfunction of the human body in time to save a life.

Chapter 2

Radiation Physics

2.1 Atomic Structure

The intention here is to stress those aspects which have the closest association with the apparatus used for production and application of X-rays. The model of an atom, in which the nucleus occupies a central position surrounded by electrons in orbit, is well known to the student of elementary physics (See 2 Fig. 1.). Perhaps it is as well to stress that this model is by no means perfect as the following description illustrates. The nucleus of the atom has a positive electrical charge upon it both equal and opposite to the sum of charges on all the electrons of that atom. So it would seem that, unless energy is continually supplied to the atom, the electrons would eventually move towards the nucleus under electrostatic (and gravitational) attraction. Yet this does not happen and so the quantum theory is put forward as an explanation which produces a more complex mathematical model. However, we will employ the simpler orbital one as our image of the atom.

It is accepted that electrons move around the nucleus so that electro-static attraction balances with the centrifugal force. The electron moves in these paths without loss of energy by radiation and only well defined paths are allowed. If we imagine a space-ship in orbit around the earth it is a fact that, by expenditure of energy, the orbit radius is increased. So too the electron can "jump" from one orbital path to another by absorbing or emitting energy. If it moves closer to the nucleus it emits energy: if it

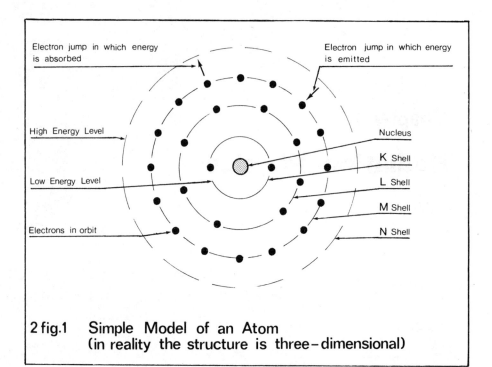

Electron jump in which energy is absorbed

Electron jump in which energy is emitted

High Energy Level

Nucleus

K Shell

Low Energy Level

L Shell

M Shell

Electrons in orbit

N Shell

2 fig.1   Simple Model of an Atom
(in reality the structure is three-dimensional)

moves away from the nucleus it absorbs energy. It is found that each
orbital path can be assigned an energy level and that the energy absorbed
or emitted when the electron "jumps" is equal to the difference in energy
levels between the two paths. So the electrons can be made to absorb or
emit energy. The radiated energy will be characteristic of the atom
involved and is thus referred to as characteristic radiation. It will have a
well defined wavelength which we will see is related to its energy. Energy
is also emitted when a free electron is retarded and travels at a reduced
velocity after a collision. This will produce radiated energy of many
different wavelengths.

The electron paths or shells described above have been labelled
K, L, M, etc., as shown in 2 Fig. 1 and each shell is known to contain a
specific maximum number of electrons. Atomic physics now uses a more
detailed nomenclature to identify the electron shell, as it is known that no
two electrons within the atom can have the same energy.

It should be noted that the energy of an electron in a particular
path (state) is constant. The shell is more like a cloud path as the electron
of one state will be found at various distances from the nucleus at different
times. However, its total energy is always constant. As it moves away
from the nucleus but within the same shell its potential energy increases
but its kinetic energy decreases. When it moves from one shell to another,
it must be supplied with energy or release energy. Although the outer

shells contain electrons with the highest energy it is electron movement between the inner-most shells which releases (or absorbs) the most energy. The reason for this is that the energy level differences between neighbouring shells are greater for those shells closest to the nucleus. When an electron changes shells the energy released (or absorbed) is a measure of the energy difference between the shells and not related directly to the energy level of the shell occupied or vacated. An electron which has absorbed energy and leaves a vacancy in an atomic shell produces an atom which is termed excited. At the earliest opportunity the electron in the excited state will re-occupy a lower vacant energy level with release of the absorbed energy.

2.2 Electromagnetic Radiations

It has been stated that the electron emits energy under certain conditions and a wavelength is assigned to the energy; but what is this energy? It is referred to as electromagnetic radiation - but why? An electric charge in motion is always accompanied by a magnetic field. So there is always a magnetic field around a wire carrying a current.

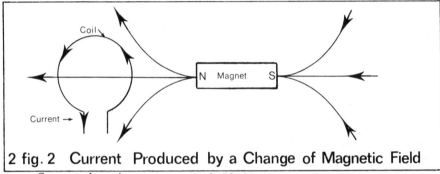

2 fig. 2   Current Produced by a Change of Magnetic Field

Conversely, when a magnetic field changes, an electric field is set up and a current can be made to flow in a wire whilst moving a magnet with respect to it (2 Fig. 2). It is also found that the direction of the electric field is perpendicular to the direction in which the magnetic field is changed and that the electric field only exists whilst the magnetic field is changing (2 Fig. 3). When an electron moves in an atom, from one orbit to another, there is a movement of electric charge as the electron is negatively charged. During transition the electron sets up a magnetic field at right angles to the electric field. The field only exists during the transition state and builds up rapidly from zero and decays rapidly to zero. It is the acceleration of the electron and its deceleration which cause changes or pulses in the fields.

When no current is flowing in a wire there is no magnetic field. It takes a finite time for a field to be set up, at a point distant from the wire by a current flowing through the wire. Similarly it takes a time to return to zero. When an electron in an atom makes a transition between two

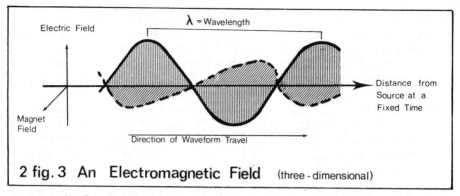

2 fig. 3 An Electromagnetic Field (three-dimensional)

states (orbital paths) the movement of the charge is roughly analogous to a short pulse of current in a wire. Again magnetic and electrical pulses are set up but not felt at a distance until a time-lapse dependent on the distance. So energy is radiated at a finite speed.

The speed of the electromagnetic disturbance in a vacuum is found to be the same as the speed of light. So we are led to conclude that light is an electromagnetic disturbance created by the motion of charges. Radio waves, infra-red waves and ultra-violet waves are also found to travel at the speed of light and so we find a family of radiations which are called electromagnetic waves. In fact the subdivision of electromagnetic waves by name is not fundamental but purely for convenience. The only difference is their wavelengths and, of course, their different effects. For example we cannot see radio waves, but we can "see" light waves. We cannot see infra-red rays but they do affect photographic emulsions.

We can now bring into perspective X-rays and gamma-rays which also belong to the same family of electromagnetic radiation. Fundamentally they are no different to light except that they are of shorter wavelength and have the property of greater penetration through media. One of their properties is also the ability to affect a photographic emulsion and produce a latent image in the same way as light. However, the eye will not respond to X-rays and so they are invisible. (See 2 Fig. 4).

Sound waves, it should be noted, do not belong to the same family.

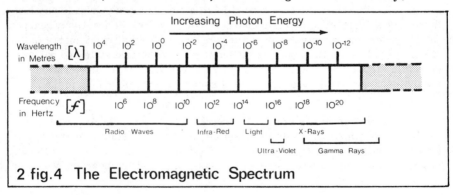

2 fig.4 The Electromagnetic Spectrum

They are not electromagnetic radiations. They require a medium in which to travel whereas light, X-ray and gamma waves can travel happily through a vacuum.

2.3 Waves and Quanta

We have referred to electromagnetic radiations as waves. Waves can be composed of particles. Waves on the sea are an example of this effect and sound waves a less obvious one. Are X-ray waves and light waves made of particles? As they do not require a medium through which to travel it seems that they are not of a particle nature. However, when they react with matter, e.g. to produce photographic effects, they do seem to act as particles, as energy and momentum are conserved in such inter-actions. On the other hand the wave theory accounts for their propagation.

From the discussion in Section 3.3 of photo-electric emission (the release of electrons from a material by an incident radiation) it will be seen that electromagnetic radiation appears to be propagated in small localised packets, which are called photons. The energy in these packets is found to be related to the wavelength of the particular radiation. The photons therefore consist of a definite burst, or quantum, of energy. As the waves travel at a constant speed in a vacuum the following relationship can be expressed :

$$V = f \lambda$$

Where V is the speed of the wave in a vacuum
λ is the distance between crests (wavelength)
f is the number of complete cycles which pass a point in one second (frequency)

The frequency, and therefore the energy, of the photon is determined by the motion of the charge. A warm body i.e. a body in which the atoms are vibrating and therefore electron charges are in motion, (temperature being a measure of the vibration), may emit infra-red radiation of low energy or long wavelength. As the body is heated photons of a higher energy are emitted: their wavelength is now shorter. If the body is heated further characteristic radiation may be emitted through electron jumps within the atom.

What actually happens is that the body absorbs energy (e.g. in form of heat) and releases it in the form of light. If we bombard an atom with a high energy electron i.e. accelerated electron , the kinetic energy may be absorbed by the atom and released in other forms such as heat or X-radiation. The energy of the bombarding electrons is converted into other forms of energy in three distinct ways.

Firstly the electron can be completely stopped or reduced in speed by progressive collisions. A complete stop will release its energy in one packet or quantum whose energy will be determined by the original velocity of the electron. A partial reduction in velocity will release a packet of lower energy. Secondly the incident electron may knock an atom's electron out of its orbit. The gap produced is then filled by an electron falling from an outer orbit which thus releases a characteristic quantum of energy. Thirdly energy from slow moving electrons which have been subjected to various collisions will be released as heat. A hot body is simply one in which the atoms are in vigorous motion. In fact a large proportion of the energy expended in the production of X-rays is formed into heat and causes problems in the design of radiographic equipment for the production of intense beams of X-radiation. More than 99% of the electrical energy required for the production of X-rays is converted into heat.

2.4   General Properties of Electromagnetic Radiation

Electromagnetic radiation has the following properties:-

a)   It travels in straight lines.
b)   Its intensity obeys the inverse square law (discussed in 5.11).
c)   It is not deflected by a magnetic field.
d)   It can be transmitted through a vacuum.
e)   It is subject to diffraction and interference effects.

X-radiation has a wavelength in the region of 10^{-10} metres or a frequency of 10^{18} Hz (cycles per second). The wavelengths and frequencies for other types of electromagnetic radiation are given in 2 Fig. 4 . The interference phenomenon exhibited by X-radiation makes holographic radiography to be possible

Holography is a modern imaging technique which produces a truly three-dimensional recorded image. In an ordinary photographic camera a lens is used to focus the light rays which have spread out from an object (See 2 Fig. 5a). It is not possible to obtain a recognisable image on the film if we dispense with the lens. For example, no image is produced if we place the film behind the shutter but without a lens. We must be losing something in the registering process as the light there does contain all the information, which is proved by the image formed on the insertion of a lens. In holography a monochromatic coherent reference wave (light or X-ray radiation of one wavelength) is superimposed on the scattered wave from the object and the resultant interference pattern recorded on film (See 2 Fig.5b). This film, after development, is called a hologram but still does not display a recognisable image. If the hologram is illuminated with the same wavelength used initially, an observer looking through it, will see a virtual image of the object. Contrary to a normal stereoscopic image (a technique also used in radiography), the hologram produces a truly three-dimensional image, whereby the observer can change the perspective by altering his direction of viewing. By moving his head he can look around an object and see parts of the background which would otherwise be obscured. Future 3-D television sets may well adopt this principle.

However, the application of this technique is in its infancy so far as medical radiography goes.

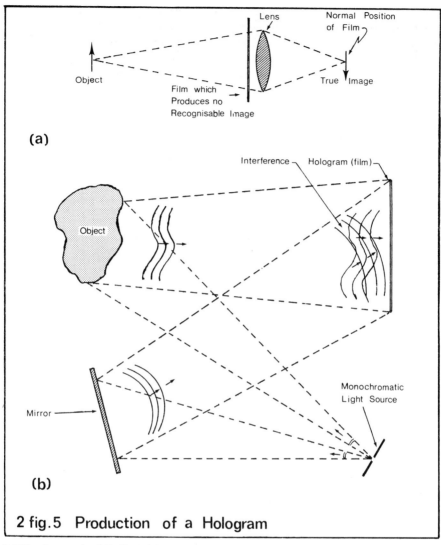

(a)

(b)

2 fig.5 Production of a Hologram

2.5 Fundamentals of Radioactivity

X-rays are also emitted in certain natural radioactive processes. Electromagnetic radiation of a higher energy and thus shorter wavelength than X-radiation is often released during the disintegration of unstable nuclei. Broadly speaking, the radiation emitted by the atomic nucleus is known as gamma radiation and the radiation originating outside the nucleus is known as X-radiation.   Today X-rays can be generated in such apparatus as betatrons, synchrotrons and linear accelerators with energies equal to those of gamma rays.

Unstable nuclei disintegrate spontaneously and emit both electro-magnetic radiation and particles. The nucleus of the atom is very small

25

but carries most of the mass of the atom. The nucleus is composed of neutrons and protons which occupy energy levels in much the same way as electrons. When a nucleon (i.e. neutron or proton) jumps from one energy level to a lower one, a gamma-ray photon is released. The energy difference between levels is, however, much larger than that between electron levels.

The rate of emission is unaffected by the chemical or physical state of the atom. It is only dependent on the kind and number of nuclei. In a particular radioactive sample, the rate continually decreases and the time it takes for the rate to halve is often quoted. The specific activity is the number of disintegrations per unit mass per unit time.

Chapter 3

Light

3.1 <u>Intensity and Quality of Light</u>

Light is the name given to a small band of wavelengths in the electromagnetic spectrum to which our eyes are sensitive.

An incandescent source, i.e. a hot body, will emit light photons of energies dependent on the temperature of the body and in intensity dependent on the wavelength being considered (See 3 Fig. 1). From a cooler body less energy is given out at each wavelength and also the wavelength at which most energy is emitted is moved towards the infra-red region.

3.2 <u>The Light Spectrum</u>

In a non-incandescent source, e.g. a sodium lamp as opposed to a filament lamp, the energy is emitted at well defined wavelengths. In such a source the electron changes its state from one energy level to another and produces line spectra. In other words it emits light at specific frequencies (colours) and not in a continuous spectrum of all wavelengths (as white light).

It has been noted that the speed of propagation of electromagnetic radiation is constant in a particular medium and a maximum in a vacuum. In fact it is in a vacuum approximately equal to 3×10^8 metres per second. The wavelength, according to colour, lies in the region of 10^{-6} metres. Instead of quoting a wavelength, a frequency could be quoted.

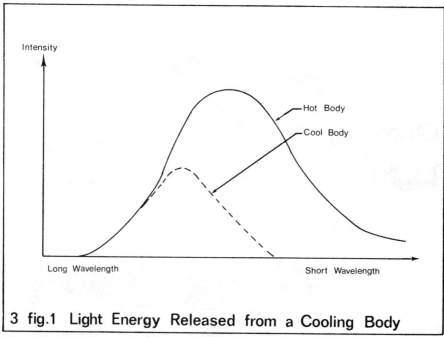

Intensity

Hot Body

Cool Body

Long Wavelength   Short Wavelength

3 fig.1 Light Energy Released from a Cooling Body

If a wave travels at a certain velocity, V, and has a wavelength of, λ ,

then its frequency f is given by :- $f = \dfrac{V}{\lambda}$

Light is a form of energy - both the incandescent source and the non-incandescent source requiring an energy input in order to produce a light output.

The intensity of light falling on a surface is determined by the number of photons arriving per unit area per second.

Light radiates from its source and doubling the distance between the illuminated area and the source produces a fourfold reduction in intensity at the surface. In other words the illumination is reduced or increased according to the inverse square law in relation to the distance. (See Section 5.11).

The quality of the light is purely dependent on the wavelength (or frequency) which determines its colour. Light is readily absorbed by most matter. It may even be selectively absorbed. (A red object only appears red as it has absorbed all the incident white light except the red wavelength which is reflected.) It will, however, pass through some materials such as glass.

Among the many properties of light(such as reflection and refraction) one property of importance is its propagation in straight lines. It is this property of X-rays which also is of importance.

28

The photographic emulsion of an X-ray film is sensitive to both X-rays and visible light. Advantage is taken of this property and is discussed in section 3.5. However, the emulsion is not so sensitive to some specific wavelengths of visible light and emulsions have been prepared which, when handled in a room illuminated with special lighting (i.e. lighting of narrow wavelength band), make dark procedures unnecessary.

3.3   Photo-electric Emission

Electrons move from one atom to another and will, for example, leave the surface of a metal plate thus creating a positive charge on the plate preventing the release of more electrons. Energy can be applied in the form of heat to release more electrons. This principle is applied in a thermionic valve. Light energy can also have the same effect. This phenomenon is called photo-electric emission.

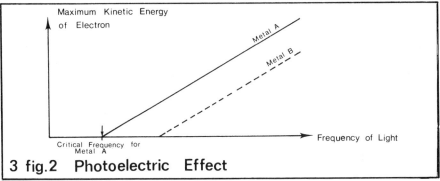

3 fig.2   Photoelectric   Effect

If we conduct an experiment involving a variation in the frequency of the incident light and measure the maximum kinetic energy of the released electrons we obtain a result as shown in 3 Fig. 2.

The following is also found : —

a) The number of electrons emitted per second is proportional to the intensity of incident light.

b) Emitted electrons have a range of kinetic energies from zero to some maximum value.

c) The maximum value of kinetic energy is dependent on the frequency of incident light and not its intensity.

d) Below a certain frequency of incident light no electrons are emitted regardless of the intensity of the light.

e) Above this frequency electrons are immediately liberated in quantity

f) The critical frequency depends on the type of metal.

From the observations listed above it is concluded that light energy falls on the metal in small localised packets. Individual electrons absorb these packets. The energy in each packet is proportional to the frequency of the light. The intensity is proportional to the number of packets or photons.

The electrons being struck by a photon gain energy - some of this energy is expended in escaping and the rest appears as kinetic energy. The least tightly bound electrons emerge with the maximum kinetic energy.

There is seen to be a linear relationship between the frequency of the incident light photon and the energy of emitted electron.

It can be shown that the energy of the incident photon is given by : -

$$E = h f$$

where f = frequency of photon and h = (Planck's) Constant.

As is shown on the graph (3 Fig. 2) for a different metal B (electrons more tightly bound) - more energy is required to escape and less is available from the photon for conversion into kinetic energy. So it is seen that energy is conserved when there is an interaction between electro-magnetic radiation and particles (i.e. when light is absorbed).

As electrons transfer from one atomic state to another, the light is again emitted in the form of discrete packets. These photons are also found to have energy hf.

3.4   The Photocell

A device in which we make use of the photo-electric effect is called a photocell. It can take a variety of forms but principally produces an electrical current when acted upon by light, X-radiation or gamma radiation. The electrical current generated can be used for a variety of purposes. One use is the automatic termination of a radiographic exposure. It may be operated directly by the action of light photons or by X-ray photons causing a special material to emit light which in turn acts on the photocell. This material is discussed in the next section. It should be pointed out here that the device may not respond linearly to all levels of electromagnetic energy and compensations may have to be incorporated to achieve a more linear response.

A photomultiplier tube is often used to control exposure times, particularly where a light image is normally produced for other reasons in the system. This tube is simply a specialised photocell in which a cascade of electrons is formed by photoemission of primary electrons generated by the incident light. The device is thus very sensitive. It is described in more detail in Chapter 10. (10.5.1)

3.5   Fluorescence

The eye is not sensitive to X-rays in that it cannot form an image in the way it can with light. At times we would like to observe a dynamic image produced by X-rays. This requires conversion of the X-ray energy into light energy. This can be done in a variety of ways but the simplest is by means of a fluorescent screen.

Various substances, such as calcium tungstate, zinc sulphide or barium platino-cyanide, emit light when bombarded by X-rays (or fast moving electrons). This phenomenon is known as fluorescence. Some of these materials will continue to emit light for a short period after irradiation has ceased. This phenomenon is called phosphorescence or afterglow. Luminescence is a term covering both these phenomena.

The same mechanism, as was discussed in the production of light from heat, is operating in the fluorescent screen except that the energy is in the form of X-radiation. The X-ray photon energy is absorbed by the atoms in the screen causing the atoms to be raised to an excited state. By an excited state we mean that electrons move to a higher energy level. Some moments, or even minutes, later the electrons will jump to a lower energy level and emit energy in the form of light. The colour of the light will depend on the atomic structure of the screen as we know that the energy jump is dependent on the particular atoms. The wavelength in turn is dependent on the energy. The intensity is dependent on the X-ray input, i.e. rate of absorption of X-ray quanta. In this way a light image is produced. Fluoroscopy is one form of utilising this effect.

It was mentioned above that fast moving electrons will produce fluorescence when allowed to bombard a suitable material. This principle is used in the image intensifier and television picture tube.

Fluorescent screens are also used to enhance image production on the radiographic film. It has already been mentioned that X-rays will produce a latent image in a photographic emulsion. To increase the image formation radiographic film is coated with emulsion on both sides of the base. However, it is not surprising to expect that X-radiation which has managed completely to penetrate the body under examination will happily pass through the X-ray film with little absorption. This is wasted energy and to retrieve some of it we can place fluorescent screens, normally called intensifying screens, both sides of the film. These screens fluoresce and add to the image produced directly by X-ray photons by the superimposition of an image produced by light. As room light would also affect the emulsion, the film and screens must be kept in a light tight cassette. Good contact must be maintained between the film and screens to produce a sharp image.

Phosphorescence, the release of light for a period after the incident radiation has ceased, will cause a lag in the image of moving objects. So a suitable luminescent material has to be selected for a specific application. As the film is often in a cassette some minutes after the exposure it may not be a problem there as the stored image is static with respect to the film. However, too much afterglow (lag) on a television picture tube would be a problem.

There is a variety of grades of screens available. Some produce a higher light output for a certain X-ray input than others, and are described as "fast" when used as intensifying screens, for they reduce the exposure time considerably. However, slower screens often have the advantage of producing more detail in the image as their grain size is smaller.

Another important point to note is that the fluorescent screen emits light of a characteristic colour due to the mechanism by which the light is produced. Consequently, when used together with photographic film, it is important to select a screen and emulsion combination which match. The film will be colour sensitive, i.e. may react more efficiently to a certain colour of light, and so must be chosen to match the colour of the light emitted by the fluorescent screen. Screens which emit a green or blue light are in use. As the cones and the rods of the eye respond more efficiently to green a screen emitting this colour is chosen for applications requiring direct viewing. On the other hand, the strongest photographic effect is produced by the shortest wavelength of visible light plus the adjoining ultra-violet radiation. Therefore intensifying screens used in combination with photographic emulsions usually fluoresce with a bluish light.

Chapter 4

X-Ray Production

4.1   Production of X-Rays

In common with many discoveries, X-rays were produced accidentally as we have seen in the first chapter. The production of X-rays has been discussed at the atomic level in Chapter 2. The technological aspects in their production, particularly in high intensities, is covered by Chapter 8 where the X-ray tube is described in detail. We have seen that X-rays are generated when electrons, travelling at a high velocity, collide with atoms. The X-ray tube is purely a device in which the electrons can first be produced, accelerated,and made to collide with a suitable material which will liberate X-radiation. Here we will confine ourselves to the basic principles of the production of X-rays (See 4 Fig. 1).

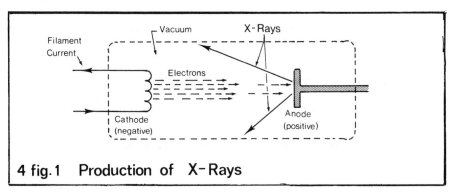

4 fig. 1   Production of X-Rays

Firstly, we have to provide a copious supply of electrons. This is easily achieved by heating a wire filament to about 2,000°C, by passing a current through it, in a vacuum. The atoms in the wire will vibrate so much by the heating effect of the current that electrons will be able to free themselves and leave the wire at its surface. The electrons, being negatively charged, will leave behind a positive charge on the filament (which is called the cathode). So a cloud of electrons will be held around the cathode which will inhibit the release of any more electrons.

Secondly, we need to accelerate the free electrons and this is done by placing in the tube a second electrode, called the anode, which has a voltage positive with respect to the cathode. This will attract the negatively charged electrons in the cloud and allow others to leave the filament. A current will now flow between the cathode and anode. By increasing the temperature of the cathode we can increase this current.

If we make the anode of a suitable material and accelerate the electrons sufficiently, requiring at least 1,000 volts, X-rays will be produced on collision of the electrons with the atoms of the anode. The atomic number of the material of the anode, i.e. the number of electrons rotating around the nucleus, determines the X-ray output. The higher the atomic number the greater the output will be. However, to cope with the heat which is simultaneously generated the anode material must have a high melting-point. Other methods of alleviating this heat problem are discussed in Chapter 8. These desired features plus a high thermal conductivity and high thermal capacity per unit volume leads us generally to select tungsten, atomic number 74, melting point 3410°C for the anode material. Various ways of improving tungsten's role include:- addition of rhenium to maintain a smoother surface for a longer period (a rough surface would re-absorb a large proportion of the X-radiation produced) or coating the surface with carbon to improve the heat dissipated by radiation. In order to employ the characteristic radiation of the anode for special applications other materials can be selected. Molybdenum is often chosen for radiography of soft tissue. Normally with the tungsten anode use is made of the white radiation (i.e. multiwavelength radiation) although the characteristic radiation is of practical importance.

4.2   Intensity of X-radiation and its relation to continuous and characteristic spectra

Let us consider the variations made in the X-ray beam by alterations to the electrical factors applied to the X-ray tube.

A beam of X-radiation represents an energy flow. We can measure radiation by its associated energy. The intensity of an X-ray beam is defined as the energy flowing through an imaginary surface of unit area in unit time. It can be measured in terms of watts per cm^2, for example.

It is shown in 4 Fig. 2 that, as the tube current is increased, the proportion of different wavelengths remains the same but that the intensity

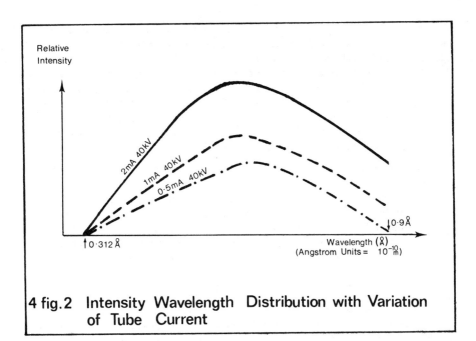

**4 fig.2 Intensity Wavelength Distribution with Variation
of Tube Current**

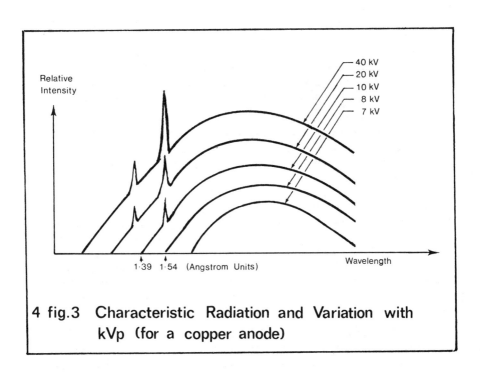

**4 fig.3 Characteristic Radiation and Variation with
kVp (for a copper anode)**

of radiation is directly proportional to the tube current. It can also be seen that there is a minimum wavelength for the specific tube voltage applied, whereas there is no specific upper wavelength limit. Remember that the shorter the wavelength the greater is the energy of the X-ray photon and its penetrating power. It has been pointed out that we can increase the tube current by increasing the filament temperature. Note, however, that this does not increase the penetrating power. Increase of intensity will only mean that the image on the X-ray film will be produced in a shorter time or that the fluoroscopic image is brighter.

If the voltage applied to the tube is high enough, the curve of relative intensity against wavelength will show peaks. These peaks are a result of the release of characteristic radiation (electron jumps between energy levels) and their position and number will depend on the anode material. Peaks produced by a copper anode are shown in 4 Fig. 3 . The characteristic radiation of tungsten is produced above 75 kV and makes an appreciable contribution to the intensity of the X-rays emitted.

4.3 Effects of Variation of the Tube Voltage and Current

We have seen that an increase in the current produces an increase in the intensity of the output X-ray beam which issues from the spot on the anode bombarded by the electrons. It is normal to vary the tube current over a range from a few milliamperes to over 1 ampere. Unfortunately an increase in tube current produces a heating problem in the anode. The area on the anode which the electrons strike will become very hot so there is a limit which must be imposed. However, for some procedures a low intensity is required involving only a few milliamperes to pass through the tube e.g. in fluoroscopy. For radiographs to be taken in a fraction of a second, a high intensity produced by tube currents of around 1,000 milliamperes is required.

The effect of a variation in the potential difference applied to the X-ray tube can also be seen in 4 Fig. 3 . Below 7,000 volts (7kV) no characteristic radiation is produced with a copper anode. As the voltage is increased the electron kinetic energy is increased, new shorter wavelengths of radiation are introduced, and the main peak of the curve (but not the characteristic peaks) moves towards the shorter wavelength. Consequently an increase in tube voltage produces a beam of higher energy i.e. greater penetrating power. Also, the intensity of radiation is increased with an increase in kV even when the tube current is kept constant. Note that an increase in kV will increase the tube current by dragging more electrons from the space cloud but this is normally compensated for in the apparatus by automatically reducing the tube filament temperature. Thus for graph 4 Fig. 3 the tube current is kept constant for all kV settings .

It will be seen in subsequent chapters that the high voltage applied to the X-ray tube is often pulsating. When an electrical engineer refers to an alternating voltage he usually quotes a figure which is lower than the peak reached during the cycle and is referred to as the root mean square value. In the production of X-rays the maximum voltage reached during the cycle is of prime importance and so, when referring to the varying voltage, it is the peak voltage which is usually quoted. This is strictly written "kVp" but on most occasions the p is understood and omitted. When calculating power a careful note has to be made of this point. It has been noted that there is a minimum wavelength for a specific tube voltage. The highest peak voltage determines the greatest speed, and hence kinetic energy, that the electrons will attain during their acceleration towards the anode. The electrostatic force, proportional to the voltage on the anode, is responsible for the acceleration. Thus the speed of the electron is changed by varying the anode voltage. The energy attained by the electron is the maximum available for absorption, and subsequent release, as photon energy.

Maximum Photon Energy = Maximum Electron Energy

The photon energy is related to its frequency (See Section 3.3) and, therefore, to its wavelength; λ.

It can be shown that : -

λ minimum = $\dfrac{hc}{EV}$ where   h = Planck's Constant
                         c = speed of light
                         E = Electron Charge
                         V = peak voltage

and thus :

λ minimum = $\dfrac{\text{Constant}}{\text{peak voltage}}$ = $\dfrac{12.35}{\text{kVp}}$ $\overset{\circ}{A}$

(One Angstrom Unit, $\overset{\circ}{A}$, $= 10^{-10}$ metres).

Chapter 5

X-Ray Interaction with Matter

5.0   Main Properties of X-rays

The main properties of X-rays which make them suitable for the purposes of medical diagnosis and therapy are :−

a) Their capability to penetrate matter coupled with differential absorption observed in various materials.

b) Their ability to produce luminescence and their effect on photographic emulsions.

c) Their ability to ionise gases i.e. remove electrons from atoms to form ions.

d) Their ability to produce biological effects.

As we are concerned here with only diagnostic apparatus,we will not discuss the therapeutic biological effects. However, adverse biological effects which are now well known require measures for protection.

5.1   Processes of Interaction with Matter

The penetrating power is of prime importance in diagnostic radiography. Should the entire body transmit the rays to the same extent, no image other than a silhouette would be formed. X-radiation is, however, absorbed to a lesser or greater extent by different tissues. Bone is far more efficient in absorbing,whilst air-filled lungs transmit readily.

When an X-ray beam is attenuated there must have been an interaction with matter. This can take place in three basic ways :-

a) Absorption (photo-electric attenuation).

b) Scatter (Compton attenuation).

c) Pair production.

5.2 Absorption by Photo-electric Effect

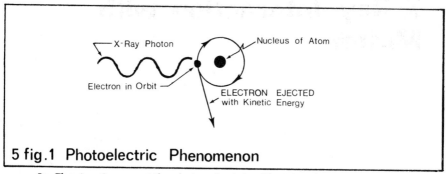

5 fig.1 Photoelectric Phenomenon

In Chapter 3 we met the photo-electric effect in which light photons produced the emission of electrons. X-ray photons can similarly be completely absorbed by an atom (See 5 Fig. 1). Their energy is used to eject an electron from its atomic orbit. Some of the energy of the X-ray photon is used to release the electron and the remainder is used to give the electron some kinetic energy. The ejected electron travels through the surrounding matter where it is slowed down by collisions which liberate secondary electrons and lower energy radiation, including X-rays. The vacancy in the electron path, left by the ejected electron, is filled by an electron from a higher energy level with the emission of its excess energy in the form of characteristic radiation. Photo-electric attenuation is found to be greater the higher the atomic number of the matter involved. Hence bones (calcium) absorb to a greater extent than soft tissue (equivalent to water). However, the photo-electric effect decreases sharply with an increase in X-ray energy. As the tube voltage is increased, greater penetration of the body is obtained as the X-ray photons are of greater energy.

5.3 Compton Effect

It has been found that scattered radiation is produced by incident X-radiation and that the scattered ray has a longer wavelength than the incident ray. (See 5 Fig. 2). Furthermore, the reduced frequency has been found to be related to the angle of scatter (See also Chapter 14).

This effect, Compton Scatter, can be accounted for by the interaction of the X-ray photon with an electron, in which some of its energy is transferred to the electron. The electron receives kinetic energy at the

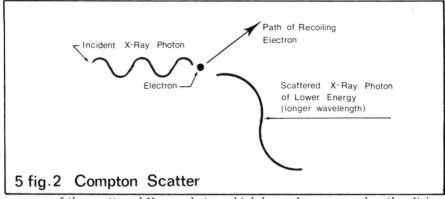

5 fig. 2 Compton Scatter

expense of the scattered X-ray photon which has a longer wavelength. It is interesting to note that in this interaction it can be shown that energy and momentum are conserved. Therefore, energy is shared between the electron and photon. There is a striking similarity between the behaviour of electro-magnetic radiation and particles such as electrons. So electromagnetic radiation is seen to have a particle nature on interaction although it has a wave property in propagation. It has also been found that particles such as electrons and photons in turn act as waves when propagated. In fact the word quantum is used to describe not only the photon but also the electron, neutron and any other "packets". Photons act in a similar manner to other particles when they interact. However, one important difference is that they have no rest mass energy. True particles have rest mass energy which we can loosely describe as matter which can be converted into energy. This is given by Einstein's equation

$$E = mc^2$$

where E = Energy
m = mass of particle
c = velocity of light

5.4 Pair Production

Electromagnetic energy and kinetic energy can in fact be transformed into rest mass energy. This leads us on to the third way in which a beam can be attenuated. If the X-ray photon possesses a very high energy (equivalent to that produced by an electron accelerated by over 1 million volts) it can be converted into an electron-positron pair i.e. it is changed into two particles. The positron is similar to an electron in mass but has a positive charge. However, in diagnostic energy levels we will not meet this effect, as the tube voltage rarely exceeds 200 kV.

5.5 Ionisation

When an incident photon removes an electron from its atom, it will produce a positively charged ion and a free negatively charged electron. The electron is normally bound to the atom but the energy surrendered by the photon enables it to free itself. The free electron may even have enough excess kinetic energy to free other electrons in a gas. So with a given quantity of X-rays (number of quanta), hardness (wavelength of quanta) and a given density of gas particles, a certain number of atoms can be ionised. This ionisation will make the gas conductive. The effect can be used to measure X-ray intensity or control exposures. We have, of course, met ionisation during the account of the photo-electric effect.

5.6   Factors Affecting the Transmission of a Homogeneous Beam

Since practically all diagnostic X-ray tubes have tungsten anodes and are operated at a range of high tensions, it should be remembered that the X-ray beams used are heterogeneous, consisting of hard (short wavelength) and soft (long wavelength) components. The radiation spectrum is continuous from the minimum wavelength determined by the maximum tension. In addition, a line spectrum of characteristic radiation (a function of the anode material) is superimposed upon the continuous spectrum.

If we have a monochromatic beam of light i.e. a beam of one wave-length or colour, then it is possible to block completely this light with a filter which absorbs that wavelength. However, if we have polychromatic light (mixture of wavelengths) the same filter would transmit most of the light except the particular colour it is designed to absorb. The same principle applies to our heterogeneous X-ray beam.

For much of the following discussion we must simplify matters by considering the X-ray beam as consisting of one wavelength. The production of X-radiation has been explained briefly. Now let us consider more deeply its absorption.

Many of us are familiar with the blue to violet colour of light which comes from a mercury vapour lamp. So let us use this to demonstrate absorption of radiation. The characteristic colour of light from the mercury lamp has its origins in the very atoms of the mercury. Electrons change to a lower energy level and emit light of a wavelength related to the energy jump. The packet of energy (photon of light) released is of the exact amount required to push an electron in any other mercury atom from that same lower level to the higher level. If it does achieve this, then the photon is absorbed. If the photon found its way into another type of atom, say sodium, its energy may not fit so conveniently. It might have insufficient energy to cause a sodium electron to change levels as the energy level differences in sodium differ to those of mercury. So we would expect mercury vapour to be the best absorber of light from a mercury vapour lamp.

We can test this theory very simply by the arrangement of apparatus shown in 5 Fig. 3 . Mercury is heated to provide mercury vapour in a beam of light provided by a mercury lamp. A clear shadow of the steam-like vapour will appear on the screen showing that the vapour is a good absorber of its own characteristic light.

If we now replace the heated mercury with heated sodium the shadow of the sodium vapour does not appear. So it appears sodium vapour is not a good absorber of light from a mercury lamp. Perhaps you are not convinced that we managed to create a sodium vapour in our experiment and hence no

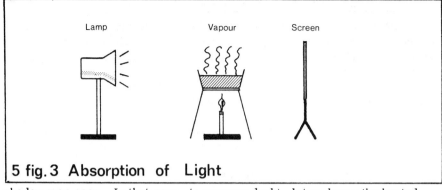

5 fig. 3 Absorption of   Light

shadow was seen. In that case, to remove doubt, let us leave the heated
sodium in place and change the lamp for a sodium lamp. The roles are now
reversed but the principles are still the same. We now find that a shadow
of the sodium vapour is produced by the characteristic sodium line spectrum.

Turning now to our X-ray beam, it follows that tungsten would be the
best absorber of the characteristic radiation produced by a tungsten anode.
However, it will be less effective in absorbing the continuous spectrum of
radiation also present.

The absorption of X-rays in matter depends on several factors : –

a) The thickness of the substance in the direction of the rays.

b) The density or concentration of the substance.

c) The nature, i.e. atomic number, of the absorbing substance.

d) The nature of the rays i.e. their wavelength or hardness.

5.7 Absorption due to Body Thickness

The thicker the body through which the X-rays must pass, the greater
is their absorption. A monochromatic beam which is attenuated 50% in a
layer 1 cm thick, will be reduced to 25% of the original beam in the next
centimetre thickness. Only $12\frac{1}{2}\%$ will pass through a thickness of 3 cm.
Theoretically the beam will penetrate any thickness under the law given
above. A few more centimetres of absorber will soon attenuate it to under
1% of its original intensity.

5.8 Absorption Related to Density of Substance

The higher the density of a substance, the greater is the number of
atomic particles per unit volume and the greater is the absorption of
X-radiation by collision with electrons.

In the body, this is demonstrated by greater transmission in the organs
which contain air (such as the lungs) as compared with the other soft tissue,
even though air and soft tissue has approximately the same atomic number.

43

5.9 Absorption due to the Atomic Number of the Substance

The higher the atom number of a substance the greater is the number of electrons contained within the atomic sphere. The atomic diameter is largely independent of the atomic number, so the greater the atomic number the greater the possibility of collisions between electrons and X-ray photons - thus the greater is the absorption. The state of the material (i.e. solid, liquid or gas) is not important in this connection, subject to the densities being the same.

Even the chemical state is unimportant. Unlike light, which is readily absorbed by sulphur and carbon but not by the carbon disulphide (compound of sulphur and carbon), X-rays are as readily absorbed by the compound as they are by the elements. Thus bone (calcium-atomic number 20) is a more efficient absorber than soft tissue (atomic number 7).

5.10 Absorption Dependence on Hardness of Rays

The softer the rays, the longer the wavelength (produced by lower tube tensions), the more readily they are absorbed. The harder they are the more easily they penetrate substances. The permeability of a substance is inversely proportional to the third power of the wavelength. The absorption is therefore directly proportional to the third power of the wavelength. If the relative permeability of bone and soft tissue at one wavelength is compared with that at a different wavelength, it is found that the relationship differs. With harder rays the bones become relatively more transparent, and relatively less transparent with softer rays.

The contrast produced on the X-ray film is determined by the relative transmission. So it follows that the harder the radiation, the less is the contrast. For example, high kV techniques (short wavelengths) are used to produce transparent ribs in a thorax radiograph.

In a radiographic exposure, we have three basic variables which will alter the density of the image produced on the film. For a certain exposure time, it is obvious that an increase in intensity of the beam will increase the density of the image. It should also be clear that the greater the penetrating power of the primary beam, the greater will be the image production.

For the human body, experiment has shown that the exposure value (E) is related to the intensity (tube current = mA), exposure time (s = seconds), and tube tension (kV) in the following way :−

$E = kV^n \times mA \times s$ (where n = an integer)

In practice it is found that "n" approximately equals 5. So for a variation in exposure time, tube tension or current, but maintaining the same exposure value, the following equation must be satisfied.

$kV^5 \times mAs = $ Constant

From this equation it can be seen that the exposure value is doubled by doubling the tube current or exposure time; but that a small increase

44

in tube tension will greatly increase the exposure value. A 15% increase in kilovoltage halves the mAs required. A 15% decrease in kilovoltage doubles the mAs required.

5.11   Reduction in Intensity due to the Inverse Square Law

So far we have considered the reduction in intensity due to absorption. For a variety of reasons the distance between the X-ray tube and the fluorescent screen or film is varied. We will not discuss these reasons here,as most relate to desired radiographic projections to eliminate distortion or to provide magnification. Sometimes,the distance is varied due to the construction of the X-ray apparatus which carries the tube and imaging device. Here we are concerned with the result of variation in this distance.

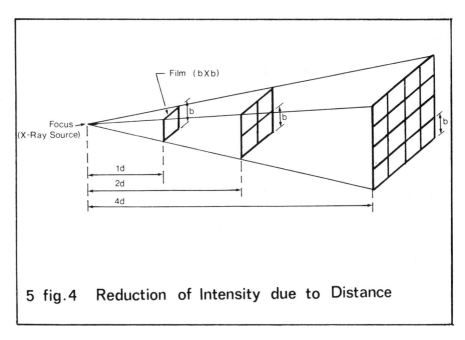

5 fig.4   Reduction of Intensity due to Distance

In 5 Fig. 4 we have a representation of a square film of area b x b which is at a distance d from the X-ray source. If we remove this film and allow the X-radiation (or light for that matter) to reach a film,which is at a distance twice that of the first film from the source, we can immediately see that the radiation per unit area is reduced. The X-ray beam is divergent; at distance 2d it now covers an area $4b^2$ which is four times greater than at distance d. The geometry in proof of this is very simple. The reader should be able to identify similar triangles with their apexes at the tube source where a common angle is shared. If the side d is increased to 2d then side b of the square film is increased to 2b.

The area the beam covers at the furthest position is four times that at half the distance. Therefore the intensity per unit area is reduced four-fold. If the distance is increased to 4d then the intensity per unit area in reduced by a factor 16. It follows then that a variation in distance has a large effect on the exposure value.

5.12 Filters

Partial absorption of rays, on passing through matter, tends to produce a more homogeneous beam. The soft rays are more easily absorbed and so it contains a higher proportion of harder rays. (See 5 Fig. 5). A filter which is simply a metal plate or a combination of plates of various metals is inserted in the beam to reduce the amount of soft radiation. It is varied in thickness according to the results desired. Soft radiation is mostly absorbed by the patient and so it is not image forming and can be removed with advantage. The filter also reduces, to a lesser extent, the intensity of the hard rays.

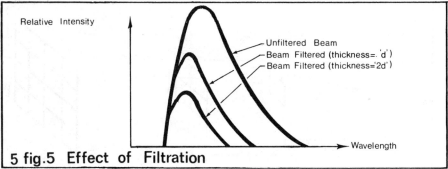

5 fig.5 Effect of Filtration

In diagnostic radiography aluminium is usually chosen. To prevent too thick a filter being necessary, copper is sometimes added. Some metals are unsuitable in relation to the photon energies in use, as characteristic absorption also takes place, which may occur at the short wavelengths required. Wedge shaped filters can also be used to even out exposures when radiographs are taken over a large area of the body which requires different exposure factors in various regions.

5.13 Scattering of X-rays

Scattering of X-rays was met in the Compton effect (5 Fig. 2). This causes an attenuation in the intensity of the primary X-ray beam in the forward direction. However, scattered photons of shorter wavelengths are produced and will be sent in many directions. Similarly, the ejected electron in the photo-electric absorption effect (5 Fig. 1) will travel in any direction and may later release its energy at a wavelength equal to the original photon but in a new direction.

One important aspect to consider is that scattered radiation is not image forming. Photons which come directly from the X-ray tube, through the patient and arrive at the film or fluorescent screen of the imaging device, produce an image of the objects in their paths by a form of a shadow process. Photons, which are generated at places other than at the origin of the primary beam, will be travelling in a variety of directions and will thus not contribute towards image formation. In fact they will cause a deterioration in the contrast of the image if allowed to arrive at the imaging device. Special measures are taken therefore to prevent them from arriving on the film or screen. This is discussed more fully in Chapter 14.

Scatter is produced in both the forward direction (i.e. in direction of the primary beam) and in the backward direction. The Compton scattering produces photons in the forward direction of the maximum energy, the back scatter having the minimum energy (longest wavelength). The wavelength increases as a function of the scattering angle. The intensity of scattered radiation is also greatest in the forward direction but its relative intensity at various scatter angles alters with the wavelength of the primary beam. For high energy photons, almost all the scatter is in the forward direction. For softer radiation, the proportion to the side and rear increases.

Attenuation of the primary beam is therefore by absorption and scatter. However, the relation between these two attenuation factors varies according to the wavelength of the primary beam and the atomic number of the absorbing body. For all objects, an increase in photon energy produces an increase in the amount of scatter, compared with the amount absorbed. For elements with a low atomic number the tendency to scatter rather than absorb, is realised at lower photon energies than is the case for heavier elements. The term preferred by the International Commission for Radiological Units for absorption is, in fact, "attenuation".

Chapter 6

X-Ray Measurements

6.1 Biological Effects of X-rays

It is generally accepted that all ionising radiation is harmful. All
life forms have been subjected to nuclear radiation since the earth was
formed and even today man-made radiation only accounts for a small part
of that received by the population. A granite house can give as much
as three times the radiation to its inhabitants compared with a brick house.
In India there is a district where the natural background radiation is 10
times as great as the world average. Yet, despite all this variance, no
one has any figures to prove that it is more dangerous to live in an area
of high natural radiation level.

The biological effects of ionising radiations are threefold:-
short term (e.g. radiation sickness), long term (e.g. leukemia) and
genetic (e.g. congenital malformation). Experiments cannot be conducted
on man but those carried out on animals seem to indicate that there is no
threshold beyond which biological effects take place. The so-called safe
dose has continually been revised downwards over the years since its
establishment by the International Commission on Radiological Protection
in 1928.

The "tolerable dose" in 1934 was   1.0 rad per week
The "tolerable dose in 1950" was   0.3 rad per week
The "maximum permissible dose" in 1956 was 0.1 rad per week

Do not worry for the moment about the mysterious unit called the rad.

It is only necessary to note that it is now important to be able to measure radiation and that the amount permitted has steadily decreased. Before considering measurement let us put into perspective the amounts of radiation to which the population is exposed.

	Dose in millirad per year
Local Gamma radiation in rocks	50
Cosmic radiation	25
Natural emitters in the body (e.g. Carbon 14)	25
Medical Radiology and other industrial sources	20
Nuclear fall-out	1
Total	121

Some illnesses can be caused by radiation or as a result of "natural causes". There is no way of differentiating between the illness produced by radiation and one arising from other causes. Only by "observation" on a statistical basis can we establish, quantitatively, an effect of radiation.

The major forms of ionising radiations are Alpha particles (Helium nuclei), Beta particles (electrons), X and Gamma rays (photons). Neutron radiation (being formed of neutral particles) causes ionisation only indirectly. The neutrons remove protons from the atomic nucleus on collision and the protons in turn cause ionisation.

The unit of energy widely used in nuclear physics is the electron-volt (eV). It is defined as the increase in energy or the work done on an electron when passing through a potential rise of 1 volt.

$$1 \text{ Electron-volt} = 1.6 \times 10^{-19} \text{ Joules}$$

This unit is often applied to ionising radiations as a measure of the total energy involved. The electron-volt itself is a very small amount of energy so keV (eV x 10^3) and MeV (eV x 10^6) are often quoted.

The photon energy (i.e. the energy contained by an individual photon) provides an indication of the penetrating power of the ionising radiation. The higher the photon energy (often termed in MeV) the greater the penetrating power.

Therapeutic apparatus, in which ionising radiation is used for treatment purposes, uses either :-

X-ray or electron beams (Beta particles from accelerators)	1 to 30 MeV
Gamma rays from a radioactive source (Cobalt 60)	1.3 MeV
Beta rays from a radioactive source	few keV to 4 MeV
Diagnostic and superficial therapy apparatus (X-rays)	few keV to 250 keV

All ionising radiations lose energy in their passage through matter by processes which produce ion pairs, either as primary or secondary effects. The major component (70%) of all biological tissue is water and the process in tissue is represented by the equation.

$$H_2O + \text{energy} \longrightarrow H\cdot + OH\cdot$$

where H• and OH•are "free radicals" and are not quite the same as normal ions, H^+ and OH^-. They have different electron configurations and are more chemically reactive. The free radicals (or ion pairs) are the sources of the biological effects of ionising radiations.

The main difference in the various radiations is their range in tissue, that is the depth of penetration and the way in which they form free radicals and thus lose energy along their paths.

In contrast with the short range of Alpha particles or low energy Beta particles, X-rays, gamma rays and neutrons can penetrate very much more deeply.

This chapter commenced with a discussion of the harmful effects of radiation but has also introduced the therapeutic side. The advantages to be gained by risking a small amount of exposure to radiation for diagnostic purposes are undeniable. Therefore a balanced attitude must be taken towards exposure to radiation. Units must be defined for its physical and biological effects and some attempts made at measuring these quantities.

Radiation terms are often meaningless to everyone but the nuclear physicist. However, terms exist and it is helpful to try to understand them.

6.2 The Curie (Ci)

A curie is the unit of radioactivity. The simplest definition is that it is the amount of radioactivity in one gramme of radium. That may be an unsatisfactory definition to those not used to handling radium.

Another definition of the curie is that it is the quantity of a radioactive substance which decays at the rate of 3.7×10^{10} disintegrations per second. Every second that number of atoms emit high velocity sub-atomic particles which form nuclear radiation.

6.3 The Roentgen (R)

The roentgen is the unit of radiation exposure. Radiation dose is a measure of the amount of energy absorbed and is not strictly the same. The roentgen is defined as the amount of X-radiation which will produce 2.08×10^9 ion pairs per cubic centimetre of air at standard temperature ($0°$ C) and pressure (760 mm Hg at sea level and latitude $45°$). The milliroentgen (mR) is 1/1000R and the microroentgen (μR) is 1/1,000,000R.

It is known that to produce each ion pair in dry air requires an energy of about 33 eV.

So 1 roentgen (R) = (2.08×10^9) (33eV) = 6.86×10^{10} eV

One electron-volt = 1.6×10^{-19} Joules, therefore the energy absorbed per cubic centimetre = (6.86×10^{10}) (1.6×10^{-19})
$$= 1.1 \times 10^{-8} \text{ J/cm}^3$$

The density of dry air is 1.29×10^{-6} Kg/cm^3. So the energy absorbed per kilogramme of air is
$$\frac{1.10 \times 10^{-8}}{1.29 \times 10^{-6}} = 0.85 \times 10^{-2} \text{ J/Kg}$$

In tissue (or water) the absorption is about 0.97×10 J/kg.
Thus a roentgen could be defined as that amount of radiation that produces absorption in tissue of 0.97×10^{-2} J/kg.
(Note. Capital R is now officially used to denote the roentgen. Older text-books used the small 'r').

6.4 The Rad

The roentgen applies only to X-rays. The rad is now the preferred unit for absorbed radiation dose and is applicable to all radiations.

One rad is the radiation dose which will result in an energy absorption of 1.0×10^{-2} J/kg in the irradiated material. For X-rays the rad and the roentgen are almost numerically the same. (It should be noted that the units employed here and throughout this book are the now preferred S.I. units. For this reason some readers may have failed to recognise the definitions of the units).

6.5 Relation Between the Roentgen and the Rad

Although the amount of X-rays expressed in roentgens is often called the dose, it should be remembered that the unit is a purely physical measure of the quantity of radiation and is not a measure of dosage in the medical sense. The International Commission on Radiological Units has defined the absorbed dose, in rads, of any radiation by the amount of energy imparted to matter by ionising particles per unit mass of irradiated material, at the place of interest.

The rad cannot be used in relation to primary radiation as an independent physical unit of quantity. One rad of absorbed X-ray energy in different kinds of material corresponds to different quantities of incident X-radiation.

The relation between the exposure in roentgens and the dose in rads is given by :-

absorbed dose in rads = exposure in roentgens x 0.834 x F

where F is a factor which is dependent on the photon energy and the absorbing material. Throughtout the conventional diagnostic X-ray energy range F is almost constant. This means that, for these energies, the absorbed dose in human tissue (expressed in rads) is constantly proportional to the exposure in roentgens. This explains why the roentgen has given adequate indication of the "biological dose" for medical purposes and is frequently used as the unit of dose in a purely biological sense.

6.6.Dose-Rate

The amount of radiation, expressed in roentgens, which is administered or produced per unit of time is termed the dose-rate. The total exposure dose is obviously the rate multiplied by the exposure time, i.e. the total dose is the integral of the dose-rate. For example, a dose-rate of 50 mR/minute given for 10 minutes gives a total dose of :-

$$50 \text{ mR/min. x } 10 \text{ min.} = 500 \text{ mR}$$

Measuring instruments can be constructed which will indicate the dose-rate or the integral dose. The dose-rate can be expressed in roentgens (or rads) per second, minute or hour.

6.7 Intensity of X-rays

It is important not to confuse the difference between the intensity and quality of X-rays. If we consider light for a moment, quality is described by the colour and intensity by the brightness. The physical definition of intensity of radiation, is based on the energy of radiation which falls on a unit-area in unit time. In general we can assume that the number of X-ray photons leaving an X-ray tube is proportional to the number of electrons passing through the tube, i.e. to the tube current. Therefore the intensity of the X-ray beam rises and falls directly with the tube current. If all else is equal, doubling the current doubles the intensity of radiation and, therefore, halves the exposure time for the same total exposure dose.

The dose-rate per unit area irradiated is a measure of the intensity of radiation. Measuring instruments, which take account of the actual area irradiated, are available for measuring the total dose integrated over the entire exposure area.

6.8 Radiation Measurement

Ionising radiations have the ability to excite and ionise matter and this property is employed in their detection and measurement. In order to determine the dose, i.e. the quantity of X-rays administered, various methods can be employed which are all based on the fundamental properties of X-radiation.

Measurement can be performed in two distinct ways. The dose-rate at a given moment may be measured or a summing of all the separate doses administered during a certain time (integrated), may be made to determine the total dose.

A dosemeter can be arranged to measure the dose-rate directly or measure the dose by integration. Many available dosemeters may be switched to dose or dose-rate measurement. To follow recent I.C.R.U. recommendations the expressions dose, dose-rate and dosemeter should be changed to exposure, exposure-rate and exposuremeter.

6.9   Radiation Detection by Optical Methods

The presence of radiation can be determined by observing a fluoroscopic screen. This optical method of detection of radiation is based on the luminescent effect of X-rays. More accurate, quantitative measurements can be made by sampling the light emitted from the screen with a photoelectric cell. This method is used for automatic exposure control and is discussed further in Chapter 10. When employed to terminate an exposure, the device integrates the dose measurements. If the principle is used to control the intensity of the beam, the dose-rate is measured.

The optical method is also the basis of scintillation counters which are used to detect radiation given out by radioactive substances. The construction of a typical scintillation sensor is shown in 6 Fig. 1.

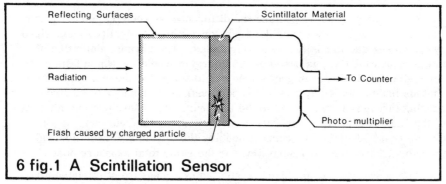

Reflecting Surfaces   Scintillator Material

Radiation

To Counter

Photo - multiplier

Flash caused by charged particle

6 fig.1 A Scintillation Sensor

The flash of light produced in a phosphor by an ionising event is detected by the photo-multiplier. The weak signal from the photo-multiplier is amplified and fed to electronic circuits in order to count the scintillations. Dose-rate can be determined (number of scintillations per unit time) as well as the integral dose.

In the scintillation detector, radiation causes excitation of the atoms of the phosphor. Light flashes are emitted when the atom spontaneously "de-excites". Scintillator material is usually solid but may be liquid, various materials being suitable for different radiations.

Certain scintillation substances have to be encouraged to "de-excite". An example is lithium fluoride which, after irradiation, shows a luminescence proportional to the dose given, only when heated (300° C). This phenomenon, called thermoluminescence, has useful application for integral dose determination as the measurement is stored and can be "read" when desired. The light emitted on heating is measured by using a photo-multiplier.

6.10 Photographic Detection of Radiation

Ionising radiation affects photographic emulsion and its presence is shown as blackening of the emulsion upon processing. In a similar manner to the thermoluminescent detector, the photographic film provides a means of storing an integrated measurement. The density of the blackening can be measured to determine the dose applied. Only a small dose of X-rays is required to cause blackening of the film. A large dose cannot be accurately measured as all the emulsion soon becomes fully activated. Thus the photographic method is suitable for demonstrating presence of or measuring very small quantities, particularly up to the maximum permissible dose range. Consequently its main application is in dose monitoring of personnel exposed to radiation. A badge is worn which contains a film. This film is developed regularly to determine the dose received. A series of filters is incorporated in the badge as the response of the emulsion not only varies with radiation type,but also with the radiation energy. The filters allow an assessment of quantity and quality to be made. The film used has a fast emulsion on one side of the base and a slow one on the other side to enable the recording of a wider range of doses.

6.11 Ionometric Detection of Radiation

One of the most accurate and convenient methods of detection of radiation is based on the ionising action of X-rays as discussed in Section 5.5. X-rays ionise gases by removing electrons from the atomic structure. The degree of ionisation depends on the quantity of X-rays, and in suitably defined circumstances can provide a reliable measure of this quantity.

Air will be ionised readily by X-rays, and this constitutes an absorption of energy. Air is chosen as the ionised medium in practical dosimetry for medical purposes as its capacity to absorb X-rays is almost equivalent to human tissue (excluding fat, bone, cartilage and brain tissue). Air, water and tissue all have approximately the same effective atomic number (7.5) although their densities differ. They all absorb an equal amount of X-ray energy per unit mass and are known as "air-equivalent".

As was mentioned the densities (i.e. mass per unit volume) of these substances differ considerably. For example, the density of water is about 775 times greater than air at $0°$ C and 760 mm Hg. Thus 775 times more X-ray energy is absorbed per unit volume, although the same energy is absorbed per unit mass.

As the absorption is proportional to the density, there is a direct relationship between ionisation of air and tissue. As there is also a relationship between the energy absorbed and the biological effect of X-rays, the degree of ionisation may be regarded as a measure of the biological effect in tissue.

55

The amount of absorption of X-rays in air has a constant relationship to the degree of ionisation and is independent of the wavelength of the radiation. In non-air-equivalent tissue, such as bone, there is not a constant relationship and the degree of ionisation (and biological effect) does depend in part on the quality of the radiation. In fact, in bone, ionisation decreases with a decrease in the wavelength, whereas with fat the biological effect of hard radiation is greater than that of soft radiation (long wavelength).

6.12 Dosemeters (Exposuremeters)

A wide range of dosemeters exist but all consist of an ionisation chamber which is charged and a metering system with which to measure the ionisation produced. A calibration system is also necessary. The ionisation of the air produces electrical current carriers which are used to determine the degree of ionisation.

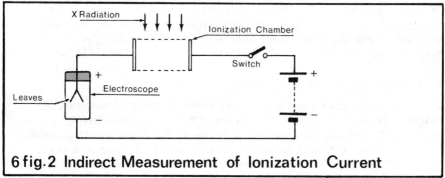

6 fig.2 Indirect Measurement of Ionization Current

An arrangement for the indirect measurement of ionisation current is shown in 6 Fig. 2. During the period that the switch is closed and radiation is allowed to fall on the chamber, the leaf electroscope will charge and the extent will be indicated by the position of the leaves. It is necessary to shield the electroscope from the radiation otherwise ionisation within itself will cause it to simultaneously discharge. Alternatively the electroscope (electrometer) can be charged initially and made to discharge via the ionisation chamber. This latter method is often used in pocket dose monitors and a reading directly made by noting the position of the electroscope leaf against a graticule.

In the direct method the very small current produced by the ionisation and potential difference across the chamber is amplified and indicated on a meter in either a rate or an integral form. The arrangement is shown in 6 Fig. 3.

The definition of the roentgen is based on the amount of radiation which will produce a certain number of ion pairs per cubic centimetre of air. The unit of exposure can also be given in terms of the charge liberated and is defined as 2.58×10^{-4} coulombs per kilogram. This may appear to be somewhat different to the first definition given in this chapter.

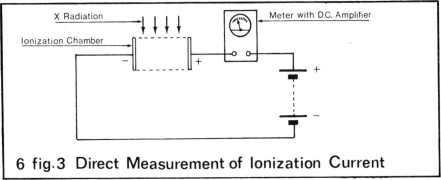

6 fig.3 Direct Measurement of Ionization Current

However, given that one coulomb is the charge contained by 6.25×10^{18} electrons and that 1 c.c. of air weighs 1.29×10^{-6} kg, it is a simple matter to calculate the charge per kilogram produced by 1 roentgen (2.08×10^9 ion pairs per c.c.). It should also be remembered that a current flow of 1 coulomb per second is one ampere. So by measuring the current through the ionisation chamber we can measure the quantity of radiation.

6.13 Ionisation Chambers

The standard ionisation chamber is constructed as shown in 6 Fig.4 and contains a known volume of air. The chamber is placed where the dose is to be determined.

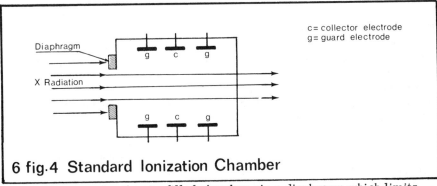

6 fig.4 Standard Ionization Chamber

X-rays enter the air-filled chamber via a diaphragm which limits the cross-sectional area of the beam. The beam forms around itself an ion cloud. Two parallel electrodes are situated inside the chamber. The outer ones, the guard electrodes, ensure that the electrical field between the electrodes is uniform in the area of the collector. The collector is insulated from the guard electrodes and a current will flow between its parallel plates when a potential difference is applied.

In the standard chamber the electrodes are placed so far from the beam that secondary electrons produced in the walls which also form ion clouds cannot reach them. Only a small part of its volume is used in the measurement of ionisation, the greater part being used to allow the radiation to reach equilibrium with its secondary radiation.

Strictly speaking the definition of the roentgen is based on the ionisation produced in a cubic centimetre of air surrounded by air. So the chamber described is called a "free air chamber" and may be used for absolute measurements. The chamber virtually has no walls to absorb radiation and so all the secondary electrons originate in the air. This apparatus is inconvenient to use as it is cumbersome and so has only specialised applications.

In practical exposure dose measuring the thimble chamber is more convenient to use. The construction is shown in 6 Fig. 5.

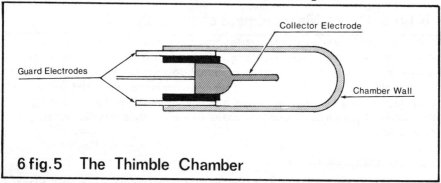

Guard Electrodes

Collector Electrode

Chamber Wall

6 fig. 5   The Thimble Chamber

In the thimble chamber, so called because of its size and shape, most of the ionisation occurs in the walls. The range of the secondary electrons is large in comparison with the dimensions of the chamber and so they contribute a large part to the ionisation of the air in the chamber. Thus the response of this type of chamber is more characteristic of the wall material than of the enclosed air. Fortunately it is possible to construct the wall from a plastic which has a similar atomic composition to air, but of higher density. The secondary radiation quickly reaches equilibrium in the dense walls and so a chamber can be made which is smaller than the free air chamber. It does not read the absolute measure of roentgens but can be calibrated using a standard source.

The true air wall chamber requires walls of sufficient thickness to absorb soft radiation such as beta rays. The thickness must be at least equal to the range of the fastest secondary electrons emitted by the X-ray photons to prevent electrons, formed in non-air-equivalent material, entering the chamber (and thereby providing an untrue measurement of radiation). If a thin-wall chamber is used, true dose measurements can only be made when there is a large air gap between the source and the chamber. When the distance is small, or when non-air-equivalent material is close to the chamber, the reading at worst will include the secondary radiation. Some chambers are provided with a removable section which exposes a thinner window for the measurement of softer radiation. The outer wall is made of a conductive plastic so that it can be used as part of the electrode assembly.

The dimensions of the chamber are dictated by the sensitivity required, which in turn depends on the distance from the source the measurement is to be made (inverse square law). If the dosemeter is to be used to measure the dose integrated over an area, the chamber must be as large as the areas irradiated. The construction of such chambers is described in Chapter 10.

Another version of chamber is the condenser type which is charged to a certain level and placed at the point where radiation is to be monitored. In use, therefore, it is not connected to the dosemeter. Ionisation causes the charge to dissipate through the chamber so that, when connected to the meter circuit, the integral dose can be determined. The condenser chamber can be used, in the same way as the electroscope type, for personnel monitoring, but has to be connected to the dosemeter for determination of the measurement. Care has to be taken that the charge is not allowed to leak in the absence of radiation.

The walls of non-free-air types of chamber cannot be made exactly air-equivalent so they are only suitable for specified X-ray energy ranges. Various versions are also made for intracavity application. However, these are mostly used in the therapeutic field and will not be discussed here.

6.14 Precautions Required in Dose Measuring

The absorbed dose is determined by the intensity of the X-ray beam, the length of time irradiation occurs and the extent to which the matter irradiated absorbs the particular radiation. The quality, or penetrating power, of the radiation is also important and this point is discussed later in this chapter. The problems of dose measuring are further complicated by the fact that the beam is heterogeneous in nature, containing both white radiation and characteristic radiation. Scattering also occurs and the beam is modified in quality by the action of material by which it is filtered. The effect of these is that it is practically impossible to calculate the dose absorbed and empirical methods are often the only way in which it can be determined.

Since ionisation is dependent on temperature and pressure, it is necessary to correct each dose measurement taken. In modern instruments this is taken care of automatically in the dosemeter, settings being made appropriate to the ambient conditions.

The dosemeter, being a delicate instrument, should be checked against a standard source periodically. Some contain a constantly radiating specimen for this purpose.

When carrying out a dose measurement "free in air", scattered radiation should be avoided by ensuring that there are no objects in the beam close to the chamber. Lead diaphragms employed to limit the beam should be flat plates rather than tubes, which tend to produce more scatter, and possibly more characteristic radiation. The characteristic secondary radiation of, for example, a copper filter which happens to be in the beam, can be reduced by a shield of aluminium placed between it and the chamber. The characteristic radiation of aluminium is so soft that it is completely absorbed in a few centimetres of air.

If the X-ray beam strikes an object close behind the chamber, lead sheets should be arranged to cover the area of the object irradiated. Lead emits considerably less scattered radiation than materials of a lower atomic number.

Thimble chambers must be fully exposed to the radiation, i.e. the beam must cover the entire air chamber. Unless otherwise stated, the dose measurement is assumed to be made with the centre of the chamber in the central axis of the beam.

If the intensity measurement cannot be made at the point of interest the dose may be measured at a different distance from the source and the desired reading calculated on a basis of the inverse square law as given in Chapter 5. However this method may well introduce inaccuracies where the rays are soft and heavily absorbed in air, where the beam is not uniform, or the chamber relatively large at the distance chosen. The dimension of the chamber should be small in relation to the distance to the source to ensure adequate cover by the divergent beam. The chamber should also be suitable for measuring both the quantity and quality of radiation under examination.

6.15 Measurement of X-ray Quality

The wavelength of radiation determines its penetrating power, this wavelength being related to the energy of the photon. In practice, every beam of X-radiation is made up of a mixture of wavelengths at different relative intensities which combine to determine its overall penetrating power - or beam quality. The minimum wavelength (hence maximum photon energy) present in the continuous spectrum of the beam is sharply defined.

The hardest radiation (maximum photon energy) is determined by the maximum X-ray tube voltage as mentioned in Chapter 4.

$$\text{Minimum Wavelength} = \frac{12.35}{\text{kVp}} \quad \text{Å}$$

With an increase in tube voltage the radiation spectrum becomes broader towards the high photon energy side. Simultaneously the intensity of radiation increases. The effective wavelength, the average wavelength of the radiation, does not change very much, however.

A filter introduced into the beam does not effect the shortest wavelength but does reduce the intensity. In fact it reduces the intensity of the longer wavelengths (low photon energy) by a greater degree than the shorter wavelengths. (See 5 Fig. 5 in the previous Chapter). The overall hardness of the beam is therefore increased by filtration. If the filter is efficient, for example a metal of high atomic number, the effective wavelength becomes shorter and the radiation more homogeneous as the filter thickness is increased.

If a beam contains a high proportion of hard rays (short wavelength) a large thickness of filter is required to reduce the intensity. If the beam is soft (high proportion of long wavelengths) a thin filter will reduce the overall intensity considerably.

The quality of the X-ray beam can be determined in a broad sense by this principle. The intensity of a beam is measured and readings taken whilst increasing the thickness of the filter in the beam. An absorption curve is then plotted of transmitted intensity against filter thickness and this gives an indication of the beam quality. (See 6 Fig. 6).

Instead of a complete absorption curve, the quality of the beam can be loosely indicated by the thickness of filter material which reduces the intensity to 50%.

The half value thickness (H.V.T), or half value layer (H.V.L) as it is often called, can be expressed in any filter material. The material chosen, to avoid very thick filters being required, depends on the range of wavelengths involved. Below X-ray tube voltages of 100 kVp aluminium is used, above 100 kVp copper is more convenient, and for very hard rays tin or even lead may be required.

In giving the H.V.T, usually expressed in millimetres, the filter material has to be specified as the thickness required will differ for each material.

Quoting the H.V.T is in effect only identifying one point on the absorption curve, the shape of which depends on the relative intensities of all the wavelengths. So two beams could have the same H.V.T but different shaped curves as shown in 6 Fig. 6.

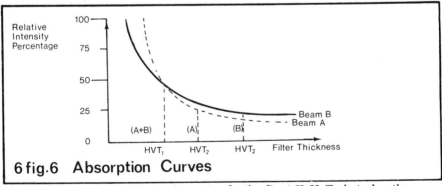

6 fig.6 Absorption Curves

It is more exact to quote, not only the first H.V.T, but also the second which is the thickness to reduce the intensity of the beam by half again (i.e. to 25% of the original).

The ratio $H.V.T_1/H.V.T_2$ is called the degree of homogeneity.

(Sometimes the reciprocal is quoted and called the degree of heterogeneity).

The quality of the beam is fully determined by the peak tube voltage, anode material and filtration (both inherent in the construction of the tube and added by filters). Thus the tube voltage, total filtration and H.V.T. are three inter-dependent factors for a certain anode material. Given two of them the third is determined.

Strictly speaking it is not only the peak value of the tube voltage but also the shape of the voltage curve which influences the quality of the beam. With a constant voltage the average hardness (and hence H.V.T) is greater than with a pulsating voltage having the same peak value.

Chapter 7

Electron Emission and Solid State Devices

7.0 Forms of Electron Emission

A good conductor contains a sea of free electrons, i.e. a large number of electrons loosely bonded to their atoms, which are able to move should a potential difference occur between the ends of the conductor. In spite of this readily available source of electrons, they do not normally leave the surface of the conductor, being bound to the material by strong surface effects.

There are, however, ways in which these effects may be overcome so that electrons can be made to leave the surface of a conductor and travel through space. This is known as "Electron Emission" and can be brought about in five ways.

(a) Thermionic emission - where heat is used to raise the energy in the conductor to a point at which electrons can leave the surface.

(b) Photo emission - where the energy level of the emitter is raised by the absorption of light.

(c) Field emission - where electrons leave the surface under the influence of an intense electrostatic field.

(d) Secondary emission - where an incident electron striking a surface ejects one or more electrons from that surface.

(e) Radioactive emission - where certain materials emit electrons by a process of nuclear disintegration. This last form of electron emission is not found in any vacuum device likely to be encountered in the field of X-ray equipment.

In air the electrons can travel only a very short distance due to the blanketing effect of the gas molecules. To construct a practical device it is necessary to enclose the electron emitter in a gas tight container and then to withdraw the air, producing as near perfect a vacuum as possible.

7.1 The Thermionic Valve

The family of devices known as vacuum tubes is dominated by the thermionic valve. This is a device which depends for its operation upon the emission of electrons from a heated surface. The heated surface often takes the form of a fine wire of high resistance metal, (known as the filament) which is heated by passing a current through it. The fact that current is used to heat the filament is incidental, the heating current being from a separate supply does not contribute to the emitted electrons. In fact the emitting surface, normally called the cathode, could equally well be heated by the application of a gas flame or the focussed rays of the sun.

The process of electron emission is analogous to the evaporation of a liquid when heated. In the case of the liquid, however, molecules are given off; whereas in the case of thermionic emission, electrons are emitted.

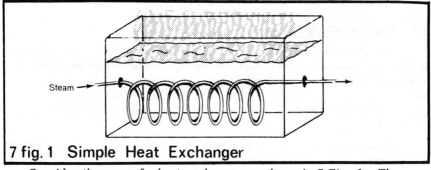

7 fig. 1 Simple Heat Exchanger

Consider the case of a heat exchanger as shown in 7 Fig. 1. The water in the tank is heated by passing steam through the coiled tube. As the temperature increases, the water will start to boil and steam will rise from the surface of the water. It might be thought that the steam is coming from the coil, but this would not be the case, unless the tube is perforated. Thus the water is indirectly heated, and would still give off steam even if the heat were to come from a gas flame or the focussed rays of the sun.

Let us leave the analogy of the water tank and return to the electron emitter, or cathode. As 7 Fig. 2 shows, each electron leaving the surface will travel out, following a curved path, to return to the surface some short time later. This is because each electron carries a negative charge, so that, as it leaves the cathode, in effect it leaves behind a positive charge which serves to attract the electron back to the surface. The energy of electrons leaving the surface will vary widely, although the maximum energy will be mainly dependent on the temperature of the emitting surface.

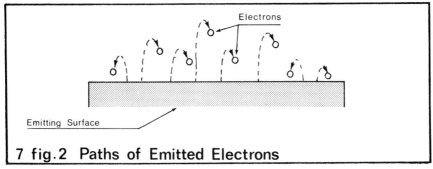

7 fig.2 Paths of Emitted Electrons

The rate at which electrons are emitted will also be dependent upon temperature. Thus a cloud of electrons will form adjacent to the surface of a heated cathode enclosed in a vacuum. This cloud of electrons is called the space charge and is depicted in 7 Fig. 3.

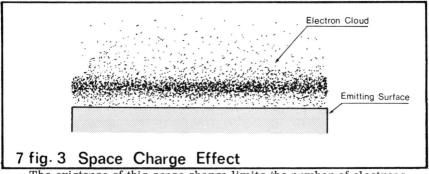

7 fig. 3 Space Charge Effect

The existence of this space charge limits the number of electrons which are able to leave the surface due to the fact that like charges repel. Thus a low velocity electron leaving the surface will be repelled by the space charge and forced to return to the cathode surface.

7.2 The Diode

If an additional electrode, called an anode, is sealed into the vacuum tube as shown in 7 Fig. 4a it will be found that some of the more energetic electrons will travel across to it so causing the anode to attain a very slight negative charge. This charge will not amount to very much since, as the anode becomes negative, it will repel any further electrons. If, however, the anode is connected back to the cathode via a sensitive current measuring device a small current will be seen to flow in the circuit (See 7 Fig. 4b).

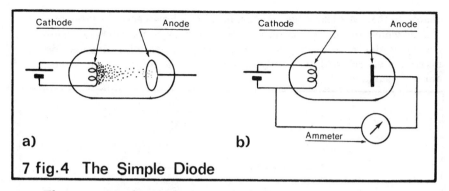

a)   b)

7 fig. 4   The Simple Diode

The current is due to electrons which, having reached the anode, flow back to the cathode via the external circuit. The amount of current will again be small since once more the anode will tend to become negative, so repelling further electrons. This negative potential can be cancelled by applying a positive potential as shown in 7 Fig. 5.

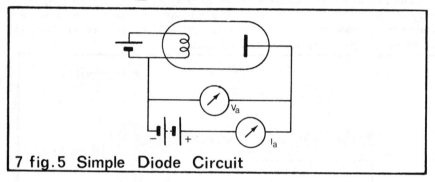

7 fig. 5   Simple Diode Circuit

If the voltage applied to the anode is varied and a set of readings taken, a graph may be drawn showing the relationship between the anode voltage (Va) and anode current (Ia). This graph always has the same basic shape but the absolute values will depend upon the construction of the individual valve. The graph is usually known as the Ia/Va curve, and an example is shown in 7 Fig. 6.

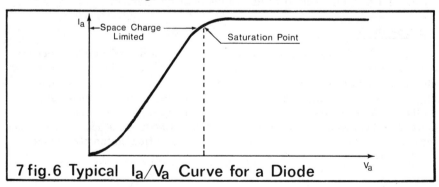

7 fig. 6 Typical I_a/V_a Curve for a Diode

The shape of the curve arises in the following way. When Va is zero very little current will flow as the anode will attain a negative voltage. As this negative voltage is overcome by the application of a positive voltage to the anode the current will start to rise. It might be assumed that, as soon as the negative potential on the anode has been overcome, the electrons would immediately move towards the anode - so giving a sharp rise in anode current. This does not happen, however, because the space charge limits the flow of current. As has already been mentioned, the cloud of negative electrons surrounding the cathode limits the number of electrons emitted. Thus when the anode first becomes positive, only the electrons which are on the tenuous outer fringe of the electron cloud move to the anode. The influence of the positive anode voltage will not be felt in the vicinity of the cathode and so the amount of emission will not change very much. As the anode voltage is raised the electron cloud will gradually thin out. Its effect upon the cathode will be reduced, so that more and more electrons will be able to leave the cathode, so giving a gradual rise in anode current.

Provided a space charge is maintained, the number of electrons emitted by the cathode is of no consequence since the anode current is determined only by the magnitude of the space charge effect. The only requirement is that the cathode should be hot enough to give slightly more electrons than the maximum needed. The valve is then said to be working under space charge limited conditions.

If the anode voltage is further increased, a point will eventually be reached at which practically all the electrons emitted by the cathode will be drawn to the anode. Once this point is reached, increasing the anode voltage further will produce only a very slight increase in anode current, and the valve is said to be working under saturation conditions. This is shown in 7 Fig. 6.

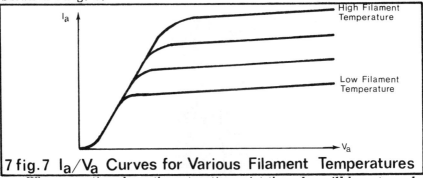

7 fig.7 I_a/V_a Curves for Various Filament Temperatures

When operating above the saturation point the valve will be extremely sensitive to cathode temperature. In fact one can draw a family of curves (See 7 Fig. 7) to show for all practical purposes that :-

(a) under space charge limited conditions the anode current is independent of filament temperature, the value of Ia being determined solely by the value of Va.

(b) Under saturation conditions the value of Ia is largely independent of Va and is determined by filament temperature.

It is perhaps worthwhile stressing the point that, if the polarity of the anode voltage is reversed so that the anode is negative, all the electrons will be repelled and no anode current will flow.

Although there is no reason why a diode should not be made in the same way as the simple example shown in 7 Fig. 4a, for reasons of efficiency it is more usual to construct the anode in the form of a cylinder. (See 7 Fig. 8).

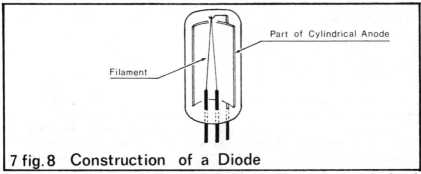

Part of Cylindrical Anode

Filament

7 fig. 8   Construction of a Diode

Since many circuits call for two diodes many examples may be found of a valve consisting of two diodes enclosed in the same envelope, and sharing the same filament. A drawing of a typical double diode is shown in 7 Fig. 9.

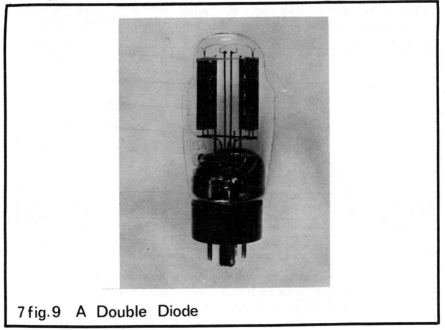

7 fig. 9   A Double Diode

For the sake of simplicity in drawing circuits, a standard symbol for a diode is used. Examples of the symbols used to denote the single and double diode are given in 7 Fig. 10.

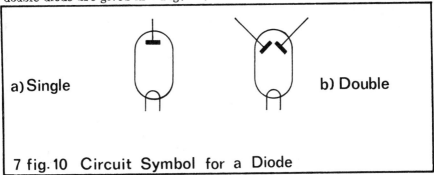

a) Single

b) Double

7 fig. 10 Circuit Symbol for a Diode

7.3 Cathode Construction

Early valves used as the filament a fine tungsten or platinum wire. This had to be heated to about 2250° C in order to get sufficient emission for practical purposes. This was inefficient in the use of power, and in addition made the valves prone to filament failure. Over the years a great deal of work has been done to produce more efficient emitters, so that, in addition to plain tungsten, one can now find thoriated tungsten and oxide coated emitters in use.

The oxide coated emitter is by far the most efficient. One can get satisfactory emission at only 900° C, so that it is possible to make use of what is known as an indirectly heated cathode. This is a cylinder, usually of nickel, coated with a mixture of barium and strontium carbonates, surrounding a heater, made of a fine wire coated with an insulating material (See 7 Fig. 11). During manufacture the cylinder is heated under vacuum conditions and the coating decomposes to form barium and strontium oxides, together with carbon dioxide which is removed by pumping. This type of construction gives a cathode isolated from the heater and its associated power supply and so gives greater flexibility of circuit design.

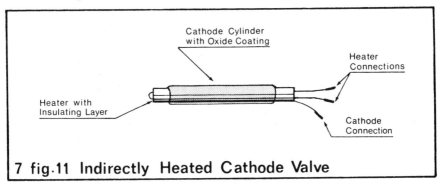

Cathode Cylinder
with Oxide Coating

Heater
Connections

Heater with
Insulating Layer

Cathode
Connection

7 fig. 11 Indirectly Heated Cathode Valve

The graph illustrated in 7 Fig. 12 shows the relative operating temperature of oxide coated, thoriated tungsten and plain tungsten cathodes.

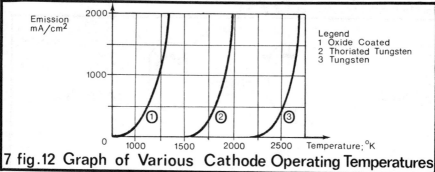

7 fig.12 Graph of Various Cathode Operating Temperatures

For low voltage rectification the oxide coated cathode is invariably used, but for high voltage work, such as in an X-ray generator, the thoriated tungsten or plain tungsten types must be employed. This is because the oxide coating is easily destroyed by the bombardment from positive ions produced by collision between the residual gas atoms and electrons. Collisions also occur at low voltage, but the energy of the ions is low, so that the space charge surrounding the cathode is able to protect the cathode from bombardment. As the voltage across the tube increases, the energy of the ions also increases, so that a point is reached at which the cathode receives bombardment, which causes permanent damage to its emissive surface.

The thoriated tungsten filament is more resistant to bombardment, but nevertheless the thin coating of thorium on the surface is slowly stripped off. By incorporating a small amount of carbon in the tungsten and forming a thin coating of carbon on the surface, the life of the thorium coating can be extended, but this results in the cathode (which is simply the valve filament in an X-ray rectifier) becoming very brittle. As the coating of thorium on the surface is stripped off, it is replaced by thorium from within the material, but the point is eventually reached when all the thorium has been used up. From then on the amount of thorium on the surface falls, which results in a fall off in the emission of the valve since the plain tungsten is not hot enough to emit electrons. As the emission falls off, the working point moves so that the valve no longer works under space charge limited conditions, but under saturation conditions. When this point is reached, the power dissipated is such that the temperature of the anode rises and failure of the valve results, due to back emission. This is discussed further in connection with the X-ray tube in Chapter 8.

If plain tungsten is used for the filament this particular problem does not occur, theoretically increasing reliability. However, the plain tungsten filament must be heated to something over 2000° C in order to give sufficient emission for X-ray use, and at this temperature evaporation of the metal takes place. As already described, the filament is the valve cathode. As the tungsten is heated some parts of the filament evaporate more quickly than others. These parts get thinner, which causes the current density through these areas to increase which results in a higher temperature at this point and a further increase in evaporation rate. Once started the process continues rapidly until a point is reached where one of the thinner areas rises to a temperature above the melting point of the metal, and the filament fails.

7.4 The Triode

The diode is used mainly for such purposes as rectification, because it will only conduct when the anode is positive with respect to the cathode. The addition of a third electrode, called the grid, permits control of the amount of current flowing from cathode to anode. Details of construction and the circuit symbol are given in 7 Fig. 13.

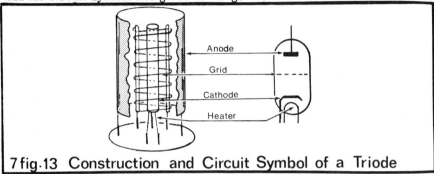

Anode

Grid

Cathode

Heater

7 fig.13 Construction and Circuit Symbol of a Triode

The Triode is normally operated with a fixed positive voltage on the anode. The amount of current flowing through the valve can be controlled by varying the voltage on the grid. The valve is normally run at such a value of Va that with zero voltage on the grid the anode current is near maximum. This means that for the grid to have control it must operate with a negative voltage.

The performance of the valve can be shown graphically by plotting the grid voltage (Vg) against anode current (Ia). This graph is popularly known as the Ia/Vg curve and an example is shown in 7 Fig. 14.

The grid is situated between the cathode and the anode and all electrons reaching the anode must pass through the grid. Since the grid is closer to the cathode than the anode, it is able to exert a much greater influence on electrons emitted from the cathode. As can be seen from the graph, the grid reduces the anode current to zero with a Vg of only −8V even though there is + 100 volts on the anode.

The grid is normally at a negative voltage and will thus repel electrons and no grid current will flow. If, however, the grid does become positive it will attract electrons as though it were an anode. Current will flow in the grid circuit and may cause the grid to heat up causing damage to the valve.

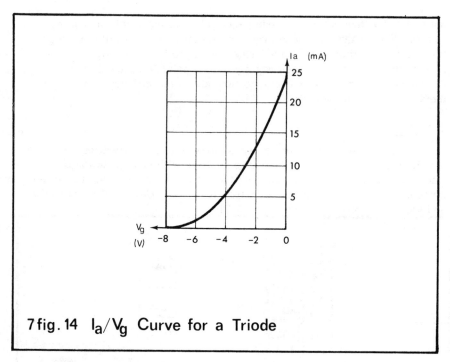

7 fig. 14 I_a/V_g Curve for a Triode

7.5 Gas Discharge Valves

There is a range of valves in use in X-ray apparatus which, although they may be classed as diodes or triodes, do not perform in the usual way. This is because, following the normal evacuation process, a small amount of gas is introduced. The gas used is important since different types and combinations of filling have a marked effect on the characteristics of the final device. The gases used include neon, argon, hydrogen, and mercury vapour.

In any vacuum device there is inevitably a small amount of residual gas, since it is simply not possible to remove every last trace. Sooner or later an electron will strike a gas atom stripping off one or more electrons, so producing a positive ion which will move towards the cathode. Before reaching the cathode surface, the ion must first pass through the space charge where it will usually re-combine with some of the electrons. Providing the number of such ions is low, no adverse effects should be produced. However if the partial pressure of the impurity is increased to about 10^{-3} mm mercury the number of collisions is sufficient to produce noticeable effects.

As the gas pressure increases the first noticeable effect is that current will now flow in the negative electrodes, e.g. (the grid). Unless steps are taken to counteract this, the grid will become increasingly positive, so causing a shift in the working point of the valve.

As the gas pressure is further increased sufficient ionisation and re-combination will occur to produce visible light. At this point the number of ions reaching the region of the cathode causes partial neutralisation of the space charge so that a sharp rise in anode current occurs up to the emission limit of the cathode. Unless the current is limited by means of the external circuit, the valve will be destroyed. Under these conditions it is not possible to control the amount of current flowing through the valve by means of the grid.

Initially sufficient negative voltage is applied to the grid to ensure that no anode current flows. If now the grid is made less negative, a point is reached at which anode current begins to flow. Ionisation now occurs and neutralisation of the space charge takes place. This causes a rise in anode current up to the maximum permitted by the external circuit. The valve is now conducting hard and will continue to do so even if the grid voltage is returned to its original negative value. To turn the valve off it is necessary to drop the anode voltage to a point at which ionisation ceases. The anode must be held at this point for long enough for all the ions to re-combine (usually a few microseconds). If at this point the grid voltage is sufficiently negative to prevent the flow of electrons to the anode, the valve will remain non-conducting when the anode is returned to the original voltage. The valve thus acts as a simple switch, the switching-on point being set by the grid voltage.

The two symbols for this type of valve, which are often referred to as thyratrons, are shown in 7 Fig. 15. The "dot" or shading denotes gas filled.

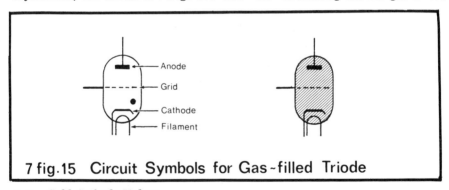

7 fig. 15 Circuit Symbols for Gas-filled Triode

7.6 Cold Cathode Valves

Some gas filled valves have no heater and so are known as cold cathode types. The most common of these is the neon filled tube, which is often used simply as an indicator, but can, with the addition of a few simple components perform a number of additional functions.

A simple neon tube, such as the one shown in 7 Fig. 16 consists of a small glass tube into which are sealed two wires. When sufficient voltage is applied between the electrodes, a small electron flow takes place due to field emission. The gas is then ionised and so gives rise to a considerable current flow unless limited by some external means. The voltage at which

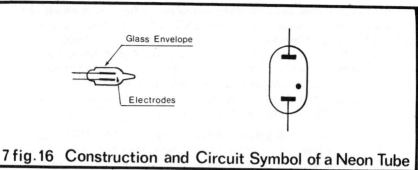

7 fig.16 Construction and Circuit Symbol of a Neon Tube

this takes place is largely a function of the secondary emission
characteristics of the cathode material and may vary between 150V, for a
clean metal cathode (i.e. nickel) and as low as 60V where a specially
treated cathode is used. Careful choice of electrode configuration and
filling, together with a range of cathode material, gives a wide range of
tubes of differing striking and maintaining voltages. The relationship
between striking and maintaining voltage can be seen on the graph 7 Fig.17.

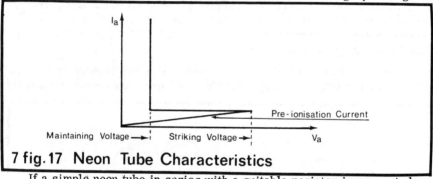

7 fig.17 Neon Tube Characteristics

If a simple neon tube in series with a suitable resistor is connected
across a supply, such as shown in 7 Fig. 18, it will be found that the tube
can be used to produce a constant voltage.

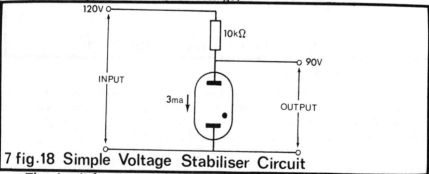

7 fig.18 Simple Voltage Stabiliser Circuit

The circuit functions as follows. If one assumes that the tube will
strike at some voltage under 120V, as soon as the supply is connected, the
tube will pass current causing a voltage drop across the 10kΩ resistor.

Since the internal resistance of the neon tube when struck is only about 50Ω, this should cause the voltage to fall to less than a volt, but in fact, if the voltage across this particular tube falls to below 90V the tube will no longer remain in a conducting state and the current will fall to zero. The voltage across the tube is thus unable to fall below 90V and so will remain at this level, the tube passing 3 mA. If a load is placed across the output the amount of current drawn through the load may be varied from zero up to almost 3 mA without producing a noticeable change in the output voltage.

The stabilising action of a cold cathode discharge tube may be improved by increasing the cathode area. This is often achieved by making the cathode in the form of a cylinder with the anode at the centre. The anode need only be a wire since it will normally only have to withstand electron bombardment.

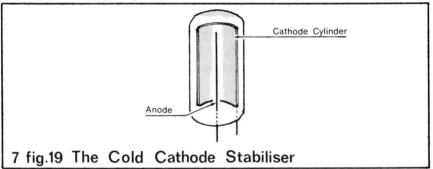

7 fig.19 The Cold Cathode Stabiliser

7.7 The Cold Cathode Trigger Tube

The addition of one or more electrodes permits the tube to perform switching functions. The circuit symbol and the construction of a simple trigger tube are shown in 7 Fig. 20. This type of tube is constructed so that there is a large difference between the striking and the maintaining voltages. Thus a voltage applied between the anode and cathode which is above the maintaining voltage but below the striking voltage will cause no anode current to flow. The tube also has a third electrode so placed as to require a lower voltage to strike a discharge between it and the cathode.(K) This electrode is called the trigger. (T)

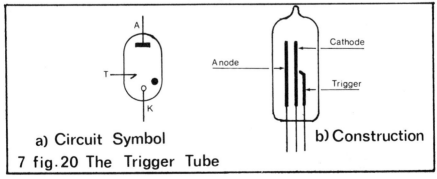

a) Circuit Symbol   b) Construction
7 fig.20 The Trigger Tube

If the voltage on the trigger is raised to above its striking voltage a discharge will take place to the cathode. Some of these electrons will be attracted to the anode, so initiating a discharge between anode and cathode. This discharge cannot be turned off by means of the trigger electrode. To turn the tube off the anode voltage must be reduced to below the maintaining voltage.

Some trigger tubes have a fourth electrode called the priming electrode to give faster and more constant results. The priming electrode maintains a constant discharge so giving a continuous supply of electrons. In use it is exactly the same as a simple trigger tube.

The working point of many cold cathode tubes is affected by light. In order to ensure consistent operation the manufacturer's instruction with regard to ambient light must be followed. In most cases the manufacturer recommends that the tube should not be used in total darkness.

7.8 The Cathode Ray Tube

In addition to the amplifying and switching devices already described, there is a thermionic display device which is becoming increasingly important in the X-ray department. This is the cathode ray tube often referred to as either a C.R.T. or a picture tube.

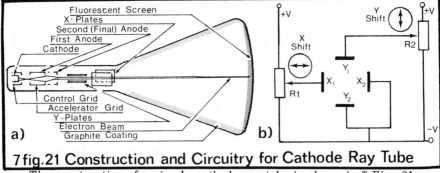

7 fig.21 Construction and Circuitry for Cathode Ray Tube

The construction of a simple cathode ray tube is shown in 7 Fig. 21a, where it can be seen that the device has a cathode and a heater, followed by a number of other electrodes which, although performing the same function as those found in conventional valves, have a somewhat different construction. In the C.R.T., a beam of electrons produced by the cathode impinges on a phosphor, coated on the inside of the glass face, and produces a spot of light. This spot can be moved about by electrostatic forces acting on the electron beam.

The grid of a cathode ray tube is usually made in the form of a cup enclosing the entire cathode surface, the electron beam emerging from a small hole. The electron beam tends to diverge due to the mutual repulsion of the electrons, so that in order to produce a fine point at the screen some means of focussing must be introduced. This is done by means of electrodes in the shape of discs or tubes, each one connected to a supply of specified voltage. High quality tubes tend to have a complex electrode arrangement although in the simpler types of tube, such as the one shown, a more elementary arrangement of electrodes is used. The final anode which is a disc with a hole at its centre through which the electron beam passes, may in many cases be connected to a layer of graphite coated onto the inside of the glass envelope. The voltage on the final anode is very high. For a small oscilloscope tube 1 to 2 kV is used, whereas some television picture tubes employ up to 25 kV. It is interesting to note that cathode ray tubes running at such high voltage give off a small amount of X-rays.

The electrode assembly is often referred to as the "electron gun". A beam of electrons emerges from the gun to strike the phosphor coating on the face of the tube. The spot of light produced can be varied in intensity by altering the negative potential on the grid. The diameter of the spot can be altered by varying the potential on the focussing anode. It will be found that, if the potential on this electrode is varied over a wide range, a point of focus occurs. Increasing or decreasing the voltage about this point will cause an increase in spot diameter.

There are four other electrodes sealed into the tube, these are the electrostatic deflection plates, which control the position of the spot; the X plates moving the spot horizontally while the Y plates move the spot vertically. The circuit shown in 7 Fig. 21b shows how the spot may be moved about by means of the variable resistors R1 and R2. In practice the spot would be moved about not by manual controls but by the magnitude of the input signals. The subject will be covered more fully under Section 7.12.2.

The cathode ray tube used in a television monitor is constructed differently since the spot is deflected by electromagnetic rather than electrostatic forces. The construction is shown in 7 Fig. 22a, where it can be seen that both focussing and deflection are by means of magnets. The use of a coil or a permanent magnet for focussing is tending to give way to electrostatic focussing as in the tubes previously discussed, but is shown here for the sake of completeness.

The use of electromagnetic deflection will not, however, give way to electrostatic deflection since it is not possible to deflect the beam through a wide enough angle by electrostatic means.

For television purposes the waveform fed to the deflection coils is always the same. The vertical deflections coils (See 7 Fig. 22b) are driven by a current waveform which changes from maximum to minimum 50 times per second. This moves the spot from the top of the screen to the bottom with each cycle of the waveform. The horizontal deflection coils are driven by a much higher frequency waveform since the spot moves from left to right 312 times during the time taken for the vertical deflection circuit to undergo one complete cycle, that is $\frac{1}{50}$ sec. (assuming a 625 line, 50 field per second, system).

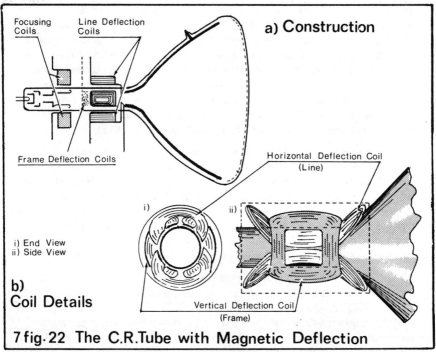

a) Construction

Focusing Coils

Line Deflection Coils

Frame Deflection Coils

Horizontal Deflection Coil (Line)

i) End View
ii) Side View

b)
Coil Details

i)
ii)

Vertical Deflection Coil (Frame)

7 fig. 22 The C.R.Tube with Magnetic Deflection

Cathode ray tubes come in a wide range of sizes. Miniature oscilloscope tubes are available from 10 mm diameter upwards, and television tubes are readily available up to 66 cm from corner to corner (this is equivalent to a 66 cm diameter tube, but the tube is squared off to save space).

A large number of phosphors are available, the type used being determined by the use to which the tube is to be put. The majority of oscilloscope tubes have a phosphor which glows with a yellow/green light since this is an extremely efficient material. The chemical composition can be varied to give a specified amount of lag, that is, the time during which the phosphor continues to glow after the electron beam has moved on. Where slow speed phenomena are to be displayed this can be a distinct advantage, but for fast waveforms a short persistance (lag) phosphor is usually preferred. Special types of tube are also available which permit the persistance to be adjusted. This variable storage facility is not, however, due to the phosphor but to the special internal construction of the tube.

Television cathode ray tubes normally have a blue/white phosphor, which has a short persistance. Colour television receivers use composite phosphors. The face is coated with a pattern of three dots, each one of a different colour phosphor, and each dot is energised by a different electron gun. The colour tube can thus be thought of as three tubes in one, each producing a different colour.

7.9 Semiconductors

In the early days of radio, long evenings were spent with headphones clamped tight on the head, carefully adjusting the "cat's whisker" in a crystal set.

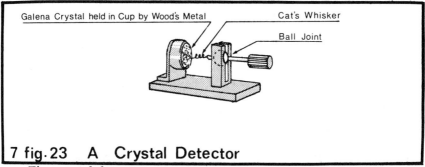

Galena Crystal held in Cup by Wood's Metal   Cat's Whisker

Ball Joint

7 fig. 23   A   Crystal Detector

The crystal detector was only one of a number of devices used in those days to convert the signal picked up by the aerial into a form that could be supplied to the headphones. In fact that crystal detector was simply a rectifier. It worked by converting the radio frequency signal picked up into a half-wave rectified voltage carrying the audio (sound) information. However, the crystal became credited with almost magical properties which have been further enhanced by the passage of time until, it seems, almost as though some crystals had the power to "pull in" radio waves like iron filings to a magnet. Nevertheless, even when shorn of its mystical properties, the crystal detector is still worth our consideration since it was the first practical semiconductor device.

In the early days the way in which the detector worked was not understood and its performance was erratic. With the introduction of the thermionic valve, the crystal detector dropped out of use until problems encountered with the development of radar during World War II brought about renewed interest in the humble crystal detector.

Thus it came about that towards the end of World War II work was being done, particularly in the Bell Telephone Company laboratories, to discover the way in which the crystal diode worked. During the course of this work, certain discoveries were made which lead to the development of the transistor and so provided the impetus to investigate the whole field of semiconductor physics. The first material to be studied was germanium; both diodes and transistors can be made using this material. The principle of operation of such semiconductor devices is entirely different to that of a thermionic device. To understand what takes place we must take a brief look at the atomic structure of a semiconductor material.

It should be remembered that all matter is made up of atoms, and these atoms consist of two parts - the nucleus in the centre and the electrons which are in orbit around the outside. These two parts have very different masses, the nucleus is about 2,000 times heavier than the electron. Electrically the nucleus has a net positive charge and the electrons have a negative charge, both charges being exactly equal, so that each atom is electrically neutral. The orbits of the electrons are arranged in a particular order around the nucleus. The innermost orbits must have the full complement of electrons before the next level can be started. A model of such an atom was discussed in Chapter 2 and shown in 2 Fig. 1.

The innermost level is known as the K shell and must contain the maximum of two electrons before the next shell can start. The next one out, the L shell, can contain up to eight electrons. The outermost electrons are known as valence electrons. It is these valence electrons which form chemical bonds with other atoms and also act as current carriers. Each atom tries to complete its outer valence shell, which it does by sharing or donating electrons. This can be seen in the case of hydrogen, where there is only one proton in the nucleus and one electron in orbit. To complete the K shell two electrons are needed. This is why hydrogen normally exists in the form of H_2 . Two atoms combine to form a molecule in which the two electrons are shared giving a more stable arrangement.

$$H = H$$

Helium has two protons in the nucleus and two electrons in the K shell. Since the K shell is now complete helium is quite stable and does not try to link up with other atoms.

$$He$$

Oxygen which has six electrons in its L shell requires two more electrons to complete its valence shell so that, if we combine hydrogen and oxygen, we get a stable material when one atom of oxygen links up with two of hydrogen, giving H_2O or water.

$$H - O - H$$

In considering how the semiconductor material works, it is worthwhile investigating how carbon atoms link up. Carbon has four valence electrons and requires four more to complete its outer ring. It can obtain these by 'joining hands' with dissimilar atoms, for example by combining with oxygen to give CO_2 in which the carbon atom shares the valence electron from two oxygen atoms.

$$O = C = O$$

Alternatively the carbon atoms can form bonds amongst themselves. This may be done in the orderly manner, which is characteristic of a crystal. In the case of carbon this involves each atom forming one bond with four nearby atoms, so that the whole mass of material is linked up by means of these co-valent bonds. Carbon in this form is known as diamond. This type of structure within any material is known as a diamond lattice. This is the type of structure to be found in semiconductor material.

For example, this type of structure is found in both silicon and germanium.

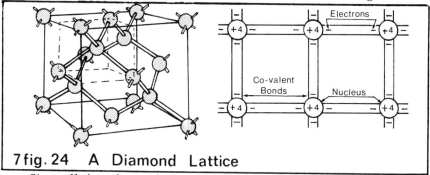

7 fig. 24   A   Diamond   Lattice

Since all the valence electrons are employed in forming these co-valent bonds, none are available to act as current carriers. It would therefore be expected that material of this type would show an infinitely high resistance. However, bonds are continually being broken due to thermal effects, so that a small number of electrons become available to act as current carriers, the number available at any one time being proportional to temperature.

In a practical semiconductor material some charge carriers are available even at a temperature of absolute zero, due to the presence of extremely small numbers of impurity atoms. In fact semiconductor devices depend for their operation upon carefully controlled amounts of impurity material. The amount of impurity added is extremely small, of the order of one part in 10^8, but the effect is considerable. The resistance of pure germanium at 25° C is approximately 60 ohm/cm^3. The addition of one part in 10^8 of a suitable impurity reduces its resistance to about 4 ohm/cm^3.

The correct choice of impurity material is also important. First of all the impurity atom must fit into the lattice structure, and secondly it must have the correct number of valence electrons. The impurities fall into two classes :-

(a) 'Donor' or N-type materials.

(b) 'Acceptor' or P-type materials.

Let us consider the properties of the 'Donor' or N-type material. It must be a penta-valent material, that is having five valency electrons, (e.g. phosphorus, antimony or arsenic). With the small amount used, each impurity atom is surrounded by atoms of germanium. Each adjacent germanium atom will form the usual system of co-valent bonds, thus linking any nearby penta-valent atoms with four germanium ones. The fifth electron will not be bonded in this way, and so can be displaced by the application of a small electrical potential thus becoming a charge carrier. A semiconductor of this type is commonly called an 'N' type semi-conductor since conduction takes place by means of negative charge carriers (electrons).

A 'P' type semiconductor can be made using tri-valent impurities such as boron, indium, aluminium or gallium, which have only three valency electrons. In the extremely low concentration used, these atoms are also completely surrounded by germanium atoms which form the normal diamond lattice structure, but since the impurity has only three electrons it is unable to form the fourth co-valent bond. It may, however, capture any free electron which happens to drift into its neighbourhood. This electron may be one which moves away from its location due for example to thermal effects. This electron will have left behind a hole elsewhere in the lattice structure, which in turn will be filled by the capture of another free electron drifting past. This gives the appearance of holes drifting about within the crystalline material. Since these holes are in fact points from which an electron is missing they have the appearance of drifting, positive charge carriers.

It must be noted that in both 'P' and 'N' type semiconductor materials there are exactly the same number of electrons as there are protons, so that the crystal is in a state of electrical equilibrium. A crystal of either 'P' or 'N' type material will act as a resistor and will conduct in any direction.

7.10 Semiconductor Diodes

To form a rectifier a single crystal of semiconductor material is used with a 'P' type impurity added at one end and an 'N' type impurity at the other. The crystal is then heated which causes the impurities to diffuse through the material until they meet somewhere in the middle, forming a 'junction' as shown in 7 Fig. 25.

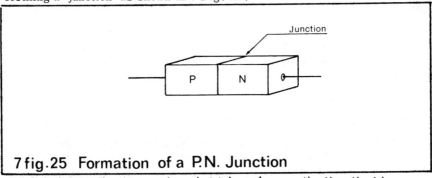

7 fig.25 Formation of a P.N. Junction

It is interesting to examine what takes place as the 'junction' is formed. As has already been said, both 'P' and 'N' types of semi-conductor material exist in a state of equilibrium, but if a 'junction' is formed between the two types of material in a single crystal this equilibrium is upset.

The 'N' type semiconductor seems to have a surplus of electrons, whereas the 'P' type seems to have a shortage. When the 'junction' forms, some electrons from the 'N' side cross the 'junction' to fill holes in the 'P' side. This produces a shortage of electrons on the 'N' side and a surplus on the 'P' side so that the 'N' side now has a positive charge and the 'P' side a negative charge, as though a small battery was connected across the region. This is illustrated in 7 Fig. 26a. This state of imbalance causes exceedingly strong forces to arise which resist any further exchange of electrons, but since these forces do not come into action until some electrons have been exchanged a small degree of imbalance is inevitable.

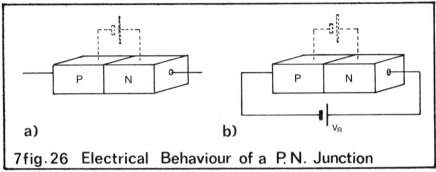

a)   b)

7fig. 26 Electrical Behaviour of a P.N. Junction

Now consider what happens when a battery is connected across the device as shown in 7 Fig. 26b. The battery is connected with the negative pole to the 'P' side of the crystal and the positive pole to the 'N' side. The 'P' side already has a surplus of electrons and the 'N' side a deficiency so the battery makes matters worse, since more electrons are being injected into the 'P' side and extracted from the 'N' side. The forces already in existence will be enhanced preventing further exchanges of electrons from taking place. The region between the 'P' and the 'N' type material will have no charge carriers since the 'N' will have lost all the free electrons to the 'P' material. This gives a very thin layer known as the depletion layer between the regions. If the voltage (V_R) is increased in the present direction this layer becomes thicker and so increases the resistance between the two conducting layers. The variation of current is as shown in 7 Fig. 27a.

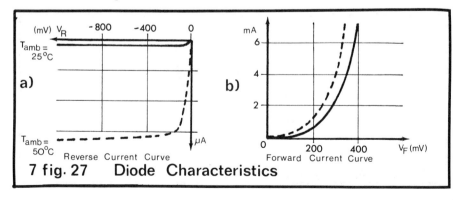

7 fig. 27   Diode Characteristics

If the battery is now reversed electrons will be extracted from the 'P' side which has a surplus and injected into the 'N' side which has a deficiency, so that the atomic forces are now working with the battery to produce a current flow. As the applied voltage rises, the depletion layer decreases in thickness, and the internal resistance falls until a very low value is reached. A graph showing the forward current flow is illustrated in 7 Fig. 27b.

It is possible to combine the curves shown in 7 Fig. 27a and 7 Fig. 27b into one to give a typical curve for a semiconductor diode, an example of which is shown in 7 Fig. 28. As can be seen a current in the order of 6 mA will flow with an applied forward voltage of about 400 mV, whereas the current with the same magnitude of reverse voltage will be only about 1μA. The reverse current does not vary to any great extent with voltage. The characteristics shown in 7 Fig. 28 are those of a germanium diode used for low power applications Larger devices may be found which have a much lower forward resistance.

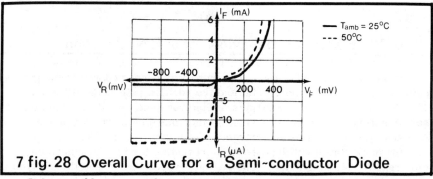

7 fig. 28 Overall Curve for a Semi~conductor Diode

It is possible to use silicon instead of germanium in the production of semiconductor diodes. The two devices are similar in their characteristics but not identical. The important differences are that in the case of silicon the reverse current is lower and the voltage required to produce a forward current is higher. In fact it is necessary to apply about 500 mV before the curve starts to take an upward turn.

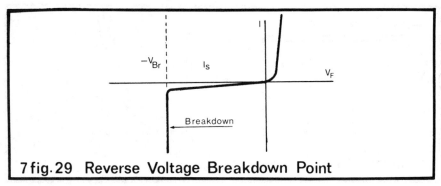

7 fig. 29 Reverse Voltage Breakdown Point

Another characteristic of interest concerns a part of the graph which has not so far been considered. As the reverse voltage is increased a point is reached at which the reverse current suddenly starts to rise. This is the point marked "Breakdown" in 7 Fig. 29. A small increase in voltage beyond this point causes a large increase in current, often causing the destruction of the device. The exact point at which this happens depends upon the properties of the semiconductor material used in the manufacture of the device and can be anywhere between 2 volts and 1000 volts. It is possible to obtain a higher breakdown voltage using silicon. In earlier types of diode the point at which breakdown took place was uncontrollable. Diodes were simply tested to ensure that they would handle more than the stated maximum reverse voltage. Nowadays the characteristics of a diode can be much more carefully planned so that a range of diodes are available with only a small spread in breakdown voltage.

Individual diodes with breakdown voltages high enough for use in an X-ray high voltage generator are quite unobtainable. However, since the physical size of each diode is small, it is a simple matter to connect a large number in series until a composite device is constructed, having a high enough breakdown voltage for the purpose.

7.11 The Junction Transistor

Just as the silicon diode has largely replaced the thermionic diode, in many applications the triode has also been replaced by a three pole semiconductor device, the transistor. The first member of the family to come into use was the junction transistor. The modern form of this is still the most widely used although there are now a number of other related devices which are becoming increasingly popular with circuit designers.

The starting point in the fabrication of a transistor is once again a thin slice of a semiconductor material, usually germanium or silicon. For the purposes of this description germanium will be taken as the material used. A thin slice of germanium containing an 'N' type impurity is carefully prepared to remove all surface contamination, after which two small pellets of indium are brought into contact with the germanium, one on each face. The whole assembly is now heated so that the indium forms an alloy with the germanium. Since indium is a 'P' type impurity this causes a region of 'P' type semiconductor to be formed around each indium pellet. A cross section through such an assembly is shown in 7 Fig. 30a. The point at which each 'P' region meets the 'N' region will form a diode, so that once again if the 'P' region is made negative and the 'N' region positive no current will flow. Whereas if the 'P' region is made positive and the 'N' region negative current will flow.

To demonstrate transistor action it is necessary to bias one junction in the forward direction and the other in reverse. In the example shown in 7 Fig. 30b the lefthand junction is biased to conduction and the righthand junction reverse biased.

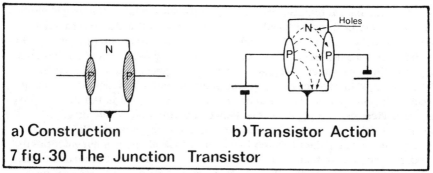

a) Construction   b) Transistor Action

7 fig. 30 The Junction Transistor

The way in which the device works is best understood by considering holes generated in the 'P' region travelling to the 'N' region. The holes drift about in the semiconductor material, and do not flow in straight lines taking the shortest path. The figure shows that some holes will travel straight to the negative contact on the semiconductor slice, whereas some others will take a longer path possibly coming into the area of the righthand 'PN' junction. This junction is reverse biased and so will have a relatively thick depletion layer, across which there will be a considerable voltage gradient. Furthermore, since the righthand 'P' region is even more negative than the 'N' region, the holes drifting into the depletion layer area will be drawn across the junction to generate a current flow in the reverse biased diode.

If the thickness of the 'N' region is reduced, the chances of a hole drifting across to the other junction is increased, so by careful design it is possible to arrive at a point where most of the holes are collected by the reverse biased junction.

At this point the three regions of a junction transistor will be named, since this will simplify further explanations. The lefthand 'P' region, which is normally forward biased is called the 'Emitter' since it is the source of the current carriers (holes in the example quoted), and this is the equivalent to the cathode of a thermionic valve. The small square of semiconductor material upon which the transistor was formed is called the 'Base', and is equivalent to the grid of a valve. The 'P' region on the right, which is reverse biased, is called the 'Collector' and is the equivalent of the anode of a valve. The circuit symbol is shown in 7 Fig. 31.

Regardless of how thin the base region is made, or how carefully the emitter or collector junctions are formed there must always be less current flowing in the collector than in the emitter. This is because, in accordance with Kirchoff's law the emitter current (Ie) is equal to the base current (Ib) plus the collector current (Ic).

$$(Ie = Ib + Ic) \text{ or } Ic = Ie - Ib.$$

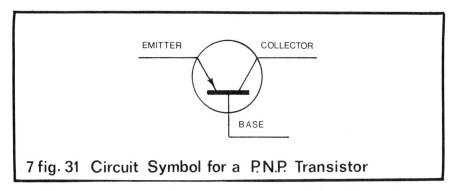

7 fig. 31   Circuit Symbol for a P.N.P. Transistor

The amount of current flowing in the base and in the collector of a given transistor will divide up according to a fixed ratio. If the current flowing into the emitter is reduced by 50% both the collector current and the base current will fall by 50%.

It may appear from the explanation given, that the device has no gain. However, one should note the differences in the operating conditions between the emitter and the collector circuits. The emitter is forward biased, so that very little voltage is needed to cause a significant amount of current to flow, in most cases the required voltage across the base/emitter junction is only about 0.5V. The collector/base junction is reverse biased so that with no current flowing the full supply voltage will appear on the collector, probably in the order of 10V. The efficiency of a transistor is expressed as the ratio of the input current to the output current or $\alpha = \frac{Ic}{Ie}$. In many cases the base current is about 2% of the emitter current, so to give the formula a practical figure, $\alpha = \frac{98}{100} = 0.98$.

The situation may be further clarified by considering an example such as that shown in 7 Fig. 32. This is known as the common base configuration.

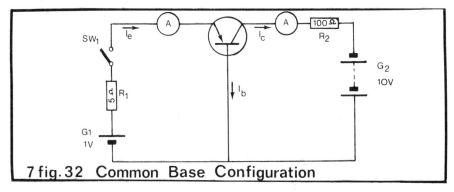

7 fig. 32   Common Base Configuration

Resistor R1 is of such a value so as to cause 100 mA to flow into the emitter when SW1 is closed. If the transistor has an α of 0.98 then the collector current will be 98 mA. The voltage from battery G2 is 10V and R2 has a value of 100Ω. The closing of SW1 puts 0.5V between base and emitter causing a current of 100 mA to flow. The total power in the emitter resistor is thus $0.5 \times 100 \times 10^{-3} = 50$ mW. When SW1 is open no current flows in the collector circuit and the voltage between collector and base is 10V. When SW1 is closed the current flowing in the collector resistor is 98 mA and the collector voltage falls to 0.2V. The total change in power caused by closing SW1 is therefore $(10 - 0.2) \times 98 \times 10^{3} \approx 960$mW. The power gain is given by $\dfrac{\text{Output Power}}{\text{Input Power}} = \dfrac{960}{50} \approx 19$

The value of α depends upon the way in which the transistor is made and, although there may be wide variation in value from one sample to another in the same batch, the value of α will remain more or less constant for a given transistor. If then we assume that α(the ratio between the emitter current and collector current) will always be the same, then it must follow that the ratio between the base current and the collector current will also be constant.

Referring once again to 7 Fig. 32 it may be seen that, if the emitter current is 100 mA and the collector current is 98 mA, then the base current must be 2 mA (Ie - Ic = Ib). One may also consider this ratio as a means of classifying the gain of a transistor.

The current gain is known as α' and is equal to $\dfrac{I_c}{I_b}$

In the example $\alpha' = \dfrac{98}{2} = 49$

7 fig.33   Common Emitter Configuration

Since we are now concerned with the current flowing in the base circuit it is convenient to move the position of R1 and SW1 to the base circuit (See 7 Fig. 33). In order to maintain the base current at 2 mA the value of R1 must now be increased, since $Ib = \dfrac{I_c}{\alpha'}$. If the voltage between base and emitter (Vbe) is once again 0.5V and that supplied by G1 is 1V then:-

$$R1 = \frac{1 - 0.5V}{2mA} = 250\Omega$$

When SW1 is closed, 2 mA will flow into the base of the transistor and cause 98 mA to flow in the collector circuit since $Ic = \alpha' Ib$. Thus there will be a true current gain and there will also be an attendant power and voltage gain.

The circuit may be further simplified by eliminating the battery G1 since careful examination of the circuit will show that the two batteries are effectively in series. The circuit may now be redrawn as shown in 7 Fig. 34.

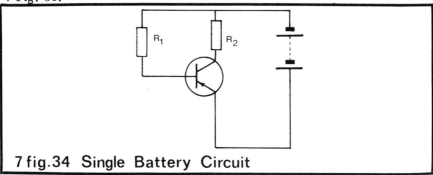

7 fig.34 Single Battery Circuit

The value of R1 must be increased to allow for the higher voltage, but apart from this, the circuit will still work in the same way. It can be seen that in this configuration the emitter circuit is common to both the base and the collector. This arrangement is therefore known as a common emitter circuit.

As in the case of a valve, the performance of a transistor can be shown graphically. The illustration 7 Fig. 35 shows that the Ic/Ib characteristic is not a straight line, so that the $\propto'$ will depend upon the point on the curve at which measurement is made.

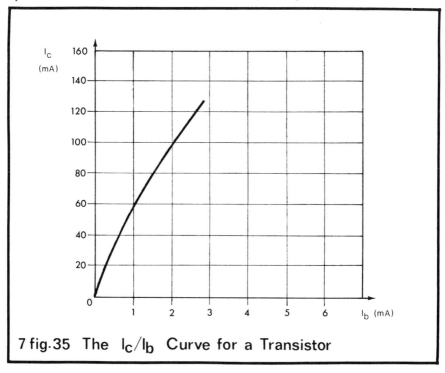

7 fig. 35 The I_c/I_b Curve for a Transistor

At present the more usual way of quoting the gain of a transistor is to talk about hf_e, that is the change (Δ) in collector current due to a change in base current under stated conditions.

$$hf_e = \frac{\Delta I_c}{\Delta I_b}$$

For example, the current gain of one popular transistor is listed in the data sheet as follows :-

> Small signal current gain
> I_E = 2 mA; V_{CB} = 5V; f = 1 kHz; T_{amb} = 25° C
> hf_e = 180

7.12 Alternative Types of Junction Transistor

The first commercially available transistors in this country used germanium. There are, however, a number of other semiconductor materials which can be used. The most popular alternative to germanium is silicon, although gallium arsenide and cadmium sulphide are also used in certain other applications.

When silicon is used as the base material of a transistor the characteristics are altered so that the design of a circuit must be changed slightly. A comparison between the silicon and germanium characteristics is given in 7 Fig. 36.

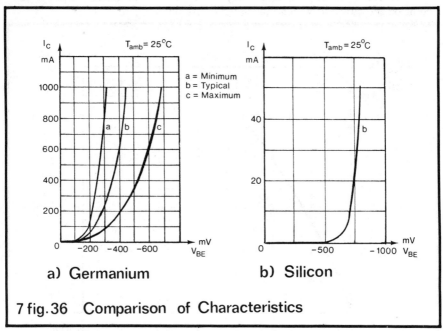

a) Germanium   b) Silicon

7 fig. 36 Comparison of Characteristics

It can be seen that Vbe for a germanium device must be increased to about 150 mV before collector current (Ic) starts to rise, whereas for a similar device using silicon, Vbe must be above 600 mV before the curve starts to take an upward turn.

The leakage current, that is the collector current which flows when there is zero voltage on the base, is much less for a silicon transistor. Typical values for a germanium transistor would be 10 μA (10 x 10^{-6} A) at 25° C with 20V on the collector, whereas for a typical silicon transistor the collector leakage current would be only 10 nano–amps (10 x 10^{-9} A) at 25° C.

A further advantage is that a silicon transistor can be safely operated at junction temperatures up to 200° C, whereas a germanium transistor must not be operated above 100° C. On the other hand, germanium devices are easy to manufacture and therefore cost less. Since the cost of silicon types may not be justified, germanium transistors are still used for many applications.

7.13 PNP and NPN Transistors

The devices so far discussed were made up of three layers; the emitter which is P-type semiconductor, the base which is N-type semiconductor and the collector which is once again a P-type semiconductor. It is possible, however, to change the order so that the emitter is N-type, the base P type and the collector N-type material.

The result of this is that the collector/base junction must now be biased so that the collector is positive with respect to the base, and the emitter/base junction biased so that the base is positive with respect to the emitter. This is achieved quite simply by reversing the polarity of the supply so that the positive line now goes to the collector.

In all other respects an NPN transistor is the same as a PNP transistor but the facility of being able to drive transistors from either a positive or a negative supply eases the task of designing complex electronic devices. Many items of equipment will be found to contain a mixture of both types and their circuit symbols are shown in 7 Fig. 37.

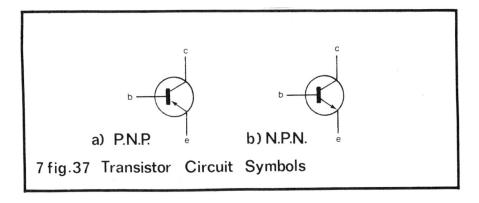

7 fig.37 Transistor Circuit Symbols

7.14 The Field Effect Transistor

The field effect transistor (F.E.T) is a semiconductor device which is voltage operated rather than current operated as is the junction transistor. Although using the same materials, the construction and mode of operation of an F.E.T. is different.

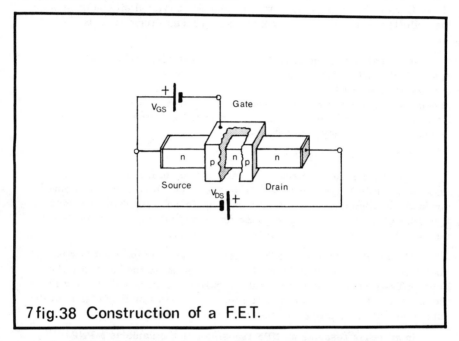

7 fig.38 **Construction of a F.E.T.**

A simplified diagram of an F.E.T. is shown in 7 Fig. 38, where the active part of the transistor is represented by a bar of semiconductor enclosed in a PN junction. This junction forms a diode which in use is reverse biased.

As has already been mentioned (Section 7.10), when a diode reverse biased a layer known as the depletion layer is formed at the junction. The thickness of the depletion layer is determined by the magnitude of the reverse voltage, the higher the voltage the thicker will be the layer.

Since the depletion layer has no charge carriers, the increase in thickness is used in the F.E.T. to restrict the cross section of the semi-conductor material which can conduct current, and thereby increases the resistance of the device, (See 7 Fig. 39). Thus the device works in a very similar manner to that of a triode valve as can be seen in 7 Fig. 40.

The three electrodes, i.e. source, gate and drain, perform similar functions to the cathode, grid and anode of a triode valve. To assist in understanding manufacturer's data, the normal designation of currents and

92

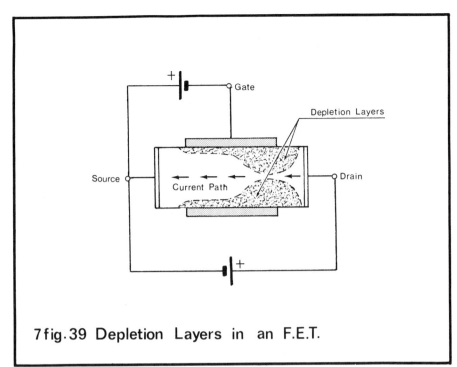

7 fig. 39 Depletion Layers in an F.E.T.

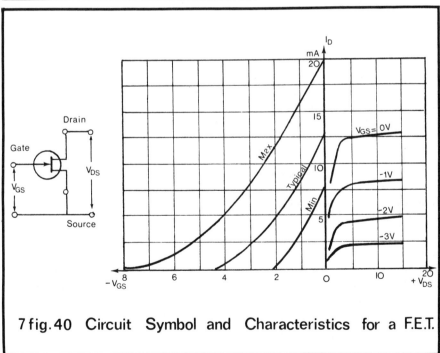

7 fig. 40 Circuit Symbol and Characteristics for a F.E.T.

voltages are given in 7 Fig. 40. Typical I_D/V_{GS} curves (equivalent to the I_a/V_g curves of a triode) and I_D/V_{DS} characteristics at various values of V_{GS} (equivalent to triode I_a/V_a curves at various values of V_g) are shown.

There are a number of other types of F.E.T. available, all working in a similar way to that described but having some differences in construction and performance. The most commonly encountered type is the metal oxide silicon transistor, often called a M.O.S. F.E.T. or MOST. This type has a higher input impedance and so is useful where extremely small input currents are involved.

7.15 The Zener Diode

The zener diode (also known as voltage regulator or reference diode) is the semiconductor equivalent of the cold cathode stabiliser (See section 7.6). The commonly adopted name, zener diode, is not strictly correct since not all the devices in this class depend upon the zener effect for their operation. Those operating above 10V depend for their effect upon avalanche breakdown.

In the avalanche breakdown condition it is found that the current carriers, due to reverse leakage currents, are accelerated by the potential across the junction until they have sufficient energy to displace other charge carriers by collision. This leads to a rapid increase in the number of charge carriers, and thus current. A small change in the amount of impurity in a sample of semiconductor will cause a large change in the resistance. The width of the junction (determined by the resistance of the base material) can be altered by changing the amount of impurity in the base material. This will, in turn, alter the potential gradient across the junction, so changing the voltage at which the charge carriers, already available, reach sufficient velocity to displace additional charge carriers by collision. So it comes about that as the impurity content of the base material is increased, the breakdown voltage of the diode falls, until a point is reached where the junction is so narrow that the chances of a charge carrier colliding with other electrons in the lattice structure become small.

It is only when the junction is very narrow that the true zener effect becomes significant. Zener breakdown occurs when the electrostatic field strength is so high that it overcomes the forces bonding the electrons to the lattice, making the electron-hole pairs available as current carriers.

There is no sharp transition between these two modes of operation, at low voltages the zener effect predominates, whereas at higher voltages avalanche breakdown takes over. Avalanche breakdown is similar to the ionisation process which takes place in a gas filled diode, whilst the zener effect is a form of internal field emission. The change of mode results in a change in shape of the characteristic curve shown in 7 Fig. 41 where it can be seen that the device exhibits a much sharper "knee" when in the

94

avalanche breakdown condition. The most important difference in the characteristics of diodes working in the zener region and those under avalanche breakdown conditions is the effect of temperature on the breakdown voltage.

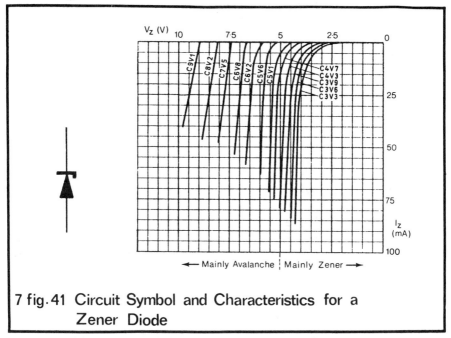

7 fig.41 Circuit Symbol and Characteristics for a Zener Diode

Diodes working entirely in the zener mode show a negative temperature co-efficient, that is, as the temperature increases the voltage falls. A diode working in the avalanche mode, however, will show a positive temperature co-efficient. Those in the middle of the range show only a very slight change in voltage with temperature, since the two effects tend to cancel. This gives a very stable device which can be used to provide an accurate reference voltage.

Zener diodes are classified according to their nominal operating voltage (V_Z) at a specified zener current (I_Z). For example, a zener diode coded C6V8 implies that its operating voltage is 6.8 volts. This is only true at a specified I_Z and in the case shown in the table below this is 5 mA. In addition there will be production tolerances of say 10% so that minimum and maximum voltages are also specified.

The table also shows the temperature coefficient (S_Z) in mV/°C for this range of diodes. The zener and avalanche effect can be seen to cancel out in the C5V6 version.

95

	Zener voltage V_Z (V) at I_Z = 5 mA			Temperature coefficient S_Z (mV/°C) at I_Z = 5 mA
	min.	nom.	max.	typ.
C3V3	3.1	3.3	3.5	-2.3
C3V6	3.4	3.6	3.8	-2.0
C3V9	3.7	3.9	4.1	-2.05
C4V3	4.0	4.3	4.5	-1.8
C4V7	4.4	4.7	5.0	-1.55
C5V1	4.8	5.1	5.4	-1.2
C5V6	5.3	5.6	6.0	-0.2
C6V2	5.8	6.2	6.6	+2.0
C6V8	6.4	6.8	7.2	+3.2
C7V5	7.1	7.5	7.9	+4.2
C8V2	7.8	8.2	8.7	+5.0
C9V1	8.6	9.1	9.6	+6.0

7.16 The Light Emitting Diode

The light emitting diode (L.E.D.) is simply a semiconductor which, when operated in the forward biased condition, emits light. Electrons from the N region are injected into the P region where light photons are generated by recombination. The wavelength of the light depends upon the energy gap between the conduction and valence band of the base material and also the impurity present.

Most light emitting diodes are made of gallium arsenide so that the light generated is in the red or near infra-red region. A great deal of work is underway in order to produce diodes which operate at other points in the spectrum, and it is now possible to purchase diodes for the green and amber regions, although these are less efficient and also cost considerably more.

Since the diodes have no filament, they have an almost infinite life. They can therefore be used with advantage to replace many of the incandescent lamps used in electronic apparatus. Their small size aids miniaturisation of apparatus, and their low current consumption and low operating voltage makes them particularly suited to transistor control.

Hole-electron pairs can be generated in semiconductor material by photon (light) energy in addition to the thermal energy already discussed. Thus photo-transistors can be made which respond to incident light and are complementary to the L.E.D.

A light emitting diode can be coupled to a photo-transistor by means of a light guide (a highly polished glass or plastic rod) in which case the power flowing in the transistor is almost directly proportioned to the power flowing in the L.E.D. Since there is no electrical connection between the L.E.D. and the photo-transistor, the input and output circuits are isolated from each other. Devices are commercially available called opto-isolators which consists of an L.E.D. coupled to a photo-transistor, the whole assembly being sealed in a package. Alternatively, the coupling between the two can take the form of a fibre optic light guide which can be a metre or more long. It thus becomes possible to feed information via a light beam from the high voltage side of an X-ray generator to the metering circuit in the control desk.

It is possible that control signals could be transmitted in this way from the desk to switch the high voltage. For this type of application the more efficient infra-red emitting diodes would be used.

Another application for the L.E.D. is in the field of data display where light emitting diodes in a matrix may be used to form characters. Read out devices on small electronic calculators are of this type and may, in future, carry out similar functions in X-ray control units.

7.17 The Thyristor

The junction transistor is used for many applications formerly carried out by the thermionic triode, but there are many other thermionic devices used in X-ray equipment which are basically different to the simple triode. One of these is the gas filled valve commonly called a thyratron. The solid state version of this device is known as a silicon controlled rectifier or thyristor. The names thyratron and thyristor are both derived from the Greek word for door. This word occurs in the New Testament where there is a reference which could be said to describe the properties of a thyristor, as it is there stated "I know your works. Behold I have set before you an open door, which no one is able to shut; I know that you have but little power."

The thyristor itself consumes very little power so that a small device is able to switch very heavy loads. Both the thyratron and the thyristor have only two states, on and off, and if used on pure D.C. once switched on,the only way to turn it off is to remove the supply.

Thyristors are now available capable of handling up to 200 amps at mains voltage. They have a fast operating time, (as little as 1 μs) and, since there are no moving parts,the life is almost infinite.

The best way to explain the operation of the thyristor is to consider an NPN and PNP transistor connected as shown in 7 Fig. 42a.

To review the operating conditions of these two types of transistors it can be said that for an NPN transistor :-

i)   it must have a positive voltage on the collector in order to operate.

ii)   with a Vbe of zero volts,the collector current will be zero.

iii)   the base voltage must be increased to more than + 600 mV in order to produce collector current.

The PNP transistor on the other hand

i) must have a negative voltage on the collector.

ii) a zero I_C with V_{BE} zero.

iii) V_{BE} more than -600 mV for collector current to flow.

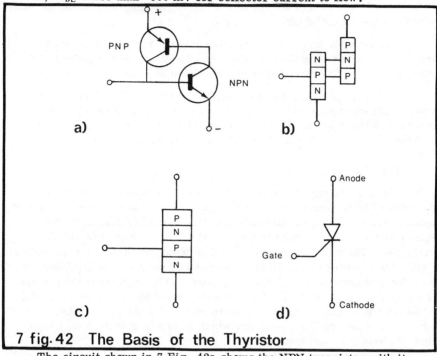

7 fig. 42   The Basis of the Thyristor

The circuit shown in 7 Fig. 42a shows the NPN transistor with its
emitter connected to the negative supply and its collector connected to the
base of the PNP transistor. The PNP transistor has its emitter connected
to the positive supply and its collector connected to the base of the NPN
transistor. When voltage is first applied between the two emitters, no
current will flow, since with zero volts on the base of the NPN transistor
the collector current will be zero. Thus the voltage on the base of the
PNP will also be zero, preventing it from conducting. The two devices
can thus be thought of as two switches in series, both of which are open.

If a short positive pulse of about 1V is applied to the base of the
NPN transistor it will start to conduct. This will apply a negative voltage
to the base of the PNP transistor, so causing this one to conduct. Thus a
positive voltage will be applied to the base of the NPN transistor which will
in turn keep the transistor in a conducting state, even when the original
pulse ends. Both transistors now act as switches which are closed, and
since both short circuit each other the circuit cannot be turned off by
means of the base voltage. The only way the circuit can be turned off is by
removing the supply as with a thyratron. Used on A.C, this will occur

naturally at the end of each half cycle.

The device as shown in 7 Fig. 42a will not conduct if the polarity of the supply is reversed.

Although it is possible to construct a device as shown by interconnecting two transistors there is a much more efficient method which can be seen by considering the diagrams 7 Fig. 42a and b together.

The circuit involves interconnecting the base of the NPN transistor, which is a P region, with the collector of the PNP transistor, which is also a P region. The collector of the NPN transistor, an N region, is also connected to the base (N region) of the PNP transistor. Thus the current flows through four layers P-N-P-N. The construction of the device can be simplified and the performance improved by fabricating the device on a single four layer chip, as illustrated in 7 Fig. 42c. The circuit symbol is shown in 7 Fig. 42d.

If the device is to be used on A.C, then some means of making it to conduct on both half cycles must be provided. Two thyristors connected as shown in 7 Fig. 43a provide a solution, but there are often problems in supplying the triggering pulse to both thyristors since the two gates must be isolated from each other.

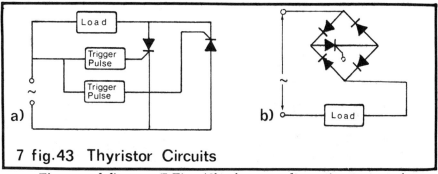

7 fig.43 Thyristor Circuits

The second diagram (7 Fig. 43b) shows an alternative system where four diodes are used to supply unidirectional current to the thyristor.

Complex circuits are necessary where it is required to switch D.C. or turn off the thyristor during a half cycle, and are becoming more common in X-ray apparatus.

Semiconductor devices may be used for many applications, such as amplifiers, switches, or rectifiers. In fact they can be used for almost all functions previously performed by thermionic valves. There are special types which have similar characteristics to those of gas filled valves. Solid state devices can also be made which respond to light, temperature, magnetic fields, radiation, sound waves and mechanical stress. They are more efficient than thermionic devices and for a given power handling capacity they occupy less space, have a longer life and are more robust. Surprisingly enough, they are also cheaper and easier to make, so that although there are some applications in which thermionic devices are still used, the number of such cases is steadily decreasing.

7.18 Integrated Circuits

When transistors first came into use, they were usually wired into conventional type circuits, in which the components were soldered between tag strips on a metal chassis (see 7 Fig. 44a). Further advances in technology led to the introduction of printed circuit boards. In this process, instead of running wires between insulated terminals mounted on a support, a plastic board is used which has a thin layer of copper bonded to the surface. The pattern of wiring is printed onto the copper using a special waterproof ink, and the board is then immersed in a bath of a solution which dissolves away the copper, except where it is protected by the ink. The remaining copper now forms the wiring. Holes are drilled in the board and the components soldered in place. This technique reduces the cost of construction and also allows the circuitry to be made more compact. An example is shown in 7 Fig. 44b.

By fashioning one edge of the board into a plug the task of replacing faulty boards is greatly simplified. The technique also lends itself to the production of ready made circuits which can be linked up into a complete system, so eliminating a great deal of design work. A further development is the encapsulation of the board plus components in plastic.

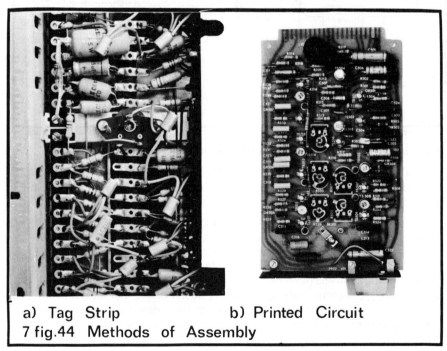

a) Tag Strip   b) Printed Circuit
7 fig.44 Methods of Assembly

From this was developed the newest device to enter the X-ray equipment field, the integrated circuit. This is simply a tiny square of semiconductor material into which are formed all the components, such as capacitors, diodes, resistors and transistors. Interconnections are made by depositing gold or aluminium onto the surface, the only additional external components required are large value capacitors, inductors and variable controls. By means of this technique extremely complex circuits may be packed into a tiny space. An example is shown in 7 Fig. 45.

The final product is very reliable and the assembly costs only a fraction of what it would be if the circuit were to be built up from separate components. One may confidently predict that the integrated circuit will have a revolutionary effect upon the design of X-ray apparatus.

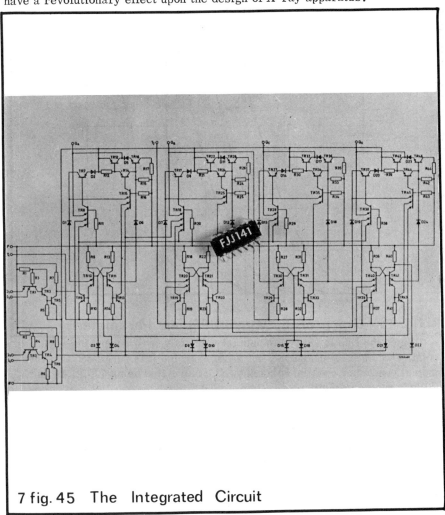

7 fig. 45   The   Integrated   Circuit

7.19 Application of Electronic Devices

Having covered the theory and construction of various electronic devices, the aim of this section is to consider the additional components required to build up complete circuits.

7.19.1 The Triode Amplifier

The efficiency of a valve as an amplifier can be stated as the change in anode current caused by a given change in grid voltage. This ratio is termed the mutual conductance (denoted g_m) and is expressed in mA/V (milliamps per volt). Thus the data sheet on the valve shown in 7 Fig. 46 gives the value of g_m as 12.5 mA/V.

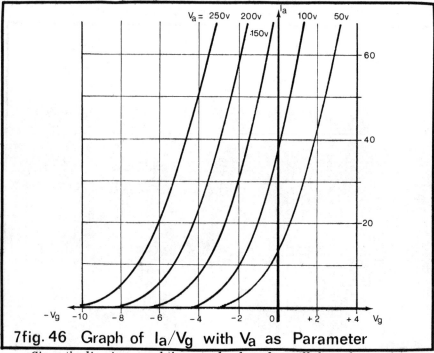

7fig. 46   Graph of I_a/V_g with V_a as Parameter

Since the line is curved the actual value of g_m will depend upon the point at which it is measured, but as an exercise it is suggested that the mutual conductance of the value shown be calculated using 7 Fig. 46 and the following parameters :-

> anode voltage (Va) = 200V
> change in grid voltage (Vg) = from -5V to -4V

Although the mutual conductance gives an impression of the gain to be obtained from a valve, one cannot express gain in terms of milliamps per volt. The gain must be expressed as a ratio between similar units. Some means is therefore required for converting the change in anode current into a change in voltage. This can be done quite simply by inserting a suitable resistor between the anode and the high voltage supply. The insertion of a resistor will however complicate things since it will lower the anode voltage by an amount depending upon current flow. To compensate for this a supply of more than 200V is needed. An example of the circuit is given in 7 Fig. 47 where it can be seen that, if a 2,000Ω (2 KΩ) resistor is used with a Vg of –4V the supply must be 250 volts since the valve will draw 25 mA causing a drop of 50V across the 2 KΩ resistor.

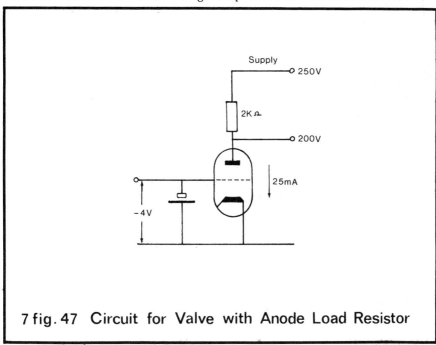

7 fig. 47 Circuit for Valve with Anode Load Resistor

If the voltage on the grid is now changed to –5V the anode current will fall to 12.5 mA. The voltage drop across the anode resistor will now be 25V giving an anode voltage of 225V. Thus a change of 1V on the grid has produced a change in anode voltage of 25V a gain of 25. More amplification can be obtained by simply increasing the value of the anode resistor. This is acceptable over wide limits providing the effect on anode voltage of the standing current is taken into account.

The simple system mentioned above will undoubtedly work, providing one is fortunate enough to have a signal which happens to have such a convenient magnitude. Most signals however are not so accommodating. Many input devices produce no output voltage until activated, whereupon a signal which swings both positively and negatively about zero is generated. With 200 volts on the anode and zero volts on the grid the valve would draw about 75 mA, which is three times the maximum recommended current. There would also be a considerable amount of grid current. To operate the valve at the correct point some means of applying the appropriate bias voltage to the grid is necessary.

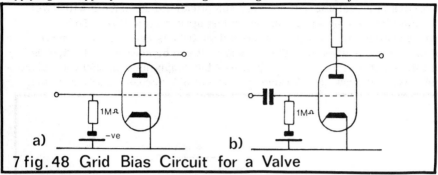

7 fig. 48 Grid Bias Circuit for a Valve

The most obvious means of obtaining the necessary bias voltage is to use a small battery connected to the grid via a high value resistor as shown in 7 Fig. 48a. Since the grid should not draw any current, the voltage drop across the 1 MΩ resistor should be virtually zero, so that the full bias voltage will be applied to the grid. The high resistance prevents the signal voltage being lost, but where the signal source has a low resistance the bias will be considerably reduced. This problem can be overcome by connecting the signal source in series with the grid resistor instead of in parallel.

Where the signal to be amplified is superimposed upon a certain voltage some means of removing the standing voltage is needed. A capacitor between the grid and the input will block the D.C, but still allow the varying voltage to pass through. This is shown in 7 Fig 48b.

The use of a battery to provide bias is simple but does have many disadvantages, not the least of which is the tendency of the battery to run down. It is therefore more convenient to derive the bias from the high voltage supply. The system most commonly used is called automatic bias. The grid must be biased negatively with respect to the cathode, which is more conveniently done by holding the grid at zero volts, and making the cathode positive. This is achieved by inserting a resistor between the cathode and the zero volt line. (R in 7 Fig. 49) which eliminates the need for a separate bias supply.

With 200 volts on the anode, a standing current of 12 mA will require -5V on the grid, calling for a 2.4kΩ cathode resistor.

The problem with this simple arrangement is that the bias will change when the grid voltage is changed, so that, if a signal is applied to the grid of +1V, the voltage between the cathode and grid will now become -4V. This should cause the anode current to increase to 25 mA, but if the valve draws 25 mA through a 2.4kΩ resistor then the voltage drop will be 6V. Now this just cannot be, since with -6V on the grid the current drawn would be only 5 mA. What really happens is that the cathode voltage follows the grid voltage and if the grid voltage is driven to +1V then the cathode voltage will increase by almost 1V so maintaining only a small

104

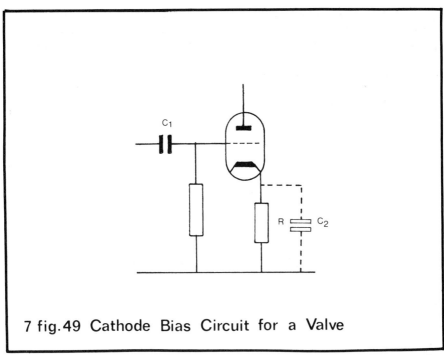

7 fig.49 Cathode Bias Circuit for a Valve

difference between cathode and grid voltage. The amplification of the valve is very low because the cathode and anode follow each other, and there is very little change in grid to cathode voltage. This is said to be due to negative feed back.

The problem may be overcome by providing a path of low impedance for the alternating signal, whilst once again blocking the D.C. A capacitor (C2 in 7 Fig. 49) is again used but since the value of the parallel resistor is now much lower the value of the capacitor must be correspondingly increased. The value of the frequency sensitive components, that is the grid resistor and capacitor, and the cathode resistor and capacitor, are chosen for the range of frequencies to be handled.

7.19.2 The Oscilloscope

In Section 7.8 the cathode ray tube was discussed and its use as a display device mentioned. This section will consider a display device called the oscilloscope in more detail and suggest some possible uses.

A set of deflection plates is shown in 7 Fig. 50. When all the plates are at zero potential the spot will be central. If for example X1 plate is made positive, then the spot will be deflected towards X1. The amount to which the spot will be deflected will depend upon the voltage applied to the plate. The deflection sensitivity is normally given in the manufacturers data, and a typical value would be 10V/cm. This indicates that for every ten volts difference across the plates the beam would be deflected by 1 cm until it strikes the plate itself and the spot on the screen disappears. A negative voltage on X2 would have a similar effect to a positive voltage on X1. Since the mass of the electron is extremely small the beam will move more or less instantaneously. The oscilloscope can therefore be used to record very fast changes in voltage.

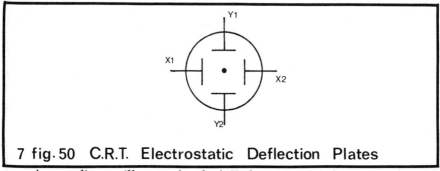

7 fig. 50   C.R.T. Electrostatic Deflection Plates

A recording oscilloscope has both X plates connected to zero volts and the potential to be measured connected across the Y plates. The applied voltage will then move the spot vertically. The spot is recorded on photographic film via a lens system. A motor drive mechanism transports the film at a predetermined speed. The result is a recording such as shown in 7 Fig. 51.

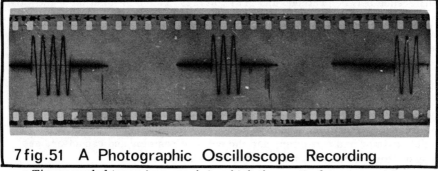

7 fig.51   A Photographic Oscilloscope Recording

The recorded trace is a graph in which the vertical component is voltage and the horizontal component time. This type of output is satisfactory where the phenomenon to be recorded is not recurrent, but has the disadvantage that the user cannot observe the phenomena under examination directly. Where a recurring event must be examined, it is more convenient to use a stroboscopic technique. This involves applying a saw-tooth waveform (See 7 Fig. 52) to the X plates so that the spot moves slowly from left to right across the tube. On reaching the right-hand side of the tube the spot is rapidly returned and the sequence restarted. The circuit responsible for generating this waveform is known as the time-base.

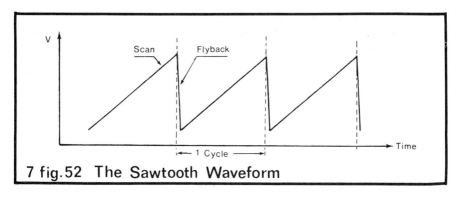

7 fig.52 The Sawtooth Waveform

While this waveform is applied to the X plates the waveform to be observed is applied to the Y plates. In order to display an apparently stationary image on the face of the tube some means of relating the sawtooth with the signal applied to the Y plates is needed.

In theory at least, it would be possible to make the speed of the timebase variable, so that it completes one cycle in a period which is some multiple of the time taken by the recurring phenomena applied to the Y plates. In practice, However, this would not be satisfactory since some small variation in frequency of either signal would cause the displayed trace to move. To prevent this some circuit is needed which brings about a positive relationship between the time-base and the displayed phenomena.

There are two ways of doing this, commonly known as synchronising and triggering, both depending upon a signal derived from the waveform to be displayed being fed to the time-base.

A synchronised time-base runs continuously but the flyback point is initiated by some feature of the Y signal (either a positive or negative excursion or a sharp spike). Thus with no X signal, the time-base may take, for example 1 second to cover the full distance of 10 cm. The synchronising signal may initiate flyback before the 1 second is up, giving a trace shorter than 10 cm. If however the synchronising signal occurs slightly after the start of flyback, the signal will be ignored and synchronism will be lost.

A triggered time-base will complete one saw-tooth, and then wait with the spot stationary on the lefthand side of the tube. The arrival of the next synchronising signal will start another scanning sequence. In this case the length of each scan will be the same, 10 cm, but the time between scans will depend upon the synchronising signal.

The time-base usually has a number of ranges. A general purpose oscilloscope may have a switched time-base ranging from 0.1 μs/cm up to 5 s/cm. The higher speeds are only required for measuring electronic waveforms such as the output signal from a television unit, (See Chapter 16) whereas the slower speeds are often needed for physiological waveforms. (See Chapter 21).

107

The deflection sensitivity of the cathode ray tube depends upon the mechanical construction of the tube and the voltage on the final anode. Although the example quoted earlier was a convenient round figure this is not always the case. Moreover the range of sensitivities quoted by manufacturers are much too low for the tube to be used for physiological measurements without some sort of amplification. In order to ensure consistent performance it is usual to build a fixed gain amplifier into the oscilloscope through which all signals must pass.

If an amplifier is to be used to display physiological signals the designer may choose a maximum sensitivity of 1 mV/cm. The cathode ray tube will require a signal of 10V to deflect the spot 1 cm so that the gain of the amplifier must be 10,000. The input to the amplifier is then attenuated by a resistor network so that a selection of switched values is obtained. The table below gives some examples.

Switch range	Attenuator
1 mV/cm	1:1
5 mV/cm	5:1
10 mV/cm	10:1
50 mV/cm	50:1
100 mV/cm	100:1
500 mV/cm	500:1
1 V/cm	1000:1
5 V/cm	5000:1
10 V/cm	10000:1
50 V/cm	50000:1
100 V/cm	100000:1

The amplifier and attenuator are designed in such a way that the instrument causes the minimum disturbance to the circuit under test regardless of the sensitivity range selected.

Oscilloscopes are available in a wide price range. Before purchasing an instrument it is advisable to read carefully through the literature to ensure that the instrument chosen has all the facilities needed for the purpose for which it is intended without unnecessary complexity (and cost).

7.20 Rectifiers for use in X-ray generators

In order to convert the alternating voltage from the X-ray high voltage transformer into D.C, a variety of devices have been used. These range from the early mechanical rectifier to the silicon rectifier now found in the latest types of apparatus. In between these two, the thermionic diode enjoyed a long period of popularity, and lest it be thought that the change from the valve to the semiconductor was made solely for reasons of fashion - this section will discuss the performance of the two classes of device and compare their characteristics.

The most outstanding reason for the adoption of solid state rectification is the improvement in reliability. A survey of valve failures shows that the most common cause of breakdown is filament failure. Thoriated tungsten filaments are brittle and so liable to break due to mechanical shock. They also lose their coating of thorium and so become less able to produce sufficient numbers of electrons. Plain tungsten, although not susceptible to these faults, must be run at such a high temperature that the tungsten slowly evaporates and causes the filament to go open circuit.

Another common cause of failure is loss of vacuum due to the release of gas trapped in the electrode structure allowing ionisation. There is also the possibility that the glass may fail. If this failure is just a minute crack the valve will once again lose its vacuum, but in most cases failure of the glass envelope is sudden and catastrophic, resulting in complete failure of the valve.

The semiconductor rectifier has no filament, is not evacuated, and does not have a fragile glass envelope, so that all of these three causes of failure are eliminated.

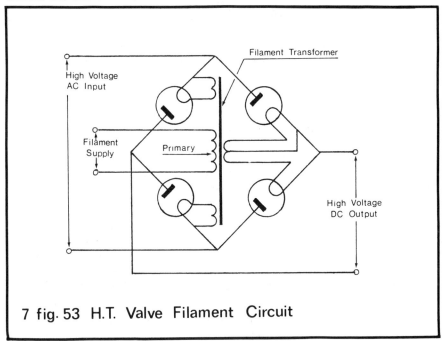

7 fig. 53 H.T. Valve Filament Circuit

A further reason for adopting solid state rectification is the reduction in both size and complexity of the generator that this makes possible. This can be seen by studying the valve filament arrangement in 7 Fig. 53. A thermionic valve must have a filament supply and since two valves have their filaments connected to opposite ends of the high voltage input, a total of three valve filament transformers are needed. At first sight this would not seem to be a great problem since a high voltage rectifying valve requires a filament current of only a few amps produced by few volts. The problem here is that the primary of the valve filament transformer is at a low potential, whilst the secondary is at a high potential. This means that the secondary windings must be heavily insulated from the primary, from the iron core, and also from each other. Just how complex this transformer is, can be seen in 7 Fig. 54. The transformer is both bulky and inefficient. Thus the elimination of the valve filament transformers permits a considerable reduction in overall size of the high voltage generator.

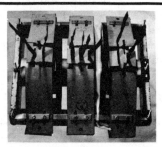

7 fig. 54 The H.T. Valve Filament Transformer

Efficiency is increased by the absence of a filament. Each valve consumes about 300 watts in the filament (a total of 1200 watts for a four valve circuit). In addition to this there is the voltage drop across the valve due to its own internal resistance. This loss is dependent upon current, so that some form of compensation is needed to ensure consistent voltage output of the generator. For the sake of convenience this is compensated together with the mains resistance losses as discussed in Chapter 9. Semiconductor rectifiers have a lower internal resistance and slightly lower power loss is produced.

For a short period of time before the appearance of silicon rectifiers, selenium rectifiers were used. In this case the voltage drop across the rectifier is greater than that found with a thermionic valve. A comparison is shown in 7 Fig. 55. Nevertheless, the selenium rectifier does give an overall improvement in reliability over the valve so that it is worthwhile to fit selenium, even though the forward voltage drop is greater.

Two different types of rectifiers are available. One is made up of six short ceramic rods. Each rod is a rectifier made up of a number of diodes to give a total working voltage of 25 kV. The complete assembly will thus work at up to 150 kV. This type of construction gives a great deal of flexibility, a rectifier suitable for 125 or 100 kV can easily be assembled. The device is used as a replacement for a thermionic valve in existing equipment. The initial cost is high, since not only are these rectifiers dearer than thermionic valves, but when the change is made to solid state rectification all four rectifiers must be changed at once. This initial expense is offset by the fact that the solid state rectifiers can normally be expected to outlast the rest of the apparatus. A range of end caps, together with a simple plastic mounting board, allows this type of rectifier to be used as a replacement for any type of existing thermionic rectifier. Where a generator is designed to be used only with solid state rectifiers, a single rod type of assembly can be used since this occupies less space and so makes a further reduction in the size of the generator possible. (see 7 Fig. 56).

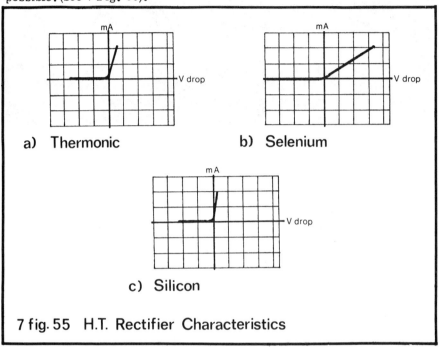

a) Thermonic

b) Selenium

c) Silicon

7 fig. 55   H.T. Rectifier Characteristics

To summarise, it can be said that it is possible in all cases to fit solid state rectifiers to any type of high voltage generator, thus giving the following advantages :-

Increased Reliability	No filament fracture
	No filament evaporation
	No loss of emission
	No flash over
	No loss of vacuum
Increased Efficiency	More consistent results
	No sudden breakdown
	No power consumption under quiescent conditions

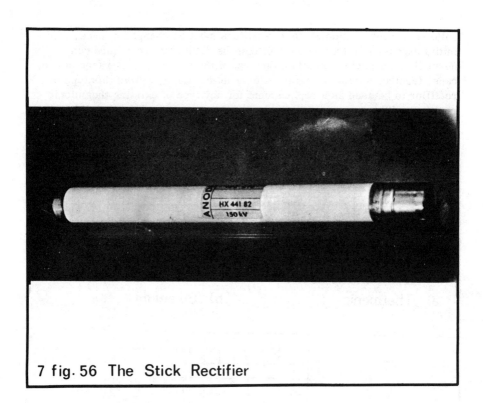

7 fig. 56 The Stick Rectifier

Chapter 8

The X-Ray Tube

8.1   Introduction

The object of this chapter is to explain in detail the design and construction of the high vacuum devices essential to the production of an X-ray beam; that is, the X-ray tube itself and the high voltage vacuum rectifiers which provided the sole practical means of rectification until a few years ago. The more recent stages of development will be traced out, and attention drawn to the materials used in the construction of tubes and valves.

A further, and vital, function of the chapter is to guide users in the safe and proper operation of a tube in order that it may give the longest possible life consistent with the task it has to perform.

8.2   A Simple Valve

The simplest thermionic diode valve that it would be possible to construct is shown in 8 Fig. 1. It consists of a metal anode and an elementary filament-type cathode sealed into opposite ends of a glass envelope. The protuberance, usually known as the "pip", is all that remains of a glass sealing tube through which the valve was pumped to a condition of high vacuum, during manufacture. The cathode is made from a simple coil of tungsten wire, each end of which is attached to a metal "pole" passing through the glass envelope via a vacuum tight seal.

The operation of this valve is based on thermionic emission. The filament, being metal and a conductor of electricity, contains free electrons

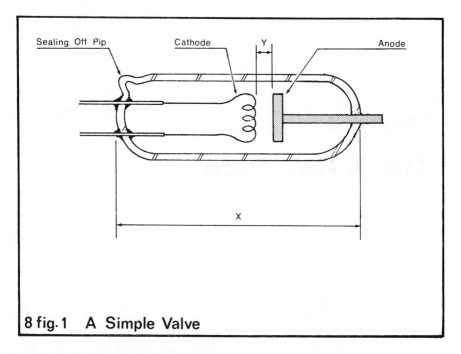

8 fig. 1   A Simple Valve

as part of the atomic structure. These electrons will flow along the wire when a small current is passed through it. If this current is increased until the filament becomes very hot, some electrons will move outside the wire itself and form a "cloud" of electrons immediately surrounding the filament. A positive potential applied to the anode with respect to the cathode will draw the electrons, which are negatively charged particles, towards the anode with an acceleration proportional to the anode voltage.

If the polarity of the voltage across the valve is now reversed, such that the anode becomes negative with respect to the cathode, the force on the electrons will be a repelling one instead of an attracting one and no electron flow will take place. Consequently, there will be no current flow in the circuit in which the valve is situated. (See 8 Fig. 2).

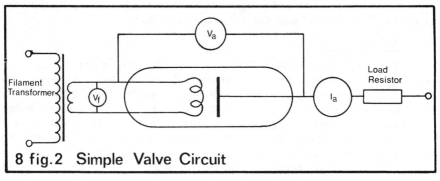

8 fig. 2   Simple Valve Circuit

In order to experiment further, consider both the current supply to the filament and the voltage across the valve to be variable, and also the valve voltage (Va) to be alternating. Let the filament current, for the moment, be as high as possible. This means that the filament will be extremely hot and that it will be very easy to attract electrons away from it. Now if the valve voltage, or to use a more correct term, the anode voltage, is increased slowly from zero, it will be noticed that quite soon a current commences to flow through the load. Furthermore, as Va is increased, the current will increase proportionally to the increase in Va. This is because the rate at which electrons are drawn away from the cathode towards the anode increases as the attracting force is increased.

The next significant stage is reached when an increase of Va no longer causes an increase in the anode current (Ia). This occurs when all the available electrons are being pulled towards the anode. This point is known as the "saturation point", and it occurs at a certain value of Va for each setting of the filament temperature.   Once the saturation point is passed, Va may be increased quite drastically with hardly any change in Ia. (See 8 Fig. 3).

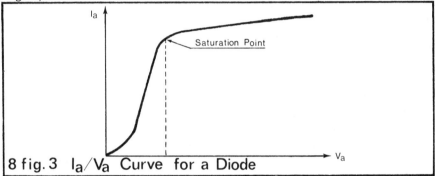

8 fig. 3 I_a/V_a Curve for a Diode

Under these conditions the anode current can only be increased by raising the filament temperature. Thus, if the filament current is increased the filament temperature will also increase and the saturation point will occur at a somewhat higher value of Va. This is because raising the temperature increases the quantity of electrons available to be attracted to the anode.

8.3   A High Voltage Rectifier

At this stage it is appropriate to modify the simple rectifier illustrated in 8 Fig. 1 in order that it may operate safely in the normal voltage range for the production of a useful X-ray beam, i.e. between 25,000 and 150,000 volts.

If such a voltage is applied to a valve of the physical size shown in 8 Fig. 1, i.e. 50 to 75 mm long, with an anode cathode separation of 3 mm, there will be an immediate electrical breakdown of the vacuum space between the anode and the cathode. Also, a breakdown of the air surrounding the valve will occur, and an electric arc will form outside the envelope between the protruding metal parts of the two electrodes. This would happen because both the anode-cathode distance "Y" and the overall length of the valve "X" are insufficient for the high voltages involved. Both media, vacuum and air, are insulators - vacuum being much superior to air - and the voltage required to break them down is proportional to the distance separating the electrodes. Thus, for example, 10 mm of a good insulator such as bakelite will withstand several times the voltage that would break down the insulation of 3 mm of the same material.

This means, of course, that in the required voltage range the valve must have a larger vacuum space between the anode and the cathode, in practice between 12 and 25 mm, and also it must have a long flashover path outside the glass envelope. For a valve designed to operate surrounded by air, this path would have to be of the order of 400 - 500 mm, but as nearly all valves and tubes nowadays operate immersed in a fluid called transformer oil, which is a much better insulator than air, a path length of 150 mm is adequate.

Further consideration can now be given to the simple diode structure of 8 Fig. 1, bearing in mind that it has now been modified to operate at a high voltage. Consider it operating in a circuit such as 8 Fig. 2, but where the supply voltage for Va is now capable of adjustment from zero to, say, 100,000 volts. The filament circuit remains the same, and a load is included such as a resistor.

If the filament is made as hot as possible, then the valve will be in a condition of maximum emission. The emission, in terms of current, will be proportional to the anode voltage below saturation point, but relatively constant above saturation point. If the load resistor is now adjusted so that the circuit current is less than the maximum possible emission of the valve, then the voltage (Va) across the valve will be less than the saturation point voltage.

This, of course, is only true when the anode is positive with respect to the cathode. When the polarity is reversed the valve does not conduct, there is no circuit current, and virtually the whole of the available voltage is applied to the valve. Hence it is necessary to design for high voltage operation although the voltage drop across the valve on the conducting half-cycle is quite low.

The subject of heat developed in the valve is now worthy of attention. Consider the valve to have the characteristics of a normal tungsten filament rectifier. If the filament is made sufficiently hot to enable the valve to pass an anode current of 500 mA then the filament is likely to be operating at about 11 volts and passing a current of 12 amperes. So about 130 watts of heat will be dissipated continuously from the cathode alone. The anode's contribution to heat developed will be proportional to the anode current (Ia) multiplied by the voltage between anode and cathode (Va). When the anode is negative, the voltage drop is very high but the current flow is virtually zero,

116

therefore no heat results. On the conducting half-cycle when the anode is positive, however, if 500 mA (0.5 amps) passes through the valve, Va will have a value of about 2,500 volts. This results in an anode heat dissipation of 0.5 amps x 2,500 volts = 1,250 watts. In practice, the X-ray tube rating will not permit a current of this order for more than about a second, so the valve under normal conditions does not have to withstand a great deal of heat.

Now if the filament temperature is reduced while the valve is passing 500 mA, the immediate result will be an increase in the voltage Va across the valve. If the temperature is reduced sufficiently this voltage will become very high indeed. As a result the velocity of the electrons flowing towards the anode will increase and eventually, if the voltage is high enough, the valve itself will emit X-rays resulting from the collision of the high speed electrons with the anode.

Another consequence would be a considerable increase in the anode heat, since this is proportional to Ia x Va.

8.4   A Simple X-ray Tube

This leads now to consideration of changes necessary to make the basic diode suitable for use as a simple, but effective, X-ray tube.

Two points stand out for immediate attention. One, the amount of heat the anode can hold is met by increasing the "heat storage capacity": the simple plate anode which sufficed in the rectifying valve must be replaced by a composite copper-tungsten structure with a high thermal capacity. Secondly, and more difficult to resolve, is the problem of image quality as a function of the size of the X-ray source. This is comparable with aperture size in a normal camera, and the principle is illustrated in 8 Fig. 4.

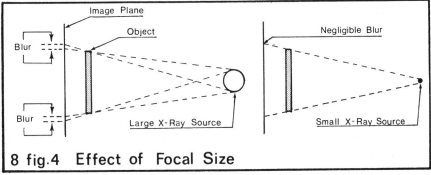

8 fig.4 Effect of Focal Size

In an X-ray tube there is a conflict of requirement in that, for good radiographic definition the smallest possible source of X-rays is required, while the high thermal loads associated with the production of X-rays demand the largest possible electron impact area. As these areas are one and the same, a compromise must be made between the size of focus really desired and the magnitude of tube current (and hence thermal load) that the radiographic technique demands, the kilovoltage in both cases being the same.

Since the X-rays emanate from a small source and are required to cover a film some distance away, it is fairly clear that the beam of radiation must be conical. This necessitates an angled face to the anode, as otherwise the anode itself would absorb at least half of the required beam. This angled face assists somewhat in resolving the conflicting requirements regarding the focal area, since to present a square focus "a x a" as viewed from the film, a rectangle of length several times the width "a" is required on the anode face.

This is illustrated in 8 Fig. 5 and is known as the "line focus" principle.

It can be seen that the apparent focal area, which determines the degree of geometric unsharpness is smaller than the actual focal area, which is the area of electron bombardment and which determines the tube rating.

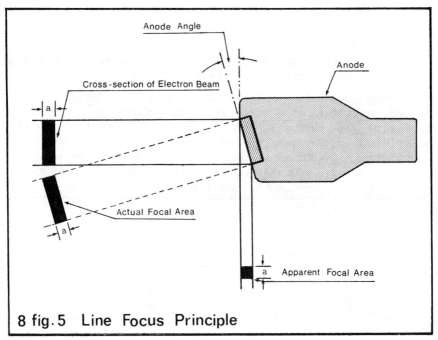

8 fig. 5   Line Focus Principle

Obviously, if the anode angle is made shallower the bombarded area is even greater for a specific size of "apparent" focus. Most target angles lie between 15° and 19°. At shallower angles the amount of X-radiation per unit of tube current falls considerably until the advantage gained in increased loading is outweighed by reduced radiation. This is discussed further in Section 8.21.

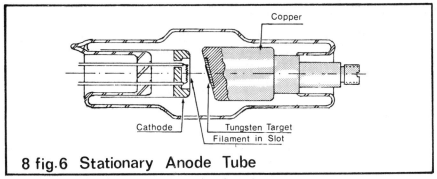

Copper

Cathode | Tungsten Target
Filament in Slot

8 fig.6 Stationary Anode Tube

8.5 Construction of a Stationary Anode Tube

The illustration 8 Fig. 6 shows a section through a typical stationary anode tube. The anode consists of a small tablet of tungsten, called the "target", soldered into a heavy block of copper.

At the rear of the anode is soldered a sealing ring of stainless steel to which the glass envelope is sealed.

The cathode is sealed into the other end of the glass envelope. It consists of a tungsten filament mounted inside a focussing slot cut in a metal block, which is mounted on a glass foot, the whole assembly being covered with a metal can for electrostatic screening.

The glass foot, such as is shown in 8 Fig. 7, is usually one of the first parts of a tube to be made. It is simply a convenient way of passing the conductors carrying the filament heating current through the glass envelope of the tube. Such a device is used in ordinary electric light bulbs, although as the current is much higher for a tube, the metal poles are somewhat larger.

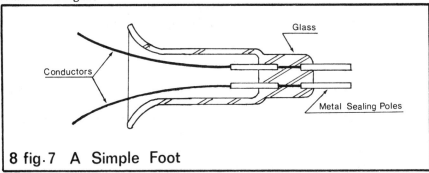

Glass

Conductors

Metal Sealing Poles

8 fig.7 A Simple Foot

The glass from which a foot is made has to be chosen to match the glass of the main envelope, since they will be later sealed together. If the coefficients of expansion of the two glasses differed, the seal would crack whilst cooling. Similarly, the metal poles have to be of a special alloy with a comparable coefficient of expansion. If a perfect match cannot be made with the glass required for the main envelope, an intermediate glass is used with a coefficient between the two. This will reduce to a tolerable degree the stress caused by the mismatch.

The cathode block, which contains the filament, is mounted above the foot, either mechanically attached to the poles or supported by the electrostatic screening can. The cathode block is usually made from nickel or a form of stainless steel, as is also the screening can.

The filament is a closely wound helix of tungsten wire, about 0.2 mm thick, the helix diameter being about 1.0 - 1.5 mm. One end of the filament is connected electrically to the block, the other passes through the block via a small insulator of ceramic material. (See 8 Fig 8a). The height of the filament in relation to the edges of the slot in the block is very critical, since this is an important factor in the focussing of the electron beam and consequently in determining the size of the focal area.

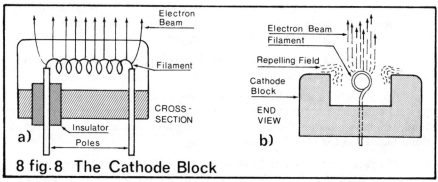

8 fig. 8 The Cathode Block

In the main, the focussing mechanism is the strong negative field existing on the edges of the slot (See 8 Fig. 8b). This field exists because the cathode is negative with respect to the anode and it is more intense with increasing sharpness of the slot edges. A radiused edge would still present a strong field, but not as strong as that from a sharp edge. This field exerts a repelling force on the electrons being drawn away from the filament. Design and experiment provides the right shape of cathode block to form the electron stream into a beam giving the required focal area where it impacts on the target.

The focussing effect of the slot edges controls the width of the electron beam. Focussing in the other dimension is determined, to a large extent, by the length of the filament itself. In some designs small tags or bars are placed at the ends of the filament to strengthen the focussing in the longitudinal plane.

The electron beam strikes the area known as the target, normally comprised of a small tablet of tungsten about 15 mm wide x 20 mm long x 3 mm thick soldered into a block of copper. Tungsten is chosen since it combines a high atomic number(74) - making it comparatively efficient in the production of X-rays - with a high melting point enabling it to withstand the heavy thermal loads.

Tungsten, however, has disadvantages. It is a poor conductor of heat and is prone to surface cracking due to high internal stresses resulting from repeated thermal loads. Nevertheless, for general diagnostic tubes it is the best compromise material considering factors such as availability, cost, and ease of forming. The melting point is about 3410° C, but the working temperature has to be kept well below this to avoid damage, and is usually limited to a surface temperature of 2,200° C. With a stationary anode tube, even this temperature is only permissible over the focal spot area since the tungsten is imbedded in copper. Loading of the tube, therefore, has to be arranged so that the boundary of the tungsten - where it meets the copper - is well below the melting point of copper (1083° C).

If the tube is to work in self-rectified circuits (see Chapter 9) a lower temperature limit must be set for the focal spot otherwise reverse emission will take place from the target. This would very quickly destroy the filament and cathode.

The copper, being an excellent thermal conductor, performs the vital function of carrying the heat rapidly away from the tungsten target. The heat flows through the anode to the outside of the tube, where it is removed normally by convection. This is discussed in the next section.

Onto the anode a ring of stainless steel is soldered. This, like the poles through the foot, has to be of a metal closely matched in coefficient of expansion to the glass itself. Two or three rings of intermediate glass are first placed on the steel ring to reduce the effect of any mismatch. Such a combination is known as a "graded seal". See 8 Fig. 9.

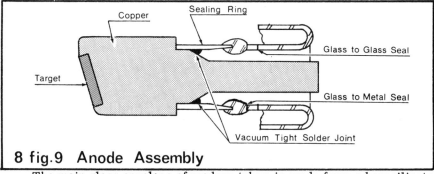

8 fig.9 Anode Assembly

The main glass envelope of modern tubes is made from a borosilicate glass such as, or similar to, Pyrex. This is known as a "hard" glass, and is very resistant to thermal shock. In this way it differs from the lead, or soda, "soft" glasses used to manufacture the earlier air insulated tubes. In those days, if a warm tube was picked up with a cold hand, it was quite possible that the tube would shatter.

8.6   A Stationary Anode Tube Shield

Before considering any further sophistication of the tube, some thought must be given to the working environment. In the form just considered two points stand out.

(a) The electrodes have open high voltage on them and must be shielded.

(b) The tube will emit X-rays in all directions and protection must be provided except where the useful beam emerges from the tube.

In addition, an oil environment must be provided for insulation and convection current cooling. To contain this oil, and meet the two points mentioned above, the obvious requirement is for a metal container completely surrounding the tube. Such a container, known as a "shield". is shown in 8 Fig. 10.

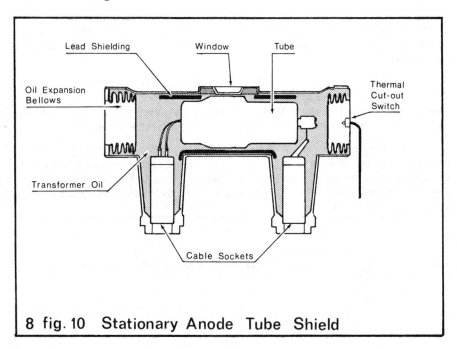

8 fig. 10   Stationary Anode Tube Shield

The main part of the shield is the metal shell, sometimes made as an aluminium casting and sometimes as a formed sheet metal structure. This is lined where necessary with 3 or 4 mm of lead to prevent the exit of any radiation except the required useful beam which emerges through a plastic window of very low filtration.

Since a lot of heat will be generated by the tube, and this heat will cause the oil temperature to rise, the oil will expand. Oil, being a liquid, is incompressible, hence a bellows, either of oil resistant rubber or thin metal, has to be provided to accommodate the expansion. When it has expanded as much as the bellows will permit, any further rise of oil temperature would mean a risk of the shield being forced open by oil pressure. To avoid this, an electrical switch is usually fitted inside the bellows to prevent further operation of the tube just before the bellows reach maximum stroke. A temperature on the outside of the shield of between 60° and 70° C is usually attained before this happens.

Special sockets, made from very high quality insulating materials, are fitted into the legs of the shield to receive the plugs of the high voltage cables passing the voltage to the tube. The plugs and sockets used are now internationally standard, although several different designs exist, e.g. for 100 kVp, 125 kVp, and 150 kVp operation.

Fortunately, the high voltage supply for almost every diagnostic X-ray shield is symmetrical about earth. That is, a 100 kVp supply across the tube means that the anode is at a potential of + 50 kVp with respect to earth and the cathode is at - 50 kVp with respect to earth. Thus a lower voltage to earth has to be insulated, and this reduces the dimension of the plugs and sockets, and also the insulation distances to earth within the shield.

Due to the very penetrating nature of transformer oil, particularly when hot, every joint on a shield has to be hermetically sealed, either soldered or with a rubber gasket.

Finally, and this is very important, to make the shield shockproof it must be very efficiently earthed. Although the cables have an earthed braiding along the outside, nowadays the amount of copper has had to be reduced to achieve cable flexibility so that it must never be relied upon as an earth for the shield. This means that a separate earth connection must be made to the shield.

8.7   Limitations of a Stationary Anode Tube

The tube so far described is representative of most modern stationary anode tubes.

Now this type of tube has very definite limitations in use. To understand them the following points should be considered:-

(a) To obtain a clear radiograph with minimum loss of detail, the smallest possible focus should be used.

(b) To withstand the thermal load associated with a radiograph, the largest possible focus should be used.

(c) Since film blackening is proportional to the product of tube current and exposure time, a blackening resulting from 100 milliampere seconds (mAs) will be identical whether the radiograph is made from a load of 100 milliamperes for 1 second or for 1 milliampere for 100 seconds. However, there is a limitation to the shortest time during which a 100 mAs can be applied since with high currents due to the finite time taken for heat to travel from the bombarded face of the tungsten, localised overheating occurs. In fact, the front face of the target could be vapourised before the temperature at the back of the target had risen significantly.

(d) If the radiograph is of a part of the body which can be held stationary, such as a hand or a foot, there is no objection to a long exposure time. However, most radiographs are of parts of the body which are affected by involuntary organic movement, such as heart, lungs, etc., and to obtain a clear image, relatively free from "movement blur", the radiograph must be taken in the shortest possible time.

Hence the requirements are very contradictory, and with the type of tube so far described (the stationary anode tube) all work done has to be a compromise between the duration of exposure and the minimum possible focal size.

Most tubes made are, in fact, double-focus tubes, having two filaments side by side, one providing a small and the other a large focus.

On the target, the foci are also sometimes side by side but can be superimposed.

8.8   The Rotating Anode Tube

The limitation previously discussed basically stems from the melting point of the tungsten forming the focal spot. If the small piece of tungsten embedded in copper is now replaced by a disc of tungsten, free to rotate such that the edge of the disc is placed over the cathode block, much greater loading per unit of focal area can be achieved. (See 8 Fig. 11).

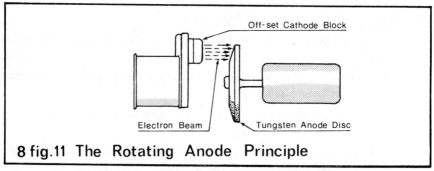

Off-set Cathode Block

Electron Beam

Tungsten Anode Disc

8 fig.11 The Rotating Anode Principle

If the anode rotates during a radiographic exposure, the thermal load will be spread over a ring of tungsten while the focal spot, considered photographically, remains stationary.

Consider a radiographic exposure during which the tungsten disc rotates once. In the example drawn in 8 Fig. 12, the apparent focal size which determines the degree of unsharpness, measures 3 mm x 3 mm, but the area over which the thermal load is spread is $9 \times 60 \times \pi = 1693$ mm^2.

With the same apparent focus on a stationary anode tube the thermal load would be distributed over an area only $3 \times 9 = 27$ mm^2.

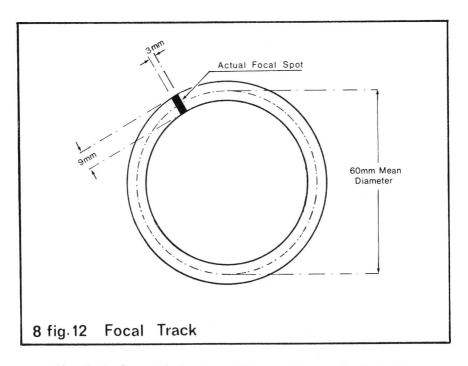

3mm

Actual Focal Spot

9mm

60mm Mean
Diameter

8 fig. 12   Focal   Track

Thus the fundamental advantage of the rotating anode tube is that a much higher thermal loading can be applied per unit of focal area.

The loading is related to the diameter of the focal track, the mass of the anode disc, and the speed of rotation. This increased loading makes possible :-

(a) a considerably greater load in terms of mA per unit time for a given focus size

or (b) a reduced focal size for a given mA load per unit time

or (c) a reduction of time for a given value of milliampere seconds for a given focus.

The rotating anode tube shown in 8 Fig. 13 is typical of the many thousands in use throughout the world. There exist several major manufacturers, but in the main their product resembles the example here as closely as different manufacturers' bicycles resemble each other.

Nowadays a range of tube sizes is available. These vary from small tubes with tungsten discs about 50 mm diameter, basically designed to replace stationary anode tubes on light mobile units, to much larger **versions** with discs of 100 or 110 mm diameter used on the very powerful sets for angiography, etc. The most common size in use is that with a disc diameter of about 75 to 80 mm and a maximum operating voltage of 150 kVp.

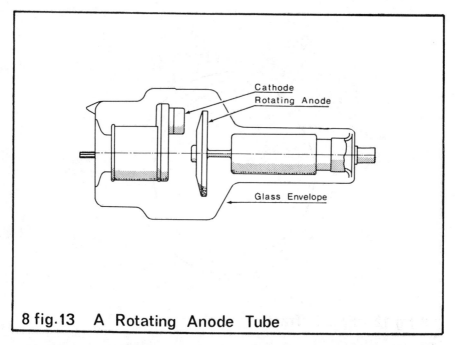

Cathode

Rotating Anode

Glass Envelope

8 fig.13   A Rotating Anode Tube

The particular design feature which distinguishes the modern tube is the mounting of the anode disc on a spindle of high melting point metal, such as molybdenum, so that the disc is a significant distance from any metal or material with a low melting point such as steel or copper. In contrast to the stationary anode tube, where the tungsten temperature is restricted by the comparatively low melting point of the surrounding copper, the tungsten disc can safely rise to a background temperature of about 1200°C at which the heat radiation presents a very efficient method of cooling. In fact, radiation cooling is the principle used for modern rotating anode tubes, just as conduction cooling is the principle for the stationary anode tube. In both cases, the heat is removed from the immediate vicinity of the tube by convection currents in the oil.

8.9   Constructional Details of a Rotating Anode Tube

The glass envelope and the cathode of the rotating anode tube are very similar to those in the stationary anode tube. The anodes, however, are very different. The only significant point regarding the cathode is that the block containing the filaments is offset to lie under the edge of the anode disc, as shown in 8 Fig. 11.

To appreciate the construction of the anode it is shown both in an assembled and a dissembled condition in 8 Fig. 14.

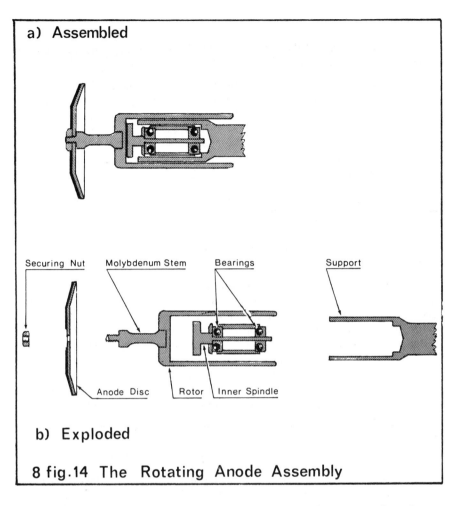

a) Assembled

Securing Nut   Molybdenum Stem   Bearings   Support

Anode Disc   Rotor   Inner Spindle

b) Exploded

8 fig.14 The Rotating Anode Assembly

The rotor is made from copper, either cast or from special quality rod. The molybdenum stem projecting from the rotor is either soldered in with eutectic silver-copper alloy or the copper of the rotor may be cast round it. In either case, the final machining is carried out afterwards to ensure true axial alignment.

The choice of molybdenum is dictated by the need for a strong metal with a melting point high enough to permit contact with the very hot tungsten disc. Molybdenum melts at 2630° C and thus is suitable. In addition, it must be sufficiently machineable to permit shaping and cutting of threads for the securing nut. Tungsten would fail in this respect, and also is too brittle. A nut screws onto the threaded portion of the rotor stem to hold the anode disc in position. It is made of molybdenum for the same reasons as the rotor stem.

The copper part of the rotor is normally blackened to increase the heat emissivity of its surface.

Manufacture of the early tungsten discs before the Second World War necessitated the development of special methods such as sintering. This involves passing a heavy electric current through a compacted mass of tungsten powder moulded into the final shape until the whole fuses together. Some machining is possible with special tools, but is difficult. In recent years discs have become more complex in design, but this is discussed in connection with high speed tubes in Section 8.20

The inner spindle on which the bearings are mounted is made from a high grade stainless steel. This component has to be machined with meticulous accuracy to ensure true running of the anode.

Two ballrace bearings are mounted on it, either separated by a distance piece or secured by circlips.

Since the bearings have to operate in a high vacuum environment, lubrication of the bearings is somewhat unorthodox. The high temperature environment precludes most normal lubricants, which would have the additional disadvantage of releasing enough vapour to spoil the condition of high vacuum imperative to the proper functioning of the tube. It is true that the earliest rotating anode tubes used highly refined vacuum greases of very low vapour pressure, but it was not a satisfactory solution. An interesting side effect was the tendency of the tungsten filaments to deform in the presence of hydrocarbon vapour released by the lubricant.

Fortunately, this situation was remedied by the successful development of metal lubricants. Lead and silver are both in common use, and are usually applied in the form of a thin film to the bearing surfaces.

The support, so called because it holds the outer, or stationary race of the bearing and consequently the whole anode,is a stainless steel component. It is fitted with a sealing ring in just the same manner as the stationary anode.

8.10 Rotating Anode Tube Shield

The shield for a rotating anode tube serves the same functions as the stationary anode tube shield, but differs in that it must contain a means of rotating the anode. It is also of necessity larger.

A cross-section through such a shield is depicted in 8 Fig. 15. The motor coils embracing the anode neck of the tube comprise the "stator", which is virtually the same as the stator winding of a single phase squirrel cage induction motor. There is no winding on, or electrical supply to,the rotor itself, other than the plain copper cylinder which forms the main part of the rotor.

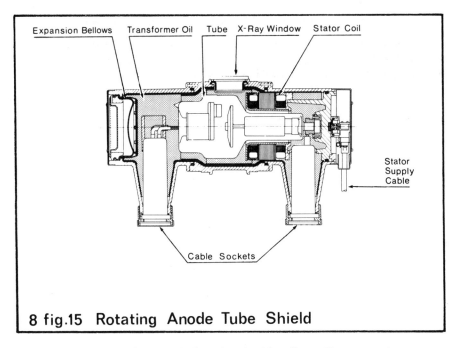

Expansion Bellows Transformer Oil Tube X-Ray Window Stator Coil

Stator
Supply
Cable

Cable Sockets

8 fig.15 Rotating Anode Tube Shield

The stator can be attached to the shield wall itself, or may be mounted cantilever fashion from an end plate at the anode end of the shield. The supply voltage for the stator, which varies according to type but is usually between 100 and 300 volts A.C., is fed in through oil-tight insulators either in the body or end of the shield.

It is important to realise that the stator core, being attached to the shield, is near earth potential, and the rotor, being part of the anode, is at a very high potential (half the operating voltage of the tube). They cannot therefore be as close together as would be the rotor-stator combination of an ordinary squirrel cage motor. In fact, they have to be separated by an oil gap and an insulating flange lining the inside of the stator assembly. The effect of this is to reduce the efficiency of the inductive coupling, but a little extra electrical power puts this right.

8.11 Anode Speed and Rotation

The anode rotational speed is purely a function of the number of magnetic poles in the stator coil and the frequency of the alternating supply, with a very slight loss of speed due to friction and other losses. X-ray tubes are nowadays classified as "standard speed" or "high speed". "Standard speed" refers to the tube which has an anode rotated slightly less than 3000 R.P.M. on a frequency of 50 Hz, and this, of course comprises most of the tubes which have been made. However, in the last decade high speed tubes operating at about 9000 R.P.M. have been coming more commonly used. These tubes will be dealt with later in this section.

The means by which anode rotation is achieved is rather complex and for a fuller understanding a text-book on induction motors is recommended. However, a brief explanation will be given here.

If the stator coil circuit is simplified, it breaks down to the equivalent form shown in 8 Fig. 16.

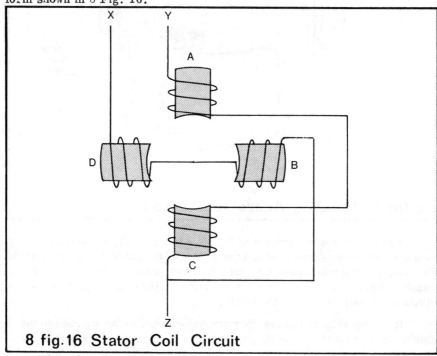

8 fig.16 Stator Coil Circuit

Now, if an A.C. voltage is applied across X and Z a current flows through path D and B. A magnetic flux is produced proportional to the current and the number of turns making up the coils. Provided that coil D is connected to coil B properly, one pole will be of north polarity when the other is south. As the current changes its direction of flow in the normal alternating fashion these polarities will reverse.

If the two paths are connected in parallel by joining X and Y, and the coils are similar in type, similar currents will flow through A and C as flow through B and D. In fact, in each path the current will have the same phase relationship to the voltage. If, however, a capacitor is included in the circuit of one path only, say B and D, the phase relationship will alter. The result of this will be that in sequence a north pole grows in strength at A and reaches maximum strength, and commences to diminish. At this point a north pole grows in B. This is followed by the growth of a north pole at C as A becomes south. The effect of this will be a resultant magnetic field rotating at 3000 R.P.M.

As this magnetic field rotates it will induce eddy currents in the rotor, since the rotor is a conductor and is being cut by the flux. The currents induced will set up their own magnetic fields, and the rotor will itself behave like a magnet, react with the magnetic field produced by the stator, and will be rotated.

To achieve the 9000 R.P.M. required for high speed tubes special stator equipment is necessary since the stator must be fed with a supply frequency of 150 Hz. Sometimes this is achieved by using a special motor alternator, or it can be produced by electronic or electrical frequency tripling.

It is vital, for reasons to be made clear later, that the anode be brought up to its operating speed very quickly. To achieve this it is normal for the stator to be of quite a high power rating, say between one and two kilowatts, but for the circuitry to be arranged so that the stator voltage, and hence the power, is reduced considerably once the anode is running at full speed. A power consumption of about 50 watts is quite sufficient to maintain the anode at speed. It must be remembered that the heat from the stator will cause the oil to expand and reduce the amount of energy which can be expended by the tube.

8.12 Tube Operation and Ratings

Before studying tube ratings, it is worth considering what actually happens to the tube when it is installed in a hospital.

There are two possible modes of operation, i.e. fluoroscopy and radiography. Fluoroscopy requires continuous use of the tube, at a low anode current, while observations are made on a fluorescent screen, or much more likely today, an image intensifier. The kilovoltage is varied according to requirement, but does not usually exceed 125 kVp. Because the anode current is low the filament current is also low.

Under these conditions the tube will go on working continuously. It will get very hot, but it may be used up to its maximum continuous rating, at which point the rate of heat loss equals the rate at which heat is put in.

It is normally only possible actually to see an insert tube working under these conditions in the factory where they are made. Testing is carried out in glass tanks in the early stages. The interesting thing is that the anode disc heats up over several minutes to a temperature between red and white heat. After about twenty minutes the whole anode is at equilibrium temperature. The disc is then at about 1200°C, the outside surface of the rotor at about 300°C, and visible heat ends about halfway down the molybdenum stem.

In contrast to fluoroscopy, radiography is the taking of an X-ray photograph for later study or for record purposes. The tube is operated for a fraction of a second at heavy anode currents, up to 1250 milliamperes, or for several seconds at lower anode currents in the order of 100 milliamps. These exposures are very different, and so is their effect on the anode disc.

Taking the case of the standard speed tube, and assuming the anode is cold, the disc will rotate less than one revolution in any exposure under $\frac{1}{50}$ sec. (0.02s). In this case, therefore, the factor limiting the amount of current through the tube is the surface, or skin, temperature of the tungsten. If the tube is observed during such an exposure the only sign of a load is a brief red flash on the focal track. The flash does not last noticeably longer than the exposure as the heat flows instantly away into the body of the disc.

During an exposure longer than 0.02 sec., the disc will complete more than one revolution and the same part of the focal track again comes under bombardment, having had a short period of time for the heat to flow away from the skin. Obviously the longer the exposure the lower the current will have to be since the track will now visibly heat up and some afterglow of the track will be noticeable.

Going to the other extreme and taking a load of, say, six seconds, the rate of heat input is much lower and the limitation will be the amount of heat the disc can hold without becoming overall too high in temperature. In other words, this is very similar to the case in fluoroscopy. A typical rating chart is given in 8 Fig. 17. It shows for a specific tube, focus size, method of rectification, and anode speed the maximum load that can be applied under various conditions for a single exposure. At low values of kV the rating is limited by the maximum temperature to which the filament can be raised. Hence the flat portion below 0.2s on the 40 kV curve.

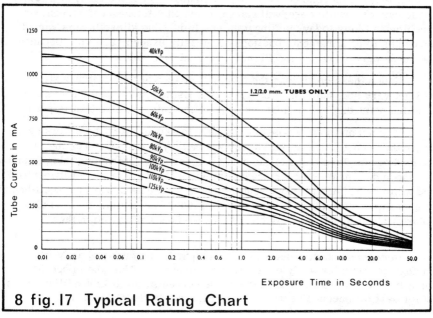

8 fig. 17 Typical Rating Chart

For any radiograph, the kVp is usually set by the type of examination. The amount of movement in the body region under examination usually dictates the exposure duration, leaving the current as the variable.

Nowadays rating charts are mainly of interest to the engineers who set up the tube on the apparatus, since nearly all modern sets incorporate overload protection systems which prevent an exposure in excess of the rating from being switched. Most sets do not have a system to prevent another exposure being switched immediately, or at any rate too soon, after the first. It is imperative that any radiographic load, or fluoroscopic session, be followed by an adequate period of cooling so that the anode disc can dissipate the heat which it has acquired.

8.13 Cooling Intervals

The length of cooling interval required, assuming the tube to be operated at its maximum rating, varies with the length of the exposure. For instance, if a load is made at 100 kVp, 125 mA, and 6 secs. the anode is virtually filled with heat and at least two and a half minutes cooling should elapse before another similar load is made. On the other hand, the application of a radiographic load of 45 kVp, 1000 mA, 0.1 sec. needs only 9 secs. cooling interval before another such exposure is made. Both the radiographic loads referred to are taken from the rating chart and are loads which utilise fully the thermal capacity of the tube for the exposure time quoted. Such loads are known as "Nomogram Loads".

To work out the cooling interval required after a load is fairly simple. Obviously, it is completely impractical to do this for each and every exposure, but if a few examples are worked out relative to the equipment in use a basic understanding is rapidly built up and use of approximately correct cooling intervals should follow.

Calculation of the cooling interval requires knowledge of the maximum continuous rating of the tube. This is expressed in terms of Heat Units per Second and for the tube on which the rating chart illustrated is based is 500 H.U./sec. The "heat unit" is a rather arbitrary unit brought into existence by the X-ray profession as a quick and simple way of expressing the energy dissipation of an X-ray tube.

The heat unit content of an exposure is calculated very simply by multiplying together the kVp, the mA, and the exposure time in secs. The first exposure mentioned, 100 kVp at 125 mA for 6 sec., therefore contains $100 \times 125 \times 6 = 75,000$ H.U. Furthermore, the exposure is made at a rate of 12,500 H.U./sec.

To work out the cooling interval needed the time required to dissipate the total 75,000 H.U. at a rate of 500 H.U./sec. must be calculated and is $\frac{75,000}{500} = 150$ secs. Subtract the time of the exposure, 6 secs., and the cooling interval is seen to be $150 - 6 = 144$ secs., or 2 mins. 24 secs.

The second exposure was based on the factors :-

$$45 \text{ kVp } 1000 \text{ mA } 0.1 \text{ secs.}$$
$$= 45 \times 100 \times 0.1$$
$$= 4500 \text{ H.U. at a rate of}$$
$$45 \times 1000 = 45,000 \text{ H.U./sec.}$$

Using the same method of calculating the cooling interval

$$\frac{4500}{500} = 9$$

Less Exp. time = 8.9 secs.

It is more difficult to assess the amount of heat in the anode after fluoroscopy. The continuous rating of 500 H.U./sec., means that the tube itself can be operated continuously at 100 kVp, 5 mA. At this rate of heat input for a period over 10 mins., the anode will effectively be full of heat and the length of cooling interval will depend on the size of the load to be applied in any subsequent radiographic exposure.

If the two exposures quoted earlier are made in succession, such that the six second exposure is applied first, then the cooling interval between these two exposures need only be sufficient to accommodate the amount of heat to be generated during the short exposure, i.e. 9 secs. Tube heating and cooling curves for a particular tube are shown in 8 Fig. 18. The heating curves are not very significant, but the cooling curve shows the comparatively high heat loss due to the increased efficiency of radiation cooling, at the high temperatures, and the much slower heat loss when the target falls below the visible heat point.

Very frequently it is required to apply a series of exposures in rapid succession to a tube. This is perfectly permissible provided that the foregoing points are borne in mind. As an additional safeguard, it is advisable to limit each separate exposure to 80% of the heat units permissible in an isolated exposure of the same duration, and also to limit the total heat unit content of the whole series, i.e. exposures + cooling periods, to 80% of an equivalent exposure of the same length.

8.14 Waveform and the Heat Unit

Earlier reference to the heat unit as an arbitrary one was because it has no fixed relationship to physical units such as volts, amps, and watts. In fact, the unit in the form "H.U./Sec." is nearest in meaning to a watt, but the factor relating the two varies according to the nature of the high voltage waveform, i.e. whether self rectified, a two or a six pulse, etc., (see Chapter 9) and various other factors such as the capacitance of cables which modify the waveform.

A watt, in its most easily considered form is the product of 1 ampere and 1 volt in a DC circuit. In an AC circuit with pure sine waves it is the same provided the values used are what is called R.M.S. (root mean square).

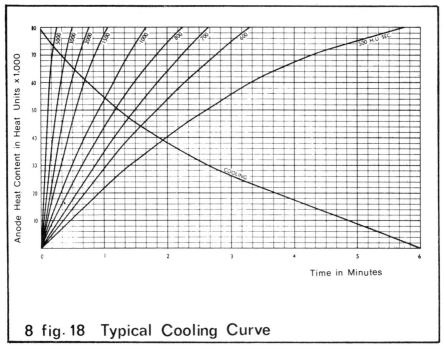

8 fig. 18   Typical Cooling Curve

The R.M.S. value of an alternating current is that value which gives the identical heating effect as the same numerical value of direct current (see 8 Fig. 19). It is, incidentally, the R.M.S. value of current (mA) which is normally quoted as part of the exposure factors.

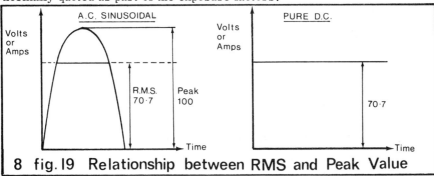

8   fig. 19   Relationship between RMS and Peak Value

A difficulty is that, with the very high voltages required to generate X-rays, measurement by meter is not very practical. Use is made, therefore, of the fact that voltages of this order will "jump" a considerable distance in air from the live electrodes to earth or between electrodes of opposite polarity. A device called a sphere-gap is used, in which the distance the voltage will jump between well polished metal spheres of about 120 or 150 mm diameter is calibrated directly in kilovoltage (see Chapter 20). Now the value this device reads is, of course, the peak voltage of the waveform, which is very significant since it determines the shortest wavelength in the X-ray beam produced.

For these reasons, tube voltages have always been expressed in terms of peak kilovoltage.

Consider the three tube voltage and current waveforms shown in 8 Fig. 20. Production of the waveforms is discussed in Chapter 9, here it is only necessary to compare the different shapes. Note that with the 6 rectifier circuit, or, to use the modern term, 6 pulse, the resultant voltage waveform is much nearer to pure D.C. than the other two cases and a H.U./sec. is consequently much nearer to being a watt. To convert H.U./sec. to watts the value of H.U./sec., must be multiplied by a factor- 0.74 for 2 pulse operation, 0.95 for 6 pulse, and 1.0 for 12 pulse or D.C. operation.

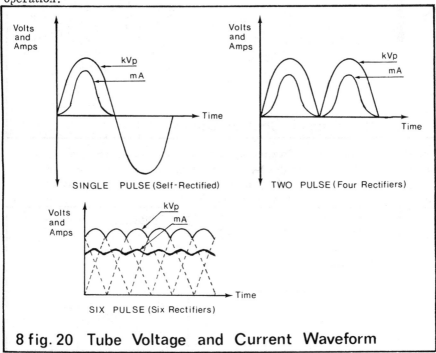

8 fig. 20 Tube Voltage and Current Waveform

A further point before leaving the subject of rating charts. On the 40 kVp curve in 8 Fig. 17, a levelling off is shown at times lower than 0.14 secs.

This is done because the filament has reached its maximum operating current, so although anode thermal capacity is available it is not possible to use it due to filament limitations.

8.15 Filament Temperature and Life

When a tube is running continuously at a few milliamperes it is not necessary to set the filament at a very high temperature. For peak loads such as 1000 mA, however, the filament has to be very hot indeed. At fluoroscopic currents a life of several thousand hours is easily attained, but the peak load temperature yields a filament life of only 2 to 3 hours.

It is vital to minimise the time that the filament runs at this temperature, and consequently for radiographic loads the filament is "boosted" shortly before the exposure begins. Simultaneously the stator is energised and the anode run up to speed. A period of about 1 sec. is sufficient for this purpose, and is ensured by applying a "preparation" delay just prior to the exposure.

While the filament is at this high temperature it is evaporating at a fast rate and depositing a film of tungsten on the inside of the glass envelope. The effect of this will be discussed later.

It is very important not to hold the set in "prep" any longer than absolutely necessary. It would be very easy, when settling a patient, to hold the set in "prep" for 10 secs. in order to make a 0.1 sec. exposure, but the preparation time would then be a hundred times more harmful than the exposure itself.

8.16 X-ray Tube Life

Two important factors in the conservation of tube life have already been discussed, i.e. cooling intervals and the unnecessary extension of preparation times.

However well a tube is treated, it is nevertheless a "wearing" thing like an automobile engine or an electric light bulb. There is bearing wear to be considered, filament evaporation, and the equally unavoidable crazing of the focal track. (See 8 Fig. 21).

Experience extending over many years has shown that the majority of tubes eventually fail due to the formation of a heavy tungsten deposit known as a mirror on the inside of the glass envelope, followed by increasing electron bombardment of the glass. This finally leads to destructive glass attack, with eventual penetration of the glass envelope. To understand this process the operation of a new tube must be reviewed.

Firstly, when a tube is switched on after a period of rest, by no means all the electrons leaving the cathode travel straight to the anode. A high percentage spray the inside of the glass. Also, those that do hit the anode frequently liberate secondary electrons. Since glass is a good insulator, and electrons are negatively charged particles, a negative charge will be built up that cannot readily leak away. This charge on the glass strongly repels further electrons, and thus forms a powerful protection against "puncture" or erosion of the glass surface by further electron bombardment.

Secondly, the focal track of the anode very soon begins to open up in

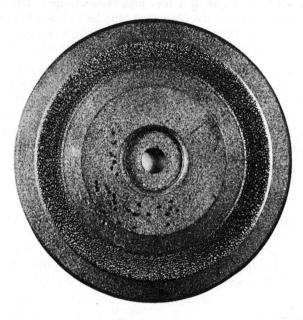

8 fig. 21 Crazing of Focal Track

a minute crazy-paving pattern (see 8 Fig. 21). This is both normal and inevitable, and provided the tube is used within its rating, this target erosion will have no significant effects for a long time. Eventually, however, the focal track crazing may reach the stage where flakes of tungsten are lifting and presenting edges to the electron beam. These edges will become molten and will add a further tungsten mirror to the one building up from filament evaporation.

Combined, the two mirrors stretch from below the cathode block to well behind the tungsten disc, and form a third, and unwanted, electrode in the tube. This causes the negative charge to leak away at an increasing rate, until eventually it has no chance to build up at all. If the mirror, as frequently happens, extends to within a few millimeters of the rotor it becomes a virtual extension of the anode.

Bombardment of the glass now becomes heavy, a first effect usually being the formation of inside surface cracks and, later, some surface melting. In either case gases are released with detriment to the vacuum and the destruction of the tube follows rapidly by actual penetration of the glass in the region of the cathode block.

8.17 X-ray Output Fall-off.

When a tube is new, the disc has only experienced those radiographic loads necessary to condition it during manufacture. The process of crazing

138

therefore, has either not commenced or is not very advanced.

Once the crazing process has commenced, some fall in radiation output is inevitable since a small proportion of the electrons are going to enter the cracks and generate X-rays that will be absorbed completely by the sides of the crack. In other words, electrons will fall into the "valleys" and then X-rays will be absorbed by the "hills".

This initial fall will cease, and the output from the tube remain consistent, unless or until the disc crazing becomes very severe. A sharp fall will then occur, usually halving the tube output. This is normally followed by tube failure within a fairly short time.

8.18   Other Reasons for X-ray Tube Failure

The X-ray tube may fail for other reasons which may include bearing failure (sometimes due to overheating on continuous running with consequential damage to the lubricant), accidental breakage, mechanical damage to the tube structure, and vacuum deterioration.

Accidental breakage is most likely to occur with mobile units when being wheeled over bumpy surfaces. Apart from advocating great care when handling tubes under any conditions it may be useful to remember how fragile the overhanging cantilever suspension of the tube anode, or its end seal really is. Whenever possible mobile units should be moved with the longitudinal axis of the shield vertical.

8.19   Further Factors Affecting X-ray Tube Rating

Earlier mention was made of a range of tube sizes available. For the same anode speed the larger the disc diameter the larger the focal track diameter and the higher is the rating. Also, the greater the mass of the disc the greater is the heat storage capacity.

In addition, the actual surface area of the disc is significant since the cooling by radiation is closely related to it. The nature of the surface also makes a great difference. Tungsten discs can be made with finishes between a bright, polished surface and a dull blackish one. The latter is very much more efficient in radiating heat.

8.20   The High Speed X-ray Tube

Mention has already been made of tubes with anodes rotating at speeds in the order of 9000 R.P.M. These are known as high speed tubes, and have been commercially available since about 1960.

If the anode rotates at this speed obviously the short time ratings improve considerably since the circumferential path swept by the electron beam is three times longer than for the standard speed tube.

The maximum benefit from the high speed occurs in loads of a duration equal to, or less than, one revolution of the disc. At multisecond exposures no benefit results from the higher 'speed since the rating limitation here is the heat storage capacity of the disc.

In fact, however, most high speed tubes available have anode discs of different design which do have higher thermal capacities. Hence a rating improvement occurs over the whole time scale.

The most important of these new designs is the composite disc. Basically this is a disc of molybdenum faced with a skin of tungsten a millimetre or so in thickness. The tungsten contains a small percentage of rhenium, which reduces the target erosion and cracking. The rhenium is not included to make possible an increase in load, nor does it extend the tube life, but it helps to maintain a more constant radiation output throughout the tube life, since the formation of "hills and valleys" previously described will be much reduced.

The composite disc is a practical proposition since the lower density of molybdenum combined with its higher specific heat and its higher thermal conductivity presents advantages over anode discs made only of tungsten. The very high cost of rhenium makes this approach less attractive, but nevertheless it is now widely used.

Standard speed tubes are permitted to slow down in their own time from 3000 R.P.M., following an exposure. High speed tubes, however pass through periods of resonance while slowing which cause high-energy vibration. They are therefore "braked" by the automatic application of a direct current to the stator winding, and in consequence pass very quickly through the resonant speeds and suffer no damage.

8.21 Anode Angle and Heel Effect

A typical distribution in X-ray output from an anode is shown in 8 Fig. 22. If a film is placed in the part of the beam normally used, it can be seen that one side of the beam will be limited by the shape and angle of the anode itself. This is true either of stationary or rotating anode tubes. No significant darkening of the film will be visible in the shadow of the anode. This is known as the "anode heel effect".

In addition to the almost total cut off in the anode's shadow, the field intensity is comparatively weak at angles adjacent to the anode face.

This is because a proportion of the electrons hitting the target penetrate either into the target material, or into the surface irregularities which exist even in a well polished surface. Radiation emanating from the impact region will be blocked or heavily filtered at angles parallel or adjacent to the anode face.

Anode angles in the main vary between 15° and 19°, but many tubes are, in fact, made with 12° or even lower angles. The object is to increase the milliampere loading for a particular focus, which is possible because the actual focus becomes longer, with a smaller anode angle, for

140

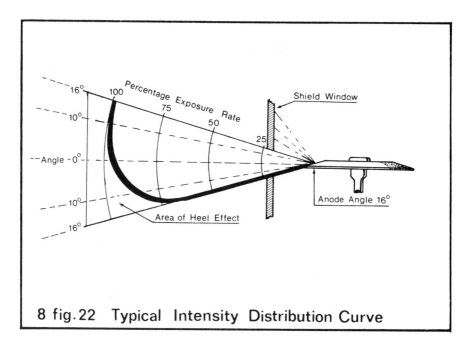

8 fig. 22 Typical Intensity Distribution Curve

the same value of apparent focus (See Section 8.4). The amount of
X-radiation per mA, however falls as the anode angle is decreased for the
reasons outlined above. Nevertheless, there is a net gain in X-ray output
provided that the angle is not too small.

A further limitation with shallow angle tubes is that the cone of
useful radiation becomes smaller, and hence the area covered at a certain
distance is less. Although this could be rectified by increasing the focus/
film distance, a corresponding increase in exposure factors would be
necessary in accordance with the inverse square law (See Section 5.10).

Many tubes today have anode discs with two different angles such
that the electron beam relative to each focus falls on a different diameter
and angle. This enables a higher mA loading to be given on one focus at
restricted beam angle, but has the disadvantage that the two focal spots
are separated along the axis of the tube.

8.22 Grid Controlled Tubes

Grid controlled tubes have been available for many years. Such a
tube is similar to the rotating anode tubes but incorporates a third
electrode called the "Grid", built into the cathode assembly to which can be
applied a negative potential sufficient to suppress the electron emission.
In practice, only the emission from the small filament is suppressed
because the amount of tube current which can be switched in this way

without upsetting other features of the tube, is limited.

Such a tube offers the advantage of very rapid switching since the whole switching action takes place within the tube itself. The switching action is effected by the removal of the negative bias of 2 to 3 kV from the grid which normally suppresses electron emission.

This system, in addition to the special equipment required in the generator, necessitates a four-conductor high voltage cable for the cathode side. One of these conductors has to be insulated for 2 or 3 kV against the others, compared with the normal 3 core high voltage cable which requires only 20 - 30 volts insulation.

8.23 Off-focal Radiation

When the main beam of electrons strikes the focal spot, some of the electrons rebound and restrike the rest of the anode,even behind the tungsten disc. X-rays will be generated by these electrons.

If a picture of the focus is taken with a pinhole camera technique, a small square image will be seen on the film . If the exposure is then increased many times, and a second picture taken, a faint image of the whole anode will appear around the very black image of the focus.

Since this off-focal radiation makes no useful contribution to image formation at all, and will, in fact, only adversely affect the quality of the picture, every effort is made to minimise it. This is done by collimating the beam as near to the focus of the tube as possible. It is achieved by fitting a lead cup with the smallest possible aperture consistent with the size of film to be covered, or alternatively by the use of a collimating device with its first pair of shutters as near the shield window as possible.

8.24 Inherent and Added Filtration

The inherent filtration of a tube - shield assembly is the filtering effect of all the components unavoidably placed in the way of the useful beam. These components include the glass envelope, a layer of insulating oil, and the plastic window. The value of filtration is expressed as the thickness of aluminium that will give the same filtration, and is usually of the order 1 mm to 2 mm aluminium. The actual figure is normally indicated on a label attached to the shield.

Since a certain amount of filtration is essential to absorb the soft radiation that would otherwise be absorbed by the skin, it is usual to add aluminium filters to the shield. Normally the amount is raised to a total, including inherent filtration, of 2.5 mm aluminium as recommended by the Code of Practice (1972).

8.25 Thermionic High Voltage Rectifiers

The era of thermionic valves for rectification of the high voltage pply to the X-ray tube is almost over. Their place has been taken by the very efficient and reliable solid state rectifiers. Initially they were made of selenium but now silicon is almost universally used.

Sufficient valve rectifiers remain in use, however, to warrant a discussion about their construction and operation. In particular, it is essential for the user to know of the hazards which can arise when valves approach the end of their useful life.

With the exception of very obsolete designs such as gas valves, the two main types to be considered are the pure tungsten filament valve and the thoriated tungsten filament valve. Really, the filament is the only difference that matters; their general construction is similar, and is typified in 8 Fig. 23.

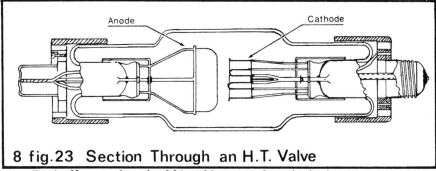

8 fig. 23 Section Through an H.T. Valve

Basically, a valve should be able to conduct the highest current demanded at the lowest possible voltage drop across the valve, and yet on the inverse half cycle be able to withstand the highest voltage available from the generator. The circuit shown in 8 Fig. 24 is probably the commonest application. It will be seen that when valve "A" is conducting, it is in series with both the X-ray tube and valve "C". The two valves that are not conducting are in parallel. Each one withstands the full potential of the generator less the volt drop across one conducting valve.

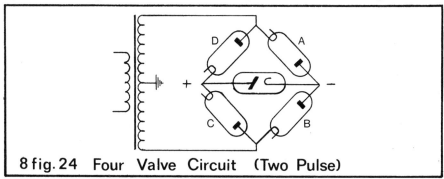

8 fig. 24   Four   Valve   Circuit   (Two Pulse)

A high proportion of the valves made in the last few years before solid state rectifiers took over were of the type known as "beaker" valves. The name was derived from the shape of the anode, which resembled a metal cup completely enclosing the filament structure. Such a valve is

143

shown in 8 Fig. 25.

Complete enclosure of the filament has two main advantages.

(a) nearly all the electrons emitted are "captured" by the anode.

(b) a negative wall charge forms less readily and even if present cannot inhibit emission since the electron flow occurs inside the anode. This is important since, while a negative wall charge is beneficial to an X-ray tube, it tends to inhibit emission and increase the "space charge" effect in a valve.

Pure tungsten filament valves contain a filament that emits electrons through sheer temperature. As with the tube filament, conservation of life is achieved by limiting peak temperature operation to very short periods - i.e. the "preparation" period plus the exposure. The filament boost is controlled by the same circuit that brings the rotating anode up to speed and boosts the tube filament.

Operating conditions of a typical pure tungsten valve filament vary from 9 volts, with a current of 10.8 amps, which is the "standby" or fluoroscopy value, to 11.5 volts with a current of 12.5 amps, which is the maximum value for short exposures. Note that even the standby figures give a filament power dissipation of nearly 100 watts.

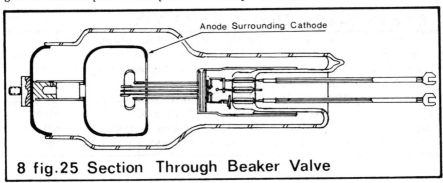

Anode Surrounding Cathode

8 fig. 25 Section Through Beaker Valve

Throughout the life of the valve, which is usually several years in the average hospital, the filament evaporates steadily and a tungsten mirror forms on the glass. Most valves of this type fail due to burn-out of the filament - much the same as an ordinary electric lamp. Such a fault is readily discernable on inspection.

Thoriated tungsten filament valves operate on a different principle. The tungsten wire contains a small percentage of thorium, which emits electrons copiously at quite a low temperature, under operating conditions of 6.5 volts 5.8 amperes. So readily does it emit that the process has to be slowed down by carburizing the outer skin of the filament, which unfortunately makes the filament about as strong as a used gas mantle.

No filament boosting is required since the temperature of the tungsten carrier wire is so low that no significant evaporation of tungsten occurs. Evaporation of thorium occurs, but only produces a slight mirror.

144

Filament burn-out, therefore, does not normally occur.

What does happen, however, is that the valve gradually loses emission, and if sufficient emission is lost the voltage drop across the valve will rise and heat will be developed in the anode. "Backfire" is then quite a common result, and often commences with a condition of "backstreaming" where the inverse current is just enough to damage the filament.

A valve in this condition can cause considerable consequential trouble, since gas release from the overheated parts can contribute to the instability of the system by causing the valve to disturb electrically. Parasitic voltage oscillations of very high frequency can be set up superimposed on the main high voltage waveform, often up to double the generator voltage. This can lead to the destruction by puncturing of other valves, the X-ray tube, and even the high voltage cables.

Unfortunately, a faulty thoriated tungsten valve, in the condition described still has the filament glowing. A superficial examination is not sufficient to suggest that the valve is faulty. The only real answer is a factory emission test, which takes time and necessitates spare valves being fitted. However, any valve which has a mirrored bulb, has brown spots on the inside surface of the glass, or has molten spots on the metal electrodes, should be regarded with grave suspicion.

In view of the consequences, it is quite essential that should any valve, which is one of a set of similar age, fail through loss of emission then the whole set should be changed. The risk of subsequent trouble by changing one valve only is far too great. These days it is a real economy to change over to a set of silicon rectifiers, which are made in "valve replacement shapes" for this very purpose.

The only time a single valve should be replaced is if the previous one has failed through a mechanical or vacuum defect, and it has been established by expert examination that no consequential damage has occurred.

Chapter 9

High Voltage Generation

9.1 <u>Direct and Alternating Current</u>

When a direct current is flowing, the electrons travel in the
same direction round the circuit from the negative terminal to the positive.
Conventional current flow is considered to be in the opposite direction.

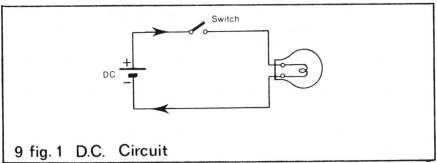

9 fig. 1 D.C. Circuit

A lamp connected across a direct current source, a battery, is shown
in 9 Fig. 1. When the switch is closed a current will flow in the direction
of the arrows causing the lamp to light.

In 9 Fig. 2 a lamp is shown connected across an alternating current
source, such as the normal 50 Hz mains supply. The voltage across the
supply terminals is changing its polarity at this frequency causing the
current through the lamp to change direction accordingly. In this circuit,

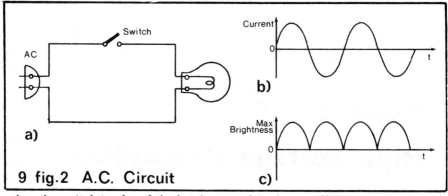

9 fig.2 A.C. Circuit

when the switch is closed the brightness of the lamp will fluctuate as the current passes from maximum in one direction through zero to maximum in the other direction (see 9 Figs. 2b and 2c). In practice the changes of current direction are so rapid that fluctuations in brightness are not apparent.

9.2   The Transformer

If a conductor is moved through the lines of force of a magnetic field, an electro-motive force will be induced in that conductor causing a current to flow through a load. A similar effect is produced if the wire is held still whilst the magnetic field is moved such that the lines of force are cut by the wire.

The transformer employs this principle and is constructed of two coils of copper wire wound on a common soft iron core. An input is applied to one coil and the output taken from the other. An alternating voltage input causes a current to flow and an alternating magnetic field to be set up in the core. The field builds up and collapses in synchronism with the polarity reversal of the input voltage. The wire forming the output coil is in the magnetic field and thus an alternating voltage is induced in it. The magnitude of this induced voltage is dependent upon the ratio of the number of turns of the input coil to the number of turns of the output coil. The input coil is called the primary winding and the output coil the secondary winding.

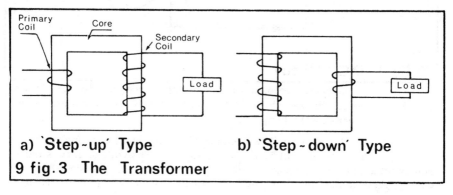

a) `Step-up` Type   b) `Step-down` Type

9 fig.3 The Transformer

The primary coil 9 Fig. 3a has three turns and the secondary coil has six turns thus the ratio is 3:6 or 1:2. This means that if ten volts are applied to the primary winding the output coil will produce twenty volts.

It should be emphasized that the total power output can never exceed the power input. In other words, ignoring losses, the product of current times voltage of the primary circuit will equal that of the secondary circuit. Thus the current drawn from the supply will be two amperes when the load current is one ampere with a turns ratio of 1:2.

The type of transformer we have considered has caused a low voltage to be increased to a high voltage and it is known as a "step up" type. It is also possible to transform a high voltage into a low one by arranging the coils as in 9 Fig. 3b, this is known as a "step down" type.

9.3   Autotransformer

The principle of operation of the autotransformer is the same as the "double wound" transformer already discussed but its construction is different, in that it has only one winding. The input is normally applied across most or all of the winding whilst the output is taken from a smaller part of it as in 9 Fig. 4a.

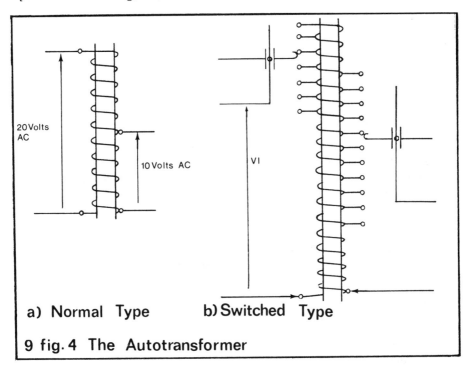

a) Normal Type   b) Switched Type

9 fig. 4 The Autotransformer

If the winding consists of 20 turns and a voltage of 20V a.c. is applied to it then each turn will have a potential of 1V a.c. If the output is taken across 10 turns then the voltage will be 10V a.c. It can be seen that the turns ratio is 20:10 or 2:1 and the transformer principle is maintained.

A more practical autotransformer which has a switched input is shown in 9 Fig. 4b. In this way a known voltage may be maintained across each turn despite variations in supply voltage V1. The output is also switched so that known voltages may be selected for use in other circuits.

9.4 High Voltage Generator

Voltages in the range 30 kV to 200 kV are required for the production of X-rays for diagnostic purposes, and they are generated by a high voltage transformer. In the interests of safety it is essential that these voltages are isolated and use is made of a "double wound" transformer contained within a housing which is earthed. A high ratio, step up transformer is used so that the voltages applied to primary winding are small in comparison with those taken from the secondary winding. Typically the ratio would be in the region of 1:400 so that an input of 250V would produce an output 100 kV.

As we have seen in Chapter 8, the X-ray tube also requires a low voltage supply for its filament and a step down transformer is also included in the transformer tank.

It should be noted that though the tube filament requires a potential across it of only a few volts, as it forms part of the cathode, one side of it must be connected to the high tension circuit.

It is normal for the high tension transformer assembly to be immersed in special oil which affords a high level of insulation.

9.5 Self Rectified Circuit

In 9 Fig. 5a the a.c. voltage is applied directly to the X-ray tube and since it can pass current in only one direction each alternate half cycle is blocked. This is known as self rectification. This type of apparatus has three distinct limitations :-

i) X-rays are produced for only half of the time that high voltage is applied to the tube.

ii) If the anode is allowed to become very hot during its conducting period it emits electrons during the reverse half cycle, causing a current which could damage the cathode.

iii) The voltage across the X-ray tube rises to a higher value during the non-conducting period because no losses occur in the generator. It is therefore necessary to ensure that the insulation of the high tension circuit can withstand the increased stress or to suppress the excess voltage.

These limitations may be accepted in simple apparatus, such as dental or portable units, in the interests of reducing size and weight, but they must be eliminated from more powerful equipment.

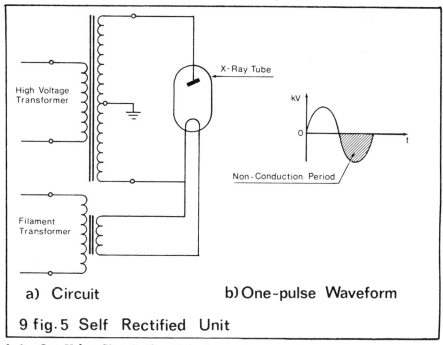

a) Circuit   b) One-pulse Waveform

9 fig. 5 Self Rectified Unit

9.6   One Valve Circuit (One Pulse)

A simple method to overcome the danger to the X-ray tube, due to
reverse current flow, is to include a diode valve in series with it so that,
even if the anode does become overheated, there will be no back-fire. The
inclusion of this valve also prevents the X-ray tube from being subjected to
the over-voltages produced during the non-conducting half cycle, though the
increased insulation to earth must be maintained. (9 Fig. 6a shows a
typical circuit).

9.7   Two Valve Circuit (One Pulse)

The size of an X-ray tube housing or shield is dependent mainly upon
the voltage stresses it has to withstand. In order to maintain small size it
is essential that the over-voltages produced during the non-conducting
period are either suppressed or blocked. In 9 Fig. 7a, valve V2 is included
at the anode side of the tube to isolate it from the high tension transformer
during the negative half cycle. It should be emphasized that the over-
voltage is still being produced and the valves must therefore be designed to
withstand it. The valves are situated in the transformer tank whose size
must therefore be increased, but this is preferable to an increase in tube
shield size.

151

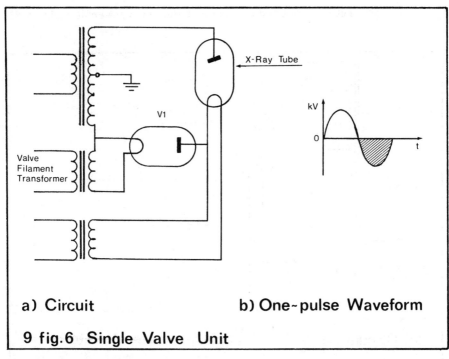

a) Circuit   b) One-pulse Waveform

9 fig.6 Single Valve Unit

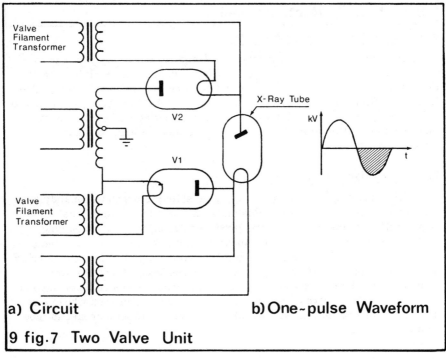

a) Circuit   b) One-pulse Waveform

9 fig.7 Two Valve Unit

9.8 Inverse Suppression

Suppression of the inverse voltage provides a better solution because it obviates the necessity for expensive high tension valves whilst maintaining a small X-ray tube shield. It may be simply achieved by the insertion of a rectifier diode in series with the primary winding of the high tension transformer. The diode is connected in such a way as to present a very high resistance, thus blocking the primary current, during the inverse half cycle, and a very low resistance during the conducting half cycle. This simple solution, however, is not sufficient on its own because it allows current in only one direction in the primary winding of the transformer which would become permanently magnetized in that direction. This in turn would lead to excessive currents being drawn. It is therefore arranged that a small current flows through a resistor connected in parallel with the diode. The value of the resistor is so chosen as to allow a small demagnetising current to flow during the inverse half cycle. The circuit is shown in 9 Fig. 8a.

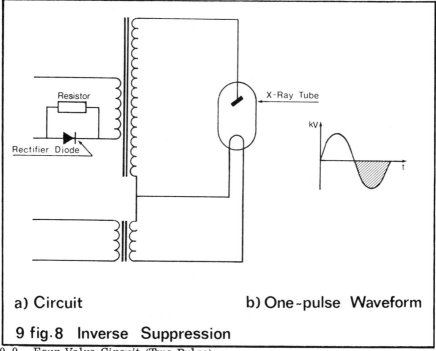

a) Circuit   b) One-pulse Waveform

9 fig.8 Inverse Suppression

9.9 Four Valve Circuit (Two Pulse)

So far we have considered self-rectified units such as mobiles, where space and weight are of paramount importance, but with high powered equipment film quality is the prime consideration. The four valve circuit produces d.c. voltage and ensures that X-rays are emitted during every half cycle. Thus the exposure time for the same radiation output is reduced by half in comparison with the one pulse system.

In 9 Fig. 9a the directions of electron flow through the rectifiers and X-ray tube are shown for successive half cycles and it can be seen that the polarity is always correct for X-ray production. Inverse suppression is no longer necessary because the tube is always drawing current and the valves, as well as rectifying the voltage, prevent a reversal of tube current.

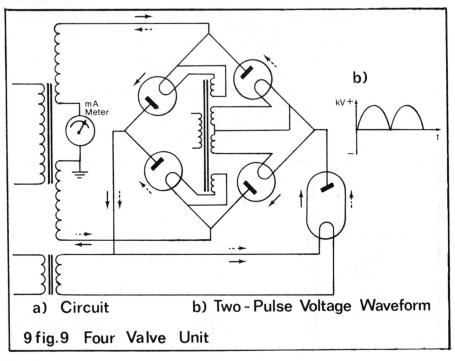

b)

a) Circuit   b) Two-Pulse Voltage Waveform

9 fig.9 Four Valve Unit

9.10 Six Valve Circuit (Six Pulse)

The six valve generator affords the opportunity of even greater utilisation of the tube during a given time, because it employs a three phase supply, which, when rectified, produces more voltage pulses. The circuit configuration of a modern six pulse generator is shown in 9 Fig. 10. The purpose of the coil L1 and capacitors C1 & C2 is to allow the centre point of the secondary windings to float with respect to earth and thus ensure that the voltage across the tube is symmetrical about earth. This means that for a 150 kV generator the maximum voltage is divided into 75 kV positive with respect to earth on the anode and 75 kV negative with respect to earth on the cathode.

Note. For the purposes of simplifying the diagram the rectifiers have been drawn as semiconductor diodes which are more commonly found in new apparatus.

154

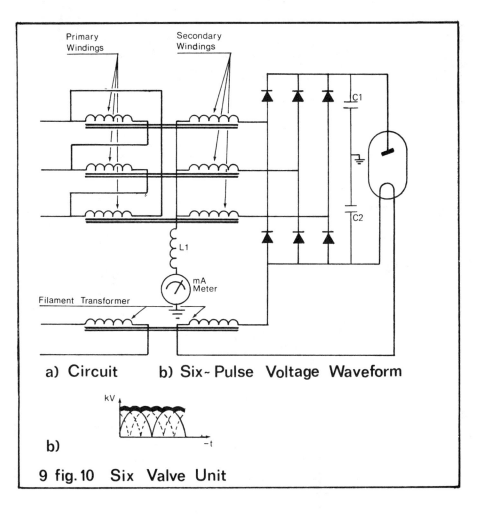

a) Circuit   b) Six-Pulse Voltage Waveform

b)

9 fig. 10   Six Valve Unit

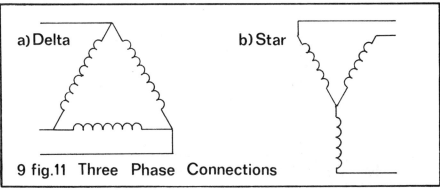

a) Delta   b) Star

9 fig. 11   Three Phase Connections

155

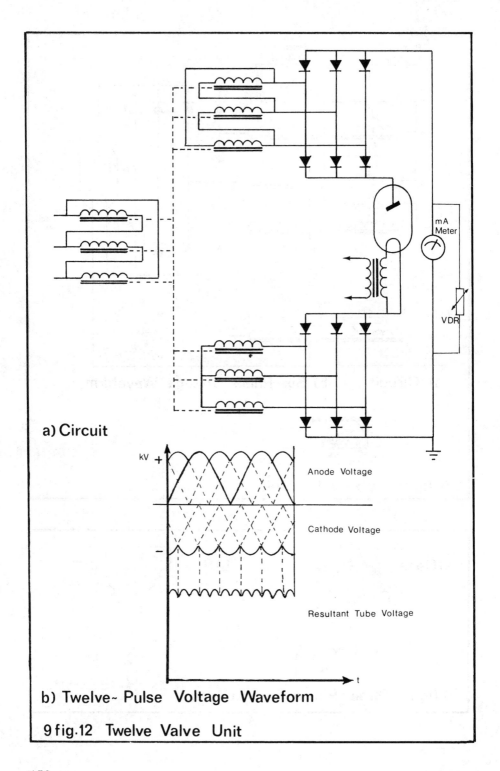

a) Circuit

kV

Anode Voltage

Cathode Voltage

Resultant Tube Voltage

t

b) Twelve-Pulse Voltage Waveform

9 fig. 12 Twelve Valve Unit

156

9.11 Twelve Valve Circuit (Twelve Pulse)

It will be noted that in 9 Fig. 10a the primary and secondary coils of the high tension transformer are interconnected in different ways. This is to take advantage of the better current and voltage characteristics of the two systems. The Delta connection used on the primary side is shown in 9 Fig. 11a and the star connection used on the secondary side in 9 Fig. 11b.

A further refinement of the three phase generator is to use a combination of both star and delta windings on the secondary side. They are connected as shown in 9 Fig. 12a and produce a voltage waveform as shown in 9 Fig. 12b which has an average value even higher than the six pulse circuit.

9.12 Meter Circuit

Another requirement of the high tension generator is some means of measuring the tube current. In 9 Figs. 9a and 12a the mA meter is connected in series with the X-ray tube at a part of the circuit which is connected to earth. In 9 Fig. 10a the meter is connected between the centre (star point) and earth but in a six pulse circuit it is also common to find a special isolating transformer in one leg of the secondary winding. In this case however, the meter will read only two thirds of the true value and a correction factor has to be applied. In the event of damage to the earth connection within the generator the high tension is prevented from reaching the control desk by including neon devices and voltage dependent resistors in the meter circuit.

9.13 High Tension Cables

In view of the very high voltages applied to the X-ray tube it is necessary to use special highly insulated cables for its connection to the generator. A cross sectional view of the cable is shown in 9 Fig. 13a.

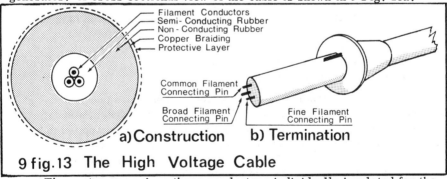

Filament Conductors
Semi-Conducting Rubber
Non-Conducting Rubber
Copper Braiding
Protective Layer

Common Filament Connecting Pin

Broad Filament Connecting Pin

Fine Filament Connecting Pin

a) Construction   b) Termination

9 fig. 13 The High Voltage Cable

The centre comprises three conductors individually insulated for the low filament voltages and surrounded by a semi-conducting rubber. This in turn is surrounded by non-conducting rubber which provides insulation against the high voltage also carried by the centre conductors. The cable is sheathed with a woven copper braiding, which is earthed, and finally covered with a protective layer, usually plastic.

For standardisation a three core cable is used for both anode and cathode sides. On the cathode side one conductor is for the broad filament, one is for the fine filament and the other is both their common connection and the high tension carrier. On the anode side the conductors are connected together within the generator. As pointed out in the last chapter a grid control tube requires a special four core cable.

The cables are terminated with a standard plug, shown in 9 Fig. 13b which fits the socket in either the high tension generator or the tube shield. Once inserted the cable ends should not be removed unless a supply of cleaning agents and silicon grease is available for application on re-fitting.

The construction of the cable is such that it acts as a capacitor, the value of which is dependent upon the length. This capacitance has various effects. Firstly, for low tube currents it tends to smooth the high voltage waveform reducing the amount of soft radiation produced by the tube. Secondly, a small capacitive current flows in addition to the actual tube current. The mA measuring circuit must be compensated to maintain accurate indication of only the tube current. Thirdly, the stored charge in the cable can lead to "afterglow" which is especially noticeable after fluoroscopy at very low tube current. This stored energy can be dangerous and should be discharged by connecting the conductors to earth prior to handling the exposed cable end.

9.14 High Tension Switch

In order to make full use of the X-ray generator it is normal to allow the connection of more than one tube. To make this possible a high tension changeover switch is included in the installation. As its name infers the switch is in the high tension circuit and therefore it is usually situated in the generator tank. Its function is to select the appropriate X-ray tube in the room for the examination to be undertaken.

The construction is shown in 9 Fig. 14. Since the switch is in the high tension circuit, it must be remotely controlled for safety reasons. It is, therefore, electromagnetically operated. There are normally three sections to the switch, each actuated by a separate coil, so that a total of three tubes may be connected.

For bi-plane examinations it is possible to energise two switches at once but limitations are imposed by the X-ray control desk. Unless the desk and generator are specially designed, the high voltage applied to each tube is the same and the exposure times are identical. It is usually possible to vary the tube current but this may not provide sufficient control for the required exposure value in the two planes. Therefore it is better to use two separate generators or one that has been specially designed for bi-plane operation.

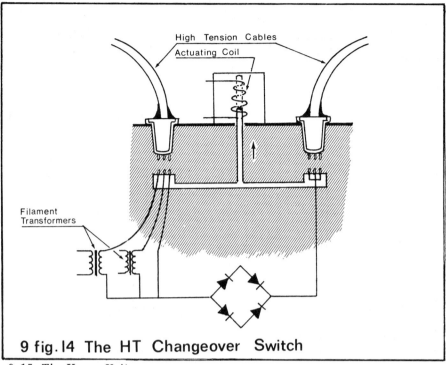

High Tension Cables

Actuating Coil

Filament Transformers

9 fig. 14 The HT Changeover Switch

9.15 The X-ray Unit

The essential requirements of an X-ray unit are as follows :-

   i) It must produce a controllable high voltage which, when applied to the X-ray tube, determines the quality (or penetrating power) of the radiation.

  ii) It must produce a controllable low voltage which, when applied to the X-ray tube filament, will determine the desired tube current and intensity of radiation.

 iii) It must provide a method of controlling the duration of emission of radiation. (An X-ray unit satisfying the above requirements is shown in 9 Fig. 15.)

The electrical input is applied via the switches S1 and S2 to the autotransformer T1. Switch S2 enables the operator to adapt the unit to a supply that may vary in voltage and the voltmeter gives an indication of correct adaption. It is now possible to adjust switch S3 to give the required high voltage applied to the X-ray tube and which will be indicated by the kV meter. The resistor R2 is provided to allow accurate calibration of the meter. In a unit of this simplicity the tube current is fixed but the resistor R1 allows setting to the correct value on installation. The mA meter is provided to indicate tube current. The timing cycle is initiated by closing a contact within the handswitch and is terminated automatically at the end of

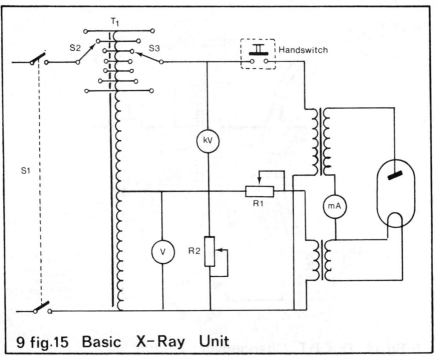

9 fig.15 Basic X–Ray Unit

a pre-selected time. The various methods of controlling the time are
discussed in Chapter 10.

This simple circuit is employed in applications where the emphasis is
on small size and light weight such as dental apparatus or portable units.
Where a wider range of examinations is envisaged a more sophisticated
form of control is required.

X-ray output is dependent upon kV (tube voltage), mA (tube current)
and t (exposure time). Since the choice of kV is governed by the nature of
the subject under examination it follows that, in order to reduce the
exposure time and minimise the effect of subject movement,the tube current
must be increased. In 9 Fig. 15 this is simply achieved by adjusting R1.
Unfortunately, when higher tube currents are involved, it is found, due to
reasons to be discussed later, that the kV is affected. Likewise, due to the
nature of the X-ray tube,any alteration in kV will produce a proportional
change in tube current.

Control of the high voltage applied to the tube is normally achieved by
means of an autotransformer which has many voltage tappings and a heavy
duty switch known as the kV control. In the diagram 9 Fig. 16 the autotransformer is represented as T1 and it is connected across the supply.
Various voltages may be selected from T1 with the kV control S2 and these
are applied to the high voltage transformer T2. The construction of T2 is
such that the number of turns on the primary winding is far exceeded by the

160

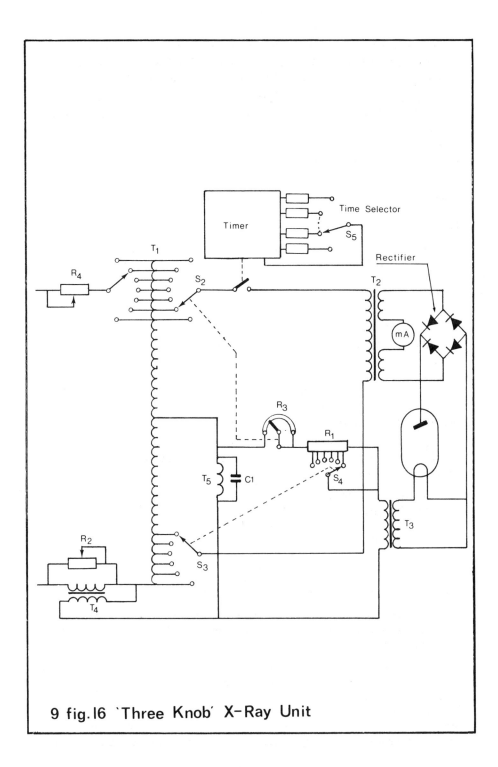

9 fig. 16 `Three Knob´ X-Ray Unit

number of turns on the secondary winding, thus providing a step up in voltage. Typically the ratio of turns would be 1:400 so 300V applied to the primary would produce 120,000V (120kV) on the secondary.

The production of X-rays in the tube is dependent upon electron bombardment of the target and a controllable supply of electrons is required. This is provided by a metal filament which emits electrons when heated. Tube current is related to the temperature of the filament and its variation will provide the necessary control of X-ray production.

The filament is supplied via a transformer T3 which, in this case, is a 'step down' type that is the number of turns on the primary winding exceeds that on the secondary winding, typically in the ratio 10:1. The resistor R1 provides control of the filament heating current.

The duration of the exposure is the next important consideration and X-ray timers fall into three main categories, namely clockwork, electro-mechanical and electronic. The function of the timer is to connect high voltage to the tube for a certain pre-determined time, selected by S5.

9.16 Compensation Circuits

When operating at higher output power the power input is correspondingly increased. This gives rise to increased losses due to the resistance of the electrical supply. Mains resistance is in fact the sum of the resistance of all the cables, terminals, etc., back to the power station. In normal domestic or industrial requirements it may be ignored but for diagnostic X-ray units it becomes significant.

For instance, if the total mains resistance (R4 in 9 Fig. 17) was one ohm (1Ω) the voltage drop across it, for various load currents (I), would be given by Ohm's Law:-

Voltage drop across R = I x R
For 1 ampere,   V = 1A x 1Ω
                   = 1 Volt
For 100 amperes,   V = 100A x 1Ω
                   = 100 Volts

It can be seen that an increase in either load current or mains resistance leads to an increase in voltage drop.

In normal circumstances the mains resistance is a fraction of an ohm, but an X-ray unit may require up to 250 amperes which produces a significant voltage drop.

The normal method of compensating for voltage losses due to mains resistance is to insert extra resistance to ensure that the unit operates from a supply whose resistance is identical to that used during initial calibration. In this way we are able to calculate the voltage loss at various tube currents and arrange that the off-load value, selected for application to the high voltage generator, is high by an amount equal to the predicted loss while on

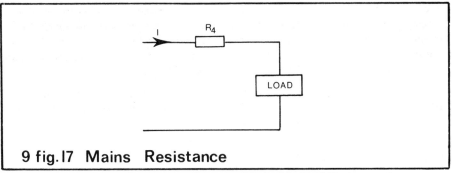

9 fig. 17 Mains Resistance

load. In 9 Fig. 18a the X-ray tube, supplied with 100 kV, is passing a current of 200 mA and in 9 Fig. 18b the same tube, operating at a higher filament temperature, is passing a current of 500 mA.

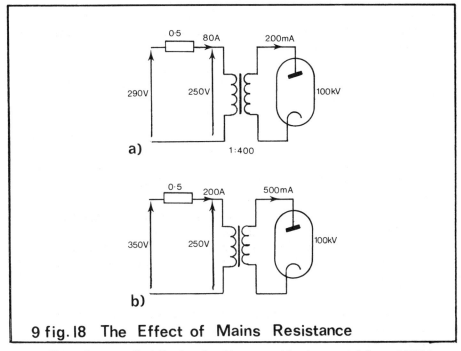

9 fig. 18 The Effect of Mains Resistance

It can be seen that the input voltage must be increased from 290V to 350V in order to maintain the high voltage at 100 kV at the increased current demand.

In 9 Fig. 16 the switch S3 is mechanically coupled to the tube current selector S4 and as the current is increased a higher compensation voltage is added.

The X-ray tube operates in a saturated condition and, as the voltage across it is altered, the current through it should remain constant within certain limits. However, in practice, as the voltage increases there is a slight increase in current. This is compensated by the potentiometer R3 in the filament circuit which is mechanically coupled to the kV control. As the kV is increased the resistance is increased, thus proportionally reducing the temperature of the tube filament and, therefore, tube current.

A further refinement is the addition of voltage stabilisation in the filament circuit to ensure that supply voltage variations are not transmitted to the filament, causing unwanted changes in tube current. Two stabilisers are shown, the first (T4 and R2) counteracts the sudden drop in voltage during an exposure and the second (T3 and C1) takes care of slow variations due to fluctuations in mains supply voltage.

9.17 Tube Overload Protection

X-ray tubes are designed to operate within defined limits of power input as published by the manufact. er. It is important, therefore, that the X-ray unit includes a device to prevent overloading of the X-ray tube. These devices take several forms, the more common of which are discussed below.

It is possible by mechanical means to interlock the kV, mA and time selectors such that they cannot be turned when this would overload the tube. This method is very complicated mechanically and is reserved for low power units which do not allow a wide range of factor selection.

The three selectors may be electrically interlocked such that, if an overload combination is selected, the exposure circuit is blocked by means of a relay. This method has been used extensively but it is now giving way to electronic circuits because they are more reliable, versatile and easier to adjust should it be necessary to cater for a different type of tube.

In the electronic type, voltages representing the logarithms of selected kV, mA and exposure time are added together and compared with voltages representing the maximum permissible product of the factors. Depending upon the resultant voltage the exposure may be blocked or allowed to take place. This method requires careful design but in operation is reliable and easy to adjust.

It should be remembered that all the above devices monitor single exposures only and tube overload is possible if the correct cooling interval is not allowed.

9.18 "Two Knob" Control

The necessity for an overload circuit may be avoided if the factor selection switches are arranged such that it is not possible to overload the tube. In this type of unit the time selector performs two functions. The first, as its name suggests, is to select the exposure time, but the second is to select a tube current. Thus it becomes an "mAs" selector. This is mechanically coupled to the kV selector such that any combination of kV and mAs will allow the maximum permissible tube load. This mode of operation

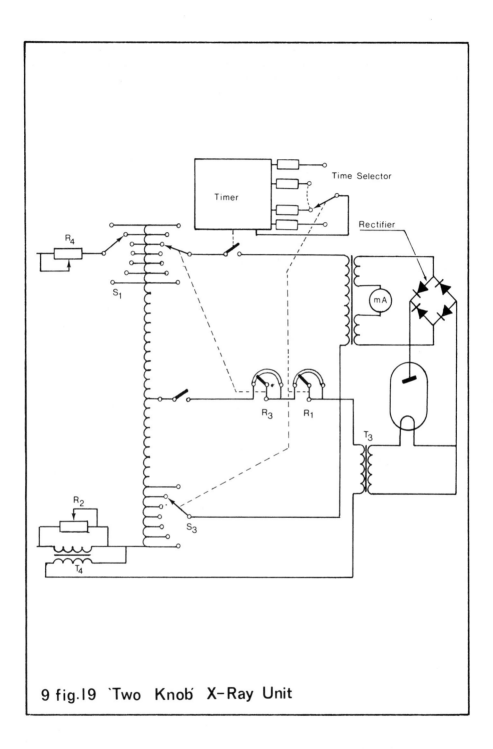

Timer

Time Selector

Rectifier

mA

R₄

S₁

R₃   R₁

T₃

R₂

S₃

T₄

9 fig.19 `Two Knob` X-Ray Unit

is known as "two knob" control or "isowatt loading". It is normal in this type of unit to allow a certain limited free mA control for special techniques, such as tomography because "three knob control" is preferable when the exposure time is determined by the auxiliary apparatus.

9.19 Falling Load Control

It is possible to terminate the exposure automatically by means of a photocell or ionisation chamber. At a fixed kV and mA, the exposure time is varied to produce the optimum film blackening. This principle is further described in Chapter 10.

When automatic exposure control is used in conjunction with either two or three knob control units complications arise in the setting of maximum factors. As the exposure time is an unknown quantity prior to the exposure, it is left to the radiographer to set an exposure time that is not likely to be exceeded by the automatic exposure control device. This in general, leads to the use of longer exposure times because the mA must be adjusted to a low value in order that a longer limit time may be selected.

This led the set designers to the conclusion that, in order to achieve the shortest possible exposure times with automatic exposure control, it was necessary to start every exposure at maximum permissible power. The tube current is then reduced during the exposure such that the rating of the tube is not exceeded. This is known as the "falling load" type of generator, or "single knob" control as only the kV is manually pre-selected.

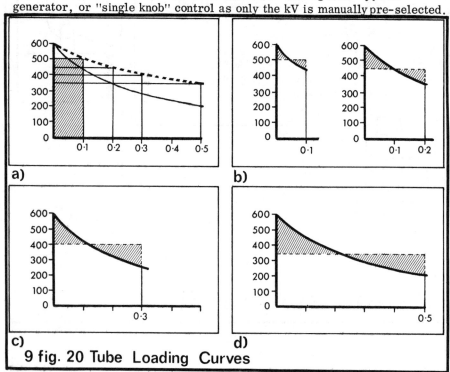

9 fig. 20 Tube Loading Curves

A simplified tube loading chart is shown in 9 Fig. 20a with various mAs values for fixed current operation depicted as rectangular areas under the dotted curve.

The solid curve is the falling load line showing the rate at which the mA decreases during the exposure. This curve is arranged so that the maximum possible input is applied to the tube. The total area below the curve at 0.1 sec. in 9 Fig. 20b is equal to the hatched area in 9 Fig. 20a. This implies that at each exp. time the hatched area below the curve in 9 Fig. 20b, c, and d equal the hatched area above the curve.

Let us now consider an exposure terminated by automatic exposure control on a conventional three knob unit. Assume that at a particular kV the correct film blackening will be achieved with approximately 50 mAs. This value may be obtained with the selection of 500 mA at 0.1 sec. as indicated in 9 Fig. 20a, but in practice it is necessary to allow a margin for error (remember that it was only assumed that 50 mAs was the required value) and a longer limit time would be required. The tube overload circuit would prohibit the selection of an increased exposure time at the same tube current, so the next lower value would be chosen. The exposure time determined by the automatic control would now be :-

$$400 \text{ mA x exp. time} = 50 \text{ mAs}$$
$$\text{exp. time} = \frac{50}{400} = 0.125 \text{ secs.}$$

However, with a falling load unit the exposure would start at the maximum permissible tube current, in this case 600 mA, and the tube current would fall until 50 mAs had been produced. Graph 9 Fig. 20b demonstrates that this would occur in 0.1 secs. Use of the falling load system has therefore resulted in a reduction in actual exposure time of more than 10%.

A simplified circuit diagram of a falling load control generator is shown in 9 Fig. 21.

Contact b closes during preparation for the exposure and completes the circuit for the X-ray tube filament which is from the main auto-transformer via contact b, R2, primary of T4, R3, R4 the secondary of transformer T2 and back to the main autotransformer. The X-ray tube filament will now boost to the temperature set by the following controls :-

R2 and R4: These resistors are set on installation to give the maximum permitted tube current with the particular focus at the kV required.

R3: This resistor is set in position of minimum resistance at the beginning of the exposure for maximum tube current.

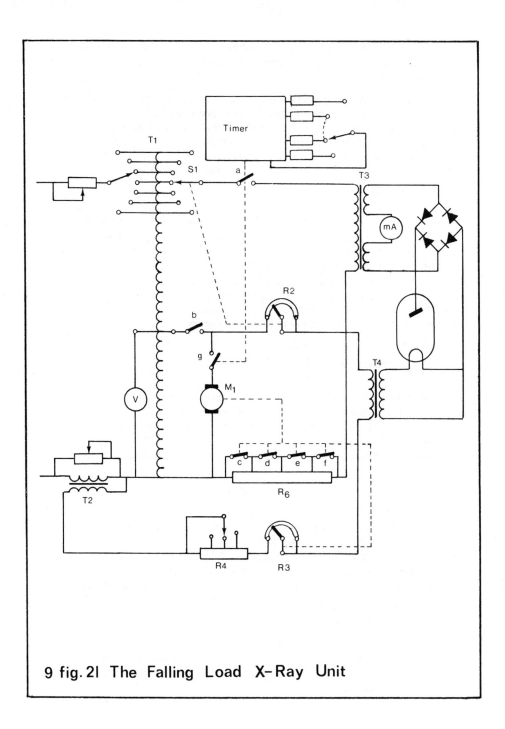

9 fig. 2I The Falling Load X-Ray Unit

Contact a: This contact of the exposure relay closes the circuit for the high voltage generator from the main autotransformer via S1, contact a, primary of T3, R6 and back to the main autotransformer. Thus high voltage is now applied to the X-ray tube.

At the same instant contact g of the exposure relay closes the circuit for the falling load motor M1 which in turn performs the following functions :-

The wiper of potentiometer R3 is rotated during the exposure such that its resistance is gradually increased, thus reducing the tube current.

At pre-determined positions of the wiper of R2 the contacts c, d, e, f open and insert parts of the resistor R6 into the circuit of the primary winding of the high voltage transformer. This ensures that, when the tube current falls, (reducing voltage losses due to mains resistance, etc.), the voltage applied to the generator is reduced, keeping the kV at a constant level.

When the exposure is terminated the falling load motor is automatically reset to the start position.

The falling load generator may be used without automatic exposure control but under these conditions no advantage is gained over the "two knob" control unit. In addition fixed current operation is provided for special techniques such as tomography where long exposure times are used.

Chapter 10

Exposure Timers

10.0 Exposure Timer Accuracy

At a certain kV, the product of tube current and exposure time, mAs, is varied to suit the object being radiographed and thus provide the required degree of film blackening. At higher tube currents the time is more critical because small errors become significant. For example, an error of 0.1 seconds is only 10% of a one second exposure but it is 50% of a 0.2 second exposure. It follows, therefore, that with high powered units greater consideration must be given to the accuracy of the exposure times in order to maintain consistency of operation. With low powered units a lesser degree of timer accuracy can be tolerated because its effect must be considered in conjunction with other, possibly greater, sources of error. For instance, there would be no point in maintaining 1% accuracy with the timer, if it was impossible to guarantee better than 5% of the tube current or even the kilovoltage, as is the case with small portable apparatus. The relative effects of kV, mA and exposure time are given in Section 5.10.

10.1 The Clockwork Timer

One simple timer consists of a clockwork mechanism controlling electrical contacts which are used to connect the high tension transformer to its energising source. The duration of closure of the contacts, thus the exposure time, is dependent upon the degree to which the spring is wound. The whole mechanism is normally contained within a handswitch with a dial calibrated in fractions of a second and a control knob which may be rotated to select the required exposure time. An accuracy of only one tenth of a second may be expected.

This method of exposure control has, up to now, been commonly employed in dental and small portable apparatus where high accuracy is not required. Even this application is now giving way to electronic control.

10.2 The Synchronous Timer

Another form of timer uses the constant speed property of a synchronous motor which is always completely in step with the mains frequency. (See 10 Fig. 1).

The motor is continuously rotated and drives a spindle connected to an electromagnetic clutch fed via slip rings. Connected to the other side of the clutch is an arm which will rotate at the same speed as the motor when the electromagnet is energised. This arm will operate a pair of contacts at the end of a pre-determined time. The time is altered by varying the position of the contacts in relation to the starting position of the arm and indicated on a calibrated dial.

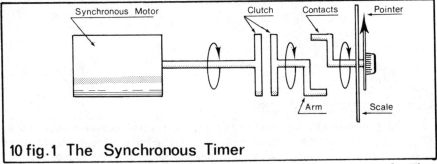

10 fig.1 The Synchronous Timer

At the beginning of the exposure period the clutch is energised. The arm starts to rotate, and after a period of time, operates the contacts which terminate the exposure. The clutch then slips until it is electrically de-energised by release of the handswitch and the arm is returned to its starting position by means of a spring.

Refinements, such as phasing circuits, were added to these timers in order to make them suitable for switching high tube currents at short exposure times. Progress in electronics has made it possible to achieve greater accuracy at a cheaper price and the synchronous timer has also become obsolete.

10.3 Phasing of the Exposure

One of the principle difficulties to overcome with controlled switching of an X-ray exposure is the sheer power involved. If we consider a normal chest examination, the power dissipated in the anode of the tube is in the region of 30 kilowatts and this must be switched on and off within a tenth of a second. In Chapter 9 we discussed alternating current and saw that its value passed through zero once every half cycle. It can be seen, therefore, that if we could arrange for the switching contacts to open and close at these points, the amount of power actually being switched would be zero and thus smaller contactors could be used. Alternatively, in low powered apparatus, a resistor may be included in the primary circuit of the high voltage generator whose function is to limit surges of current produced at the instant of applying voltage to the generator. This resistor (R in 10 Fig. 2) is short circuited by contact b which closes a fraction of a second after contact a, the main exposure contact.

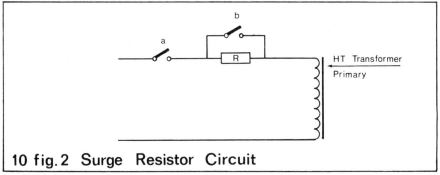

10 fig. 2 Surge Resistor Circuit

10.4 Electronic Timers

The electronic timer is based on the fact that a capacitor takes time to charge. The time that a capacitor will take to charge to a certain voltage is always constant and is determined by the supply voltage, value of the capacitor, and the resistance in series.

When the switch in 10 Fig. 3a is closed, the capacitor will start to charge. If the voltage on its terminals is plotted against time, a graph similar to 10 Fig. 3b will be obtained.

When the switch is first closed, there will be no voltage across the capacitor if it is uncharged. Therefore, the whole supply voltage will appear across the resistor until the capacitor starts to charge. The voltage across the resistor falls with the value of the charging current until both become zero when the capacitor is fully charged.

The time taken for the capacitor to charge to 63% of the supply voltage is called the time constant and is given by:-

$T = RC$

where T is time in seconds
        R is resistance in ohms
        C is capacitance in farads.

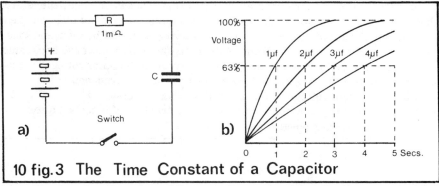

10 fig. 3   The   Time   Constant   of   a   Capacitor

By changing the value of the capacitor or resistor the time constant is altered as shown by the various curves in 10 Fig. 3b.

This principle is used in electronic timers to provide a method of control of exposure time.

10.4.1 The Thyratron

The thyratron is a gas filled triode valve which has special conduction properties. If the switch S2 in 10 Fig. 4 is closed and a positive voltage is applied to the grid, a current will flow from anode to cathode due to ionisation of the gas. Once ionisation has occurred it cannot be extinguished by opening the switch S2, but only by removal of the anode voltage, i.e. opening S1 or reducing the anode voltage to zero.

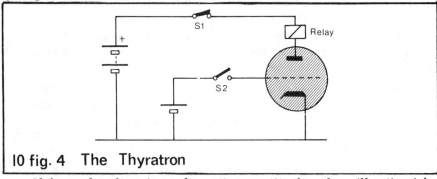

l0 fig. 4   The   Thyratron

If the anode voltage is an alternating quantity the valve will extinguish at each succeeding half-cycle, that is when the anode goes negative with respect to the cathode. This property of a thyratron makes it useful for synchronising the termination of an exposure at the zero point of the load current.

Two thyratrons which also act as a full-wave rectifier, are used for control of the relay in 10 Fig. 5. The rising d.c. voltage applied to the grids has superimposed upon it pulses, at twice the frequency of the anode voltage, produced by the phasing bridge. The phasing of these pulses with respect to the alternating voltage across the valves may be altered by varying the potentiometer in the bridge. In this way the ionisation point is

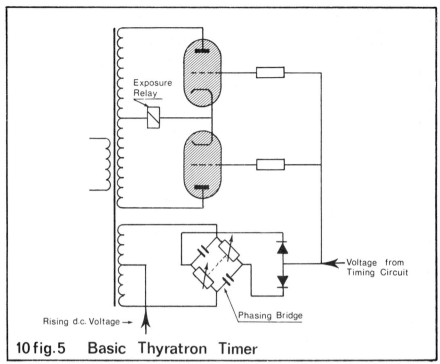

10 fig.5   Basic Thyratron Timer

controlled. Thus the start of the exposure, allowing for the pull in time of
the relay, coincides with the zero point.

When the exposure relay is energised, it connects the timing capacitor
to its charging path. After the pre-selected time has been reached, the grids
are driven negative, and the valves will not re-ignite after the anode voltage
has passed through zero. The relay itself is of special construction and its
release time is arranged to coincide with the time taken for one half-cycle
at mains frequency, i.e. 0.01 seconds at 50 Hz.

The sequence of operation is shown in 10 Fig. 6. The exposure
sequence is initiated at t_0 and the grid voltage begins to rise. At t_1 the
first synchronising pulse arrives and raises the voltage to the critical point.
At this point the grid voltage has risen sufficiently for the synchronising
pulse to be effective and the valve whose anode is positive will conduct. The
grid voltage is held at this level and the valves will conduct alternately
causing a d.c. current to flow through the exposure relay. At t_3 the relay
contacts close and begin the exposure. The time interval between t_1 and
t_2 is adjusted to suit the characteristic pull-in time of the relay. In this
way the start of the exposure is correctly phased.

At t_2 the timing sequence is initiated and after the pre-selected time,
(during which a capacitor discharges) the positive grid voltage is removed (t_3).
Thus at t_4 when the anode of the conducting valve passes through zero it will
extinguish and the other valve will not re-ignite. At this point the current

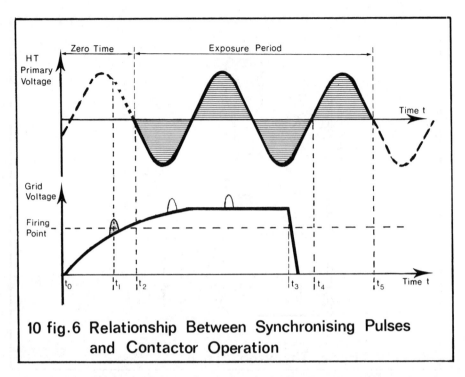

10 fig.6 Relationship Between Synchronising Pulses and Contactor Operation

will cease to flow through the relay coil and it will release. The drop out time of the relay is such that the main contacts carrying the load break at t_5 when the current has fallen to minimum. Thus the termination of the exposure is also phased.

10.4.2 Thyristor Timers

In the thyristor timer the relay and thyratron are replaced by a solid state electronic component known as a thyristor. This device is capable of switching the high currents involved without the disadvantages of moving contacts. It is similar in operation to the thyratron. Once conducting it cannot be switched off by the starting circuit but only by removal of the supply voltage or a bypass current circuit.

When exposures are to be terminated by an automatic device, the shortest exposure time with a two pulse generator under thyristor control would be one half-cycle of the supply. At 50 Hz this is 0.01 second. If a shorter exposure time is required it is necessary to introduce a high speed contactor which is capable of breaking the circuit unphased. In view of this the thyristor timer is normally reserved for 6 or 12 pulse generators where the duration of one pulse is much shorter.

10.4.3 High Tension Timers

So far we have discussed timers whose function is to switch the voltage applied to the primary winding of the high tension transformer. In some

176

cases, for instance high speed cinefluorography, the problems associated with synchronising the exposure with the film stationary period are easier to overcome by directly switching the high tension. For this purpose a high voltage triode valve is connected between each side of the high tension rectifier and the X-ray tube as in 10 Fig. 7. The capacitor C is included to remove the ripple and produce a smoother d.c. voltage.

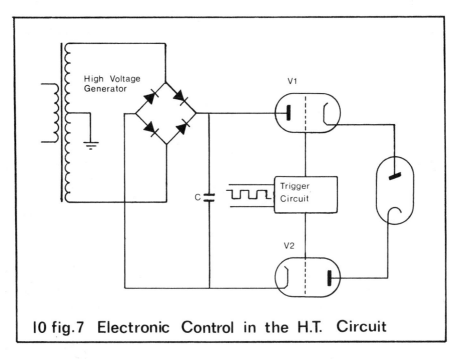

10 fig.7 Electronic Control in the H.T. Circuit

A contact in the cine camera is adjusted to close when the film is at rest and the shutter open. This signal is used to control a square wave oscillator which provides positive pulses on the grids of the valves V1 and V2 which conduct and pass a pulse of current through the X-ray tube. The length and repetition rate of the X-ray pulses may be varied by altering the on/off periods of the oscillator by resistance and capacitance circuits.

This type of circuit may be used for normal radiographic applications but is expensive and does not offer sufficient advantages over the conventional low tension timer to make it worth while for normal applications.

10.5 Automatic Exposure Control

Modern trends in radiography are to release the radiographer from unnecessary tasks so that more time may be devoted to the more important aspects, such as positioning and patient care. Automatic exposure control is a step in this direction as it obviates the need to estimate the required exposure value and reduces the number of controls.

There are two principle methods of exposure control, one employing a photomultiplier and the other an ionisation chamber.

10.5.1 The Photomultiplier System

In Chapter 3, photo-emission was discussed and it was shown that certain materials, when exposed to light, release electrons. This principle is used in the photomultiplier for converting visible light into an electrical signal. The diagram 10 Fig. 8 a and b demonstrates the operation of the device.

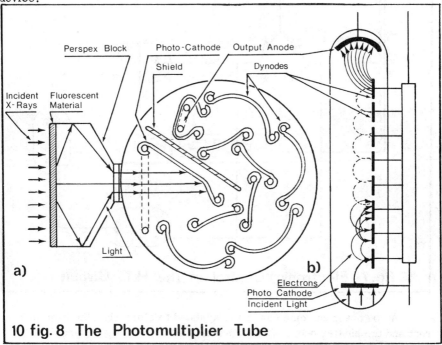

10 fig. 8 The Photomultiplier Tube

X-rays are converted into visible light by the fluorescent material and this light is directed towards the photo-cathode by a perspex block or suitable lens system. Electrons are released and accelerated towards the first dynode and their impact upon it releases more electrons. There is a potential gradient across the dynodes and the newly released electrons are subjected to even greater accelerating force towards the next dynode where they in turn release larger numbers of electrons. This process is repeated at each successive dynode and thus there is an avalanche effect through the device giving rise to an appreciable current flow. This current is proportional to the intensity of light falling on the cathode. If the current is used to charge a capacitor over a period of time the total charge is then proportional to the total light during the same period.

The voltage across the capacitor is fed into the circuits of a phototimer where it is amplified, measured and eventually used to terminate the X-ray exposure. Thus it can directly control the exposure time in accordance with the X-radiation required for correct blackening of the film.

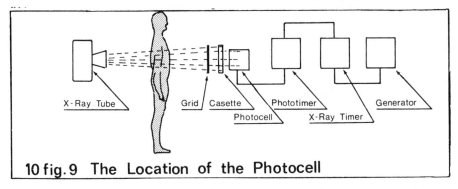

10 fig. 9 The Location of the Photocell

The position of the photomultiplier with relation to the patient is shown in 10 Fig. 9. Despite the fact that cassettes without lead backing are used the efficiency of modern high speed films and screens is such that the X-ray beam is greatly attenuated and there is very little for the photomultiplier to measure. This disadvantage, plus the difficulty in adjusting the position of the cell to monitor the dominant part to be radiographed, has led to decreasing use of phototimers for general applications. They still find a place, however, in automatic density control for photo-fluorography (Chapter 19).

10.5.2 The Ionisation Chamber System

The ionisation chamber used for automatic density control consists of two electrodes separated by air, across which d.c. voltage is applied. When subjected to X-ray bombardment some of the atoms of the enclosed air will release electrons and thus become positively charged particles or 'ions'. These ions, under the influence of the electric field across the chamber will migrate to the negative electrode causing in effect a current flow.

The chamber is placed between the patient and film and it is important, therefore, that its absorption is kept as low as possible. The centre electrode and its connection are made by spraying conducting varnish onto a plastic sheet which is then inserted between two sheets of plastic foam in which holes have been made for the measuring field area. The whole assembly is then clamped between two very thin copper plates and covered with a protective material. It is normal for one chamber to contain up to three measuring fields similarly constructed (See 10 Fig. 10).

The current in the measuring fields is very small and is used to charge a capacitor. The voltage across the capacitor is then amplified prior to its transmission through an interconnecting cable to the density control unit. There the signal is again amplified and used to control a high speed relay which terminates the exposure, when a pre-set density level has been reached.

Ionisation chambers for specific applications are designed which offer a choice of measuring fields of different shape and position.

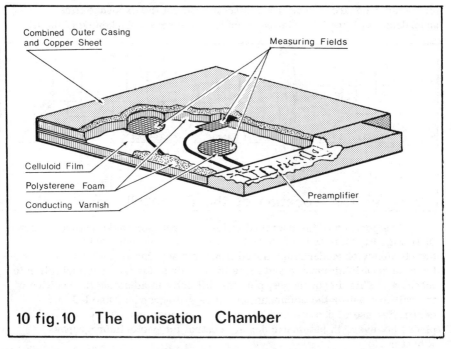

Combined Outer Casing and Copper Sheet

Measuring Fields

Celluloid Film

Polysterene Foam

Conducting Varnish

Preamplifier

10 fig.10   The Ionisation Chamber

This system offers greater flexibility of selection of measuring field than the phototimer but the position of the chamber causes an increased object to film distance. However, the chamber is very slim and this effect minimal. A further advantage is that standard lead backed cassettes may be used, reducing back scatter.

It is possible to select any combination of the measuring fields to suit the physiology of the patient and the examination to be undertaken. The chamber is very susceptible to scattered radiation and for consistency of operation correct control of the diaphragm for X-ray beam collimation is essential. It is also important to ensure that a) direct radiation does not strike the selected measuring field causing a short exposure and b) all the selected fields are subjected to the beam emerging from the patient or a long exposure will result.

In both the ionisation chamber and photomultiplier system it is important to remember that altering the film/screen combination will require a different density adjustment.

10.6 Anatomically Programmed Radiography

In order to make full use of the falling load generator, an automatic exposure control device must be employed. It is then only necessary to manually adjust the kV control.

The single knob control generator has led the way to full automation of the X-ray control desk in a unit for anatomically programmed radiography. One push button, designated to each examination is provided and controls the following functions :-

kV	– Servo controlled kV switch.
mA	– Falling load control.
Time	– Maximum time dictated by tube focus characteristic.
Auxiliary Apparatus	– Bucky, serial changer, etc.
Density	– To suit diaphragm size and user's requirement.
Dominant Measuring Fields	– To suit examination.

There are a number of selection buttons which should adequately cover the types of examination carried out in any particular room. They may be illuminated when depressed and have descriptive labels. To cater for abnormally thin or corpulent patients extra buttons may be provided to give a decrease/increase in kV and/or density level. Allowance is made for the artistic temperament of the radiographers who feel that they can do better than the machine by the provision of a button marked "OFF" which will transfer control to the main desk.

10.7 Tomographic Density Control

A recent application of the ionisation principle is found in a device for automatic density control during tomography. This is a complex problem because the exposure time is determined by the length of the blurring movement and is, therefore, pre-set. The tube voltage is largely determined by the subject and we are left with only one possibility for automatic control - namely by altering the tube current.

During the first part of the tomographic cycle an ionisation chamber is used to measure the exit dose rate from the patient. This signal is used, after amplification, to set the tube current to such a value that the film will be correctly blackened on completion of the blurring movement.

Chapter 11

Interlocks and Safety Devices

11.0 Introduction to Interlock Circuits

In order to ensure complete safety of operation of X-ray apparatus, many safety devices are included to monitor circuits which could cause a hazard if allowed to operate under fault conditions. For example, in an X-ray control desk, the selection of factors which would cause the tube to be overloaded, must prevent an exposure. This interlocking is usually achieved by means of relays.

11.1 The Relay

This is an electromagnetic device whose construction is shown in 11 Fig. 1. They fall into two main types - voltage sensitive and current sensitive.

11.1.1 Voltage Operated Relays

When the coil is connected across a voltage supply, a magnetic field is set up which has the effect of exerting a force of attraction on the armature. The armature is mounted on a knife edge and is therefore free to move causing a lever action on the contact assembly. The contacts themselves take up a new position with respect to one another, and either make contact or break contact depending upon their initial position. There is no limit to the number of contacts a relay may have, it depends upon circuit requirements.

The construction of the coil will depend upon the power required to

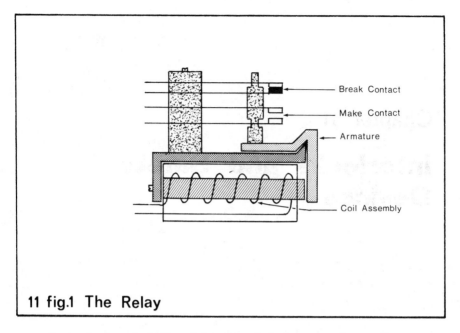

Break Contact

Make Contact

Armature

Coil Assembly

11 fig.1 The Relay

move the contacts and whether it is connected to a.c. or d.c. voltage.

11.1.2 Current Operated Relays

These are similar in operation to the voltage operated type, the only difference being they are connected in series in the circuit. The coil has a very low impedance so that the relay does not adversely affect the current it is monitoring.

11.2 Interlocks

There are some functions in the X-ray unit that require a certain time, usually of the order of one second, to reach their optimum working condition. It is customary, therefore, to prevent an exposure from being made prior to this state of readiness being reached. 11 Fig. 2 shows a typical circuit for interlocking the three conditions of operation, namely fluoroscopy, preparation and exposure.

11.2.1 Fluoroscopy Interlocks

Fluoroscopy employs very low X-ray tube current and must be prevented if the filament is not at a low enough temperature because it has been boosted for radiography by the preparation relay. Contact B of preparation relay K4 is therefore included in the circuit of the fluoroscopy relay K3 and prevents fluoroscopy occurring whilst K4 is energised.

The circuit also includes a contact that is opened by the fluoroscopy timer at the end of a pre-selected time.

184

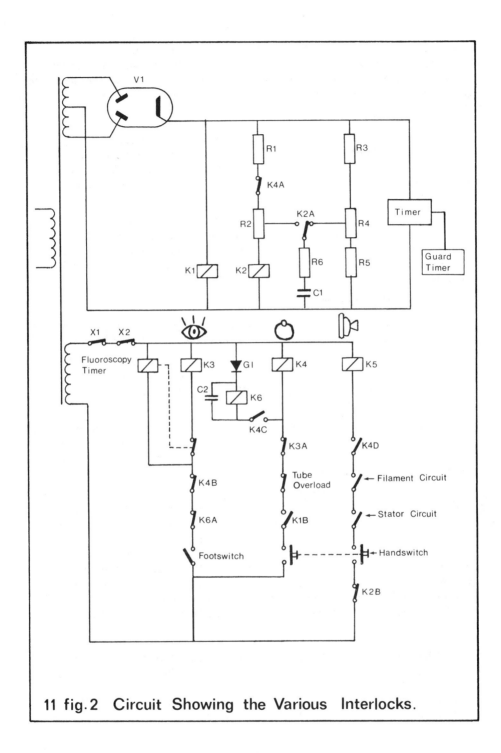

11 fig. 2 Circuit Showing the Various Interlocks.

Relay K6 is energised by a contact of the preparation relay and the capacitor C2, by providing a current from its stored charge, ensures that it does not release for some time after K4. This gives the filament a chance to cool after an exposure has been made and KCA blocks fluoroscopy.

11.2.2 Preparation Interlocks

Contact A of fluoroscopy relay K3 prevents "preparation" during fluoroscopy. It is possible that the exposure factors selected at the control desk could cause an overloading of the X-ray tube. The contact marked "tube overload" prevents the preparation relay being energised under these circumstances.

Before an exposure is started, it is essential to make sure that the timer has the correct voltage applied to it, so that its time determining circuits will function normally. Relay K1 is connected to the same source of supply as the timer and, if it does not energise, its contact K1B will prevent preparation.

11.2.3 Exposure Interlocks

The contact K4D is included in the circuit of the exposure relay K5 to prevent its operation without the prior initiation of the preparation circuits.

The actual radiographic kV only corresponds to the indicated value when the correct tube current is flowing. Therefore it is common practice to include a circuit to monitor the tube filament supply, a contact of which is connected in series with the exposure relay.

Similarly, there is a device to check that the correct current is flowing in the circuit of the motor that drives the rotating anode. A contact of this device is also included in the circuit of the exposure relay to prevent damage to the anode should it not attain the correct speed.

The function of the delay relay K2 is to prevent an exposure before the various circuits have had time to operate. In the quiescent state, its coil is energised and the capacitor C1 is connected in parallel with it by the contact K2A. At the start of preparation the contact K4A is opened but K2 will not release until C1 has discharged. This discharge time is adjusted by R2 and is normally set to one second. The resistors R3, R4 and R5 provide an alternative charging path for C1 so that the delay time will be correct despite rapid successive operations of the preparation relay. A contact of the delay relay K2B is included in the circuit of the exposure relay.

11.2.4 Tube Thermal Interlock

The X-ray tube shield usually contains a switch that is operated by expansion of the insulating oil due to excessive heating of the target. The contacts of this switch X1 are included in series with the fluoroscopy, preparation and exposure relays to prevent further input of heat to the tube before a sufficient period of cooling has been allowed.

11.2.5 Guard Timer

In order to prevent the possibility of a continuous exposure with its attendant danger to both personnel and equipment it is customary to include a secondary or guard timer. This device operates independently and terminates the exposure in the event of failure of the main timer. The time determining circuits of the guard timer are adjusted to give slightly longer times than those selected for the main timer. Once operated the guard timer disconnects the whole apparatus from the mains and prevents it from being re-connected before it has been checked by a service engineer.

11.2.6 Radiation Protection Interlocks

These interlocks are included to ensure that it is not possible to energise the tube if the protection is not adequate. For example, when the image intensifier is not coupled to the serial changer or if the serial changer is in the parked position. Their position in circuit is indicated by the switch X2.

Chapter 12

Mobile, Portable and Dental Units

12.1 Dental Units

In dentistry it is very important to recognise decay at an early stage. Moreover, it is very important to see how the teeth are located, and their internal condition during an operation. X-rays are the only media available to permit this disease to be detected at an early stage.

Since the object – film distance is rather low, and the tissue and bone thicknesses are limited, it will be evident that an X-ray machine of low power is adequate to obtain the required radiograph with sufficient contrast. In practice, it will be found that most dental units have a fixed tube voltage, in the region of 50 kV, and a fixed tube current of about 7 mA.

The model shown in 12 Fig. 1 combines the high voltage transformer and X-ray tube into a single small case, thus greatly simplifying handling and positioning, as no high voltage cables are required.

The primary windings of the transformer are fed with mains voltage via an exposure timer and the high voltage developed in the secondary windings is fed to the self-rectifying X-ray tube. The complete assembly is contained in a metal case, filled with a special insulating oil which is allowed to expand by bellows mounted in the positioning handle.

The tube is of rather a novel design employing a third electrode, called a grid, situated between the anode and cathode electrodes. The grid restricts electrons from leaving the cathode until the high voltage reaches its peak value, whereupon all electrons are released and impinge on the

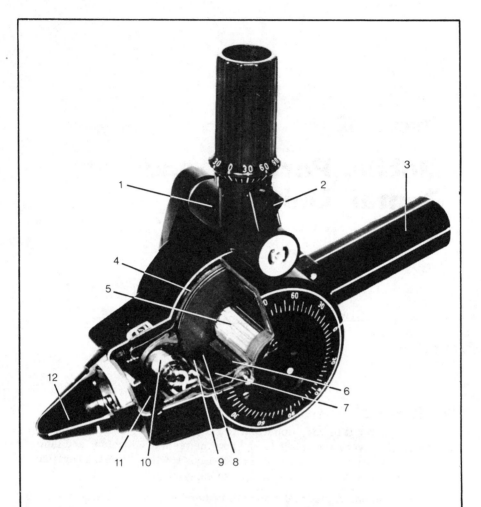

12 fig.1   Dental X-Ray Tubehead

anode at a very high velocity. Consequently, the X-radiation generated contains fewer, useless, soft rays and more hard rays. The total radiation is therefore more effective and can be compared, mathematically, to a much higher output, resulting in shorter exposure times.

In the past, the majority of dental exposure timers were clockwork, but modern units now feature electronic timing with a dental technique selector. The technique selector is designed to provide the appropriate exposure periods for each type of examination required in dental radiography, by a single switch. These techniques are arranged in a logical sequence and the exposure times are automatically compensated for fluctuations in mains supply, thus maintaining uniform film density.

For examinations requiring a longer film - focus distance, for example extra-oral views, the small cone can be removed and a longer one fitted. These cones act both as collimators and positioning aids. Further collimation is achieved by the turret diaphragm which is simply a disc containing apertures of differing sizes which can be selected at will.

Special equipment for orthodontic examinations is also available consisting of a low powered X-ray unit, but more importantly a positioning aid. With this equipment a view can be accurately repeated at a subsequent visit of the patient. Locating pieces which fit into the ears and over the nose ensure that the patient adopts the same position with respect to the apparatus. This is illustrated in 12 Fig. 2.

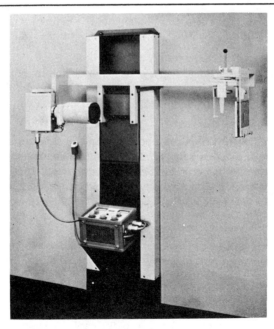

12 fig.2 Apparatus for Orthodontic Examinations

12.2. Portable and Mobile Apparatus

In many instances it is necessary to X-ray patients who, for one reason or another, are not able to go to an X-ray department. It may be that the patient is too ill to be moved from the hospital bed, is taken seriously ill at home, or is undergoing surgery in the theatre. Thus a need arises for X-ray equipment that can be taken to the patient.

12.2.1 Portable Units

A portable unit is one which can be dismantled, packed into cases and carried. It usually consists of a tubehead, some form of collapsible tube column and a control unit. (See 12 Fig. 3).

In order to make the unit lighter, more simple to operate and easier to move, it is usual for the tubehead to be constructed with the X-ray tube and its high voltage generator, enclosed in one earthed metal tank filled with oil. The X-ray tube itself is usually a small stationary anode type, operating in the self rectified mode, being connected directly across the secondary windings of the transformer. By constructing the tubehead in this way, the only connections required from the control desk are low voltage ones, which are carried in one multicore cable with a plug on each end. This cable connects to a socket in the side of the control desk and another cable connects the unit to the mains supply.

The controls provided on the desk are, of necessity, fairly limited and include a mains voltage compensator, combined kilovoltage and tube current switch, and time selector. Many units employ a clockwork hand-switch to control the exposure duration, but electronic timers are now more common.

The tubehead is mounted on a cross-arm which is carried on a vertical column. The cross-arm may be moved up and down this column by means of a rack and pinion drive. The vertical column can be taken off its base, divided into parts and packed into a carrying case for transport.

The radiographic output of a portable unit is determined by the current it can take from the mains supply. As the unit is designed to be used on a domestic supply, this current must be limited to about 15 amps. Thus the maximum radiographic output commonly found on portable units is in the order of 15 - 20 mA at 90 - 95 kV.

12.2.2 Mobile Units

The mobile unit is capable of higher outputs than the portable unit and thus is much heavier. Consequently the control table and column supporting the X-ray tube are permanently mounted on the same mobile base.

A greater selection of mA and kV values are available on the control desk which feeds a high voltage transformer often embodying a full-wave rectification circuit. Short lengths of H.T. cable connect the transformer to a normal, double focus, rotating anode X-ray tube. Most mobile units have a radiographic output of up to 300 mA and a maximum of 125 kV. This

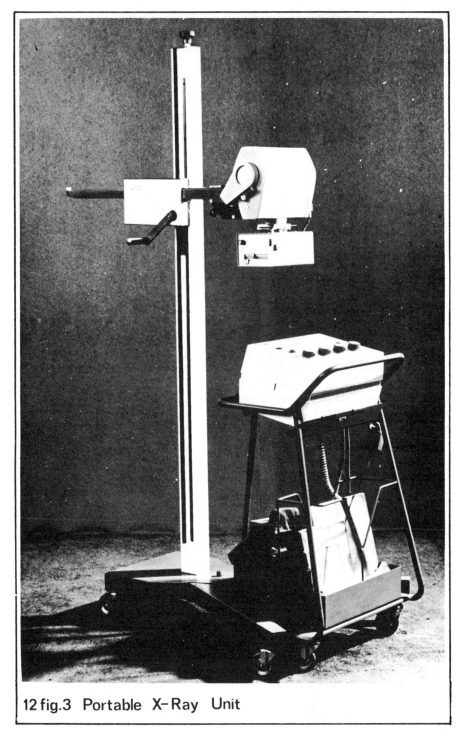

12 fig.3 Portable X-Ray Unit

level of output demands fairly high mains supply currents, in the order of 30 amps. The units are therefore usually fitted with a 30A plug and special sockets have to be provided throughout the hospital.

If the current drawn from the supply is calculated for short exposures at high power, it may be found that they are higher than the rating of the supply. This is not usually a problem as the high currents, being of short duration, do not cause overheating of supply cables. Fuses which act too quickly can be replaced by delayed action versions.

Because of the high currents demanded from the mains supply by these units, mains resistance becomes a problem, especially if the mobile is to be used in many different parts of the hospital. To ensure consistent results from one socket to another, a means for mains resistance calibration is provided and must be adjusted to suit each location before making an exposure.

Where there are limitations on the electrical supply, mobiles utilising stored energy are available. These may take the form of capacitor discharge, or battery powered inverter circuits. The former releases stored energy from the capacitor during exposure, whilst the latter converts energy stored in the battery.

12.2.3 Mobile Image Intensifier Units

Mobile intensifier units are primarily designed for use in the operating theatre and are particularly useful for hip-pinning operations where, under fluoroscopic control, the positioning of the guide wire can be checked at every stage. The number of radiographs taken can thus be reduced to a minimum, with a considerable saving in operating time. They also have many pre-operative applications.

The construction of the X-ray tubehead is very similar to that of the portable unit. As the unit is mainly used for fluoroscopy, the X-ray tube is equipped with two focii :- 0.6 mm^2 for fluoroscopy and 1.8 mm^2 for radiography. During fluoroscopy the X-ray beam is automatically limited to the size of the image intensifier by means of a motor driven diaphragm.

The tubehead is mounted on one end of a C-shaped arm (See 12 Fig.4) the other end of which is fitted to an image intensifier. Because the X-ray tubehead and image intensifier are held directly opposite each other and move together, the X-ray beam is always accurately aligned, leading to rapid and easy positioning with respect to the patient.

The C-arm is supported by a cross-arm which is mounted on a vertical column whose height above the mobile base can be varied. The base is on wheels and also carries the X-ray control unit. The control unit illustrated is very similar to the portable control desk, giving up to 5 mA for fluoroscopy and up to 25 mA for radiography at tube voltages within the range of 45 - 100 kV.

Direct viewing of the image on the intensifier can be carried out by

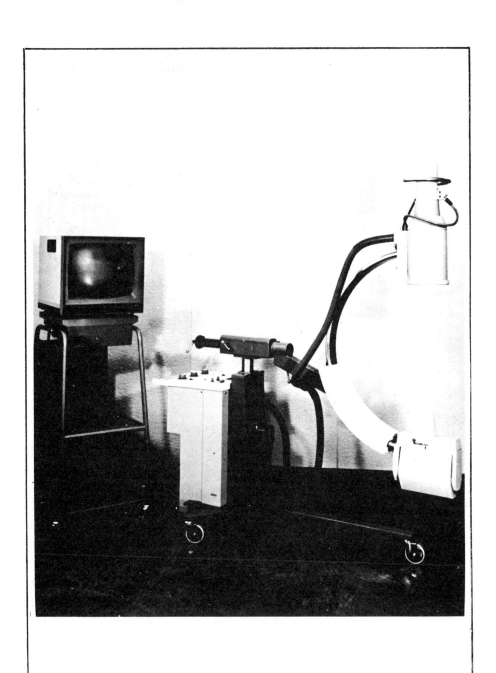

12 fig.4 Mobile Intensifier Unit

means of an articulated optical system, but it is more usual for the intensifier to be provided with a closed circuit television chain. A television camera is mounted on the intensifier and the image transmitted to one or more monitor screens. This allows more than one person to view the X-ray image simultaneously, thus giving substantial advantages over the optical viewing system.

The mobile intensifier unit may also be used for direct radiography by clipping a special cassette holder to the front of the intensifier tube.

Chapter 13

Beam Centring Devices

13.1 Introduction to Beam Centring

Beam centring devices are necessary for accurate patient positioning. They indicate the direction of the "central ray" of the X-ray beam and its point of incidence on the area under examination. The more advanced beam centring devices also provide a means of adjustment of the size of the irradiated area, and indicate the chosen area on the surface of the patient by means of light projection. Beam centring aids may be categorised as follows:-

    (i) Simple centre pointer.
    (ii) Focussed cross lights.
   (iii) Light beam diaphragms.
   (iv) Optical view finders.
    (v) Other beam centring devices.

13.2 Simple Centre Pointer

The simple centre pointer was the earliest type of beam centring device manufactured. It consists of a metal telescopic pointer on a hinged assembly, mounted in front of the window of the X-ray tube (13 Fig. 1).

During positioning, the pointer is moved into a position such that it simulates the central ray from the X-ray tube. After positioning, the pointer is swung out of the field so that it no longer obstructs the X-ray beam.

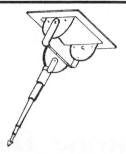

13 fig.1 Simple Centre Ray Pointer

A device using a similar principle is used on many multi-directional tomographic tables. In these devices,which are described further in Chapter 17, the central beam may not necessarily be perpendicular to the table. In units such as that shown in 13 Fig. 2, it would be necessary to ensure that the normal ray was exactly perpendicular with the table top prior to positioning with a beam centring device mounted on the X-ray tube.

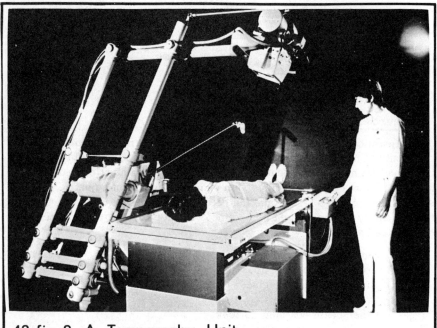

13 fig. 2 A Tomography Unit

To relieve this problem a small spot of light is projected from a lamp on the end of a moveable rod. During centring this light source is swung into a preset position such that its beam of light is coincident with a perpendicular ray. Thus the point of incidence of a perpendicular central ray is indicated on the patient without the need to centre the X-ray tube.

13.3 Focussed Cross Lights

As with the simple mechanical pointer, the focussed cross light system indicates the central beam but it is not necessary to remove the device before the radiographic exposure is made. The system consists of two focussed lamps projecting narrow slits of light. These two sources are arranged at right angles to each other, close to the X-ray tube port, such that the two beams intersect at right angles, to produce a cross of light on the surface of the patient at the point of incidence of the central beam. Such a system is shown in 13 Fig. 3 on a skull stand.

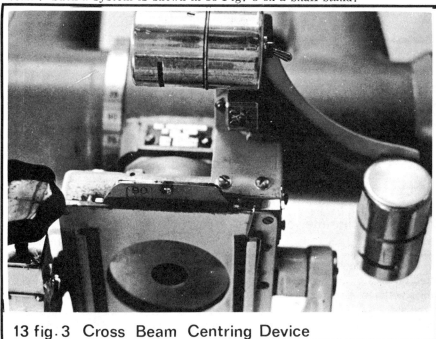

13 fig. 3 Cross Beam Centring Device

A single light source of this type may also be used to indicate the layer height on a tomographic unit. In 13 Fig. 2 is shown a mirror which reflects a line of light to the level of the selected layer on the patient. The mirror is necessary both to increase the length of the line projected and to facilitate initial calibration of the unit on installation.

13.4 Light Beam Diaphragms

The advantage of a light beam diaphragm over the centring devices already mentioned is that not only is the central ray indicated, but also the area of the irradiated field. Thus accurate collimation or "coning-down" is possible, reducing patient dose and secondary radiation. The secondary radiation aspect is described in Chapter 14.

The simplest light beam diaphragm consists of a metal cone which is fitted in front of the window of the X-ray tube. A radiolucent mirror, usually made of plastic, is fitted at an angle in front of the tube window such that light from a source outside the X-ray beam is superimposed on the irradiated area. (13 Fig. 4).

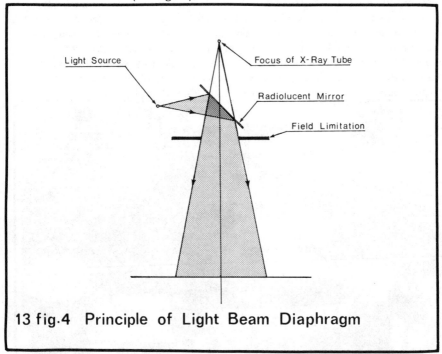

Light Source

Focus of X-Ray Tube

Radiolucent Mirror

Field Limitation

13 fig·4 Principle of Light Beam Diaphragm

In this diagram only the relevant rays have been drawn. A plate is fitted into a slot on the face of the cone. This plate, which is made of lead, limits both the size of the irradiated field, and the size of the light beam to the same area. Field limitation plates with various aperature sizes may be inserted to provide various fixed field sizes. The actual area irradiated is dependent of the focus to patient distance. As may be seen from the illustration it is necessary for the path length of the light beam to be exactly the same as that of the X-ray beam. A perspex window, with its centre marked, is fitted in front of the field limitation plate so that the point of incidence of the central ray is indicated on the patient.

In order that the light beam diaphragm may be used in daylight conditions, it is necessary for the light source to be powerful. Such lamps have a limited life and also become very hot during use. Therefore an automatic switch is fitted to limit the time during which the lamp is on. Due to the heat generated care should be taken with anaesthetised patients, for example, during hip-pinning operations when the light beam diaphragm is often touching the patient. To accommodate ambient lighting conditions the brightness of the light beam is adjustable in many types of diaphragm.

The next advance from the simple light beam diaphragm is to have adjustable lead leaves so that field size may be selected exactly according to requirements. A small, adjustable light beam diaphragm attached to a portable X-ray tubehead is shown in 13 Fig. 5. The two sliding levers adjust two pairs of lead leaves at right angles to each other. These leaves form a variable field limitation plate. As the field is rectangular the attachment of the device to the tubehead is made such that it is possible to rotate the diaphragm through 90° to allow orientation with respect to the patient.

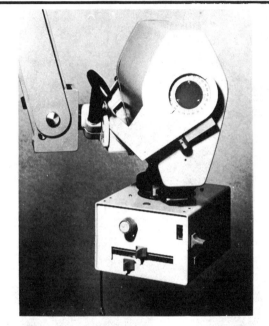

13 fig. 5 A Simple Light Beam Diaphragm

This simple system provides a beam centring device which is both small and light weight.

For general applications on static and high powered mobile X-ray units, a multi-leaf light beam is advantageous as it reduces penumbra. This is explained in Chapter 14. A multi-leaf diaphragm mounted on an overtable X-ray tube, with a handle bar device is shown in 13 Fig. 6.

Early multi-leaf light beam diaphragms were manually controlled but recently motor driven versions have become popular so that it is possible to control the diaphragm remotely. The illustration 13 Fig. 7 shows a motor-driven multi-leaf light beam diaphragm with its cover removed. The sets of leaves in each plane may be clearly seen.

Selection of opening size is made by operation of the push-buttons on the diaphragm. When it is necessary to control the diaphragm exactly to the size of a cassette in the bucky, the leaves may be adjusted according

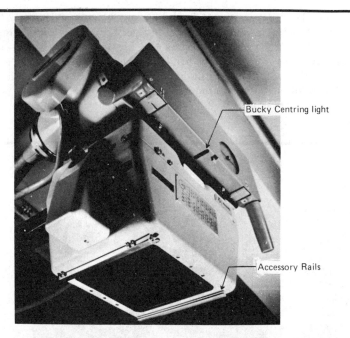

Bucky Centring light

Accessory Rails

13 fig. 6 L.B.D. and Bucky Centring Light

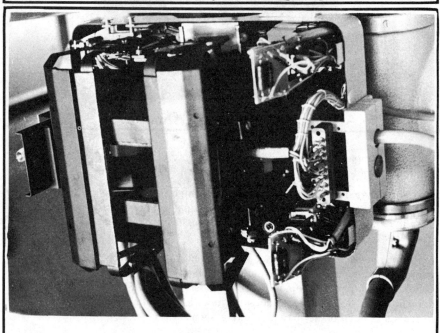

13 fig. 7 L.B.D. without Cover

to the table of settings provided, as the cassette is not visible. The leaf settings are indicated on the scales below the push buttons. Separate settings are required for different focus-to-film distances.

To facilitate the quick selection of the correct leaf opening size, automatic control may be provided. Such a control unit is shown in 13 Fig. 8. Circuitry in this unit not only adjusts for the correct opening size dependent on selection, but also corrects for different focus-to-film distances. The round knob to the right of the push buttons allows continuous adjustment other than the fixed settings provided.

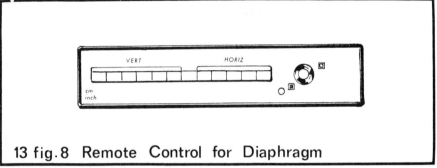

13 fig. 8   Remote   Control   for   Diaphragm

A further advance on this diaphragm selection control, is automatic selection dependent on the size of cassette placed in the bucky tray. This is done by sensing levers which "measure" the cassette when the cassette tray is advanced into the bucky and control the diaphragm accordingly.

13.5 Optical Viewfinders

In operating theatres, ambient lighting is often too bright for accurate use of a light beam diaphragm. In these cases modification of the basic light beam diaphragm designs has lead to the optical viewfinder. Here the light source is replaced by an optical system. The optical system is shown in 13 Fig. 9, and may be compared with 13 Fig. 4.

Light from the patient is reflected by the mirror and brought to a focus on a ground glass screen by a lens. An image of the area to be irradiated is thus formed on the screen and may be seen by the operator.

13.6 Other Beam Centring Devices

Whenever the overtable tube is used, centring of the bucky is conveniently carried out with the aid of a bucky centring light. This device, shown in 13 Fig. 6, projects a beam of light parallel to the central X-ray beam, at the centre of the longitudinal opening of the diaphragm. This beam projects onto the bucky tray or the handle of the tray, on the operator's side of the table, thus facilitating the centring of the bucky. This device may also be used while oblique projections are being positioned, when the beam from the diaphragm itself projects a trapezium.

203

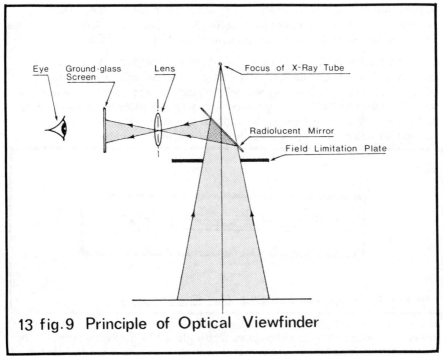

Eye Ground-glass   Lens   Focus of X-Ray Tube
      Screen

                                    Radiolucent Mirror
                                    Field Limitation Plate

13 fig.9 Principle of Optical Viewfinder

13.7 F.F.D. Scale

     With even the simplest light beam diaphragms a retractable steel
rule is usually fixed to the diaphragm so that the focus-to-film distance
(F.F.D.) may be accurately adjusted.

13.8 Centring for Automatic Exposure Control

     When using automatic exposure control units, especially those with
ionisation chambers, it is vital that the measuring fields selected are
covered by the patient and are not outside the irradiated area. To this end
a perspex plate with the measuring fields marked thereon may be placed on
the light beam diaphragm in the rails provided (13 Fig. 6). When one of
these plates is used, the areas corresponding to the measuring fields are
projected by the light beam onto the patient. They are only accurate if
used at the focus-to-film distance for which they are calibrated. This
F.F.D. is marked on each perspex plate.

13.9 T.V. Fluoroscopy Centring

     Checking of positioning may be carried out by T.V. fluoroscopy with
an image intensifier and T.V. camera mounted beneath the bucky. This is
becoming increasingly popular for quick and accurate positioning especially
for complex examinations and casualty radiography.

204

Chapter 14

Scattered Radiation

14.1 Introduction to Scatter

In Chapter 5, mention has been made of the scatter effect of an X-ray beam, as the radiation passes through matter. This Chapter deals with scatter in some detail, and how to a greater or lesser extent the detrimental effect of scatter upon the resultant film or image can be reduced.

As an analogy, the passage of light through two different types of glass will illustrate the effect of scatter. In the first example, an object is viewed through a sheet of plain glass. The light quanta will pass through the glass with very little absorption, reflection or refraction. If now, a similar object is viewed through a sheet of frosted glass, there will be so much internal reflection and refraction from the numerous ground surfaces that the image will appear distorted and obscure.

Similarly, a radiograph taken without due regard to the presence and problem of scatter, has an overall fog and severe loss of definition and contrast.

Two radiographs, one with a high degree of scatter, and one with greatly reduced scatter are illustrated in 14 Fig. 1 and 14 Fig. 2.

14.2 The Generation of Scatter

The manner in which scattered radiation arises is shown in 14 Fig. 3.

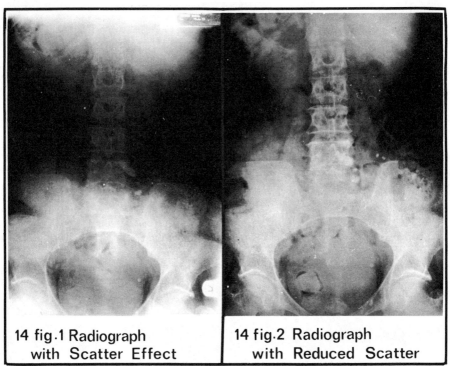

**14 fig.1 Radiograph
with Scatter Effect**

**14 fig.2 Radiograph
with Reduced Scatter**

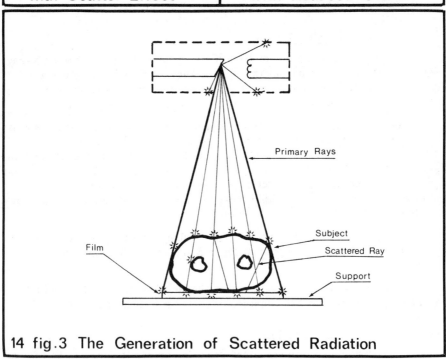

Primary Rays

Subject

Scattered Ray

Support

Film

14 fig.3 The Generation of Scattered Radiation

Scattered radiation occurs whenever an X-ray beam passes through matter. It is derived from the glass walls of the tube, from the tissue and bone of the patient, the examination table and any other patient support.

The presence of scatter must be remembered at all times, as it can be shown to be sent in all directions, and will affect a fluorescent screen or film some distance away from the primary beam. Therefore it is most important that radiological personnel make full use of the protective screens available, and be continually monitored for accumulated dosage received. For further details, it is necessary to refer to the "Code of practice for persons exposed to ionising radiations".

In 1923, A.H. Compton demonstrated that the wavelength of scattered radiation is longer than the wavelength of the primary beam. When a bombarded electron receives only part of the incident quantum energy, the result is that the scattered quantum, with a reduced momentum, and the recoil electron, with an increased momentum, can be given into vector quantities. Translating the mathematical results obtained by Compton into practical terms, the change in wavelength ($\lambda'' - \lambda'$) is independent of the wavelength of the incident ray and independent of the composition of the scattering medium, but is related to the angle of scattering.

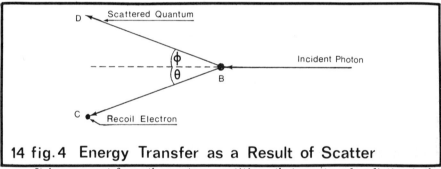

14 fig.4 Energy Transfer as a Result of Scatter

It is apparent from the vector quantities, that scattered radiation in the forward direction has the maximum energy level.

In the case of a complete energy transfer between the incident photon and an electron bound to the atomic structure, the kinetic energy of the recoil electron released is determined by the frequency of the incident photon. As the photon has to release the electron from its parent orbit within the atom, determined by the atomic structure of the substance, it follows that the emission of photo-electrons gives rise to a range of differing energy levels. Photo-electron emission can occur in all directions.

14.3 Methods of Reducing Scatter

What then can be done to minimise the effect of this scattered radiation, emanating from objects in the primary beam, and arriving at the surface of the film from all directions?

If one refers again to 14 Fig. 3, it is seen that scatter is even produced within the tube itself. All modern X-ray tubes are fitted with a rayproof shield.

The shield is fitted with a rectangular lead diaphragm which allows the emergence of the incident beam, and as seen in 14 Fig. 5, the effect of internal scatter is reduced.

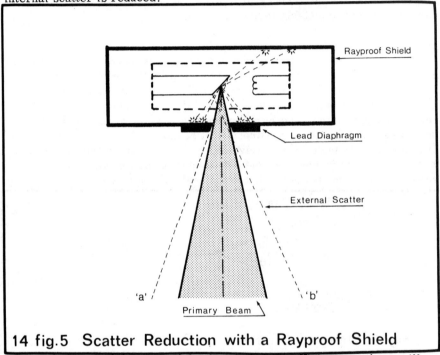

14 fig.5 Scatter Reduction with a Rayproof Shield

The fitting of this type of diaphragm is not sufficient, as there will still be scatter emitted in the directions a and b in the diagram.

A cylindrical diaphragm, sometimes referred to as a localising cone, will do much to reduce the effect of scatter (See 14 Figs. 6 and 7).

14.4 Cones and Diaphragms

The use of a cylindrical cone is of great value when fine detail is needed. A single cone however, does not fully meet the requirements for general radiographic techniques, because the area irradiated with a fixed dimension cone is a function of the Film to Focus Distance (F.F.D). For general purposes, a variable aperture device is preferable.

Such a device is known as a Light Beam Diaphragm (L.B.D.), or Collimator, and illustrations of two types are shown in 14 Figs. 8 and 9.

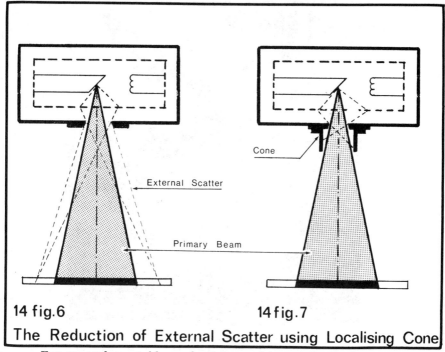

14 fig.6   14 fig.7

The Reduction of External Scatter using Localising Cone

For general overtable work, it is usual to set the diaphragm manually to the required aperture size. To assist in accurately centring the X-ray beam, and to indicate the exact irradiated area, the collimator is provided with a light source, to illuminate an area co-incident with the boundaries of the X-ray beam. (See illustration, Chapter 13 Fig. 4).

This is accomplished by directing the light from a lamp onto a thin, highly polished, radioluscent mirror, inclined at an angle, which projects the light in the same direction as the X-ray beam. As it is necessary to use a high intensity lamp, the period for which it is on is usually controlled by a time switch.

The design of a collimating diaphragm for modern fluoroscopic tables has become fairly complex in recent years. A modern examination table, often has a remotely controlled diaphragm with small electric motors driving the leaves, determining the aperture size. Modern serial changers, in general, have this control integrated with the exposure programme selector. The aperture size is then automatically determined by the exposure programme selected (film size) and the F.F.D. employed. The circuitry and design features then tend to become sophisticated.

14.5 Filters

The action of filters is explained in Section 5.12; however, one important factor here is that the filtration inherent in the X-ray tube, and that added to make a more homogeneous beam, does play a part in scatter

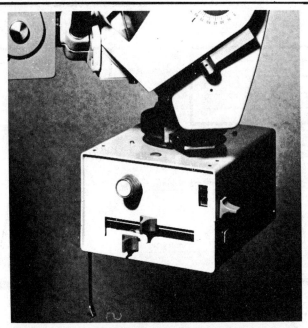

14 fig.8 A Simple Light Beam Diaphragm

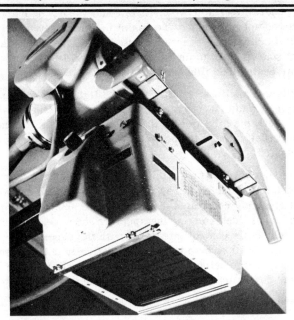

14 fig.9 A Light Beam Diaphragm Suitable for Overcouch Work

reduction. As has been stated, the wavelength of the scattered radiation is longer than that contained in the primary beam, and so will be more readily absorbed by filtration.

14.6 The Secondary Radiation Grid

It should be apparent at this stage, that the total elimination of scatter is not feasible. Thus scatter will be present in the beam, and will of course be generated in the patient and his surroundings.

There is little else that can be done to reduce scatter in the radiation before it reaches the patient and so it is necessary to consider other methods of reducing scatter radiation after the primary beam has passed through the patient. A grid is used to reduce the amount of scatter, produced in the patient, that reaches the image forming device.

Two basic types of grid are available, known as non-focussed and focussed. A grid consists of very fine radiopaque strips of lead or tungsten, interleaved with radioluscent strips, the whole assembly being bonded together to form a rigid plate a few millimetres in thickness. The number of strips vary between approximately 20 - 40 per cm. (50 - 100 per inch) dependent upon the requirements. All grids are made with high precision, and they must be treated with the utmost care.

14.7 The Non - focussed Grid

As can be seen in 14 Fig. 10, scattered radiation, deriving from the patient will usually be in a different direction to the primary rays, and so will be absorbed by the parallel strips. The central ray will pass with little attenuation through the inter strip spaces. Moving towards the periphery, the rays will be absorbed more readily by the opaque strips, the degree of absorption dependent upon the strip spacing, but scattered rays will be more efficiently absorbed.

It should be noted that scattered rays inclined in a direction parallel to the strips are not effectively absorbed, thus the grid contributes to scatter reduction and not elimination.

14.7.1 Grid Ratio

The grid ratio is the term used to express the relationship between the width of the radioluscent medium dividing the absorbing strips, and the height of the strips. The ratio is given by the height of the opaque strips divided by the distance between them.

The implication of this will be more readily appreciated by referring to 14 Fig. 11 a, b and c.

In 14 Fig. 11a, a scattered ray S will be absorbed by the metal strip, whilst the information bearing ray will pass through the grid at P.

When the distance Q is increased as in 14 Fig. 11b, a similarly angled scattered ray S will pass through the grid, and adversely affect the image.

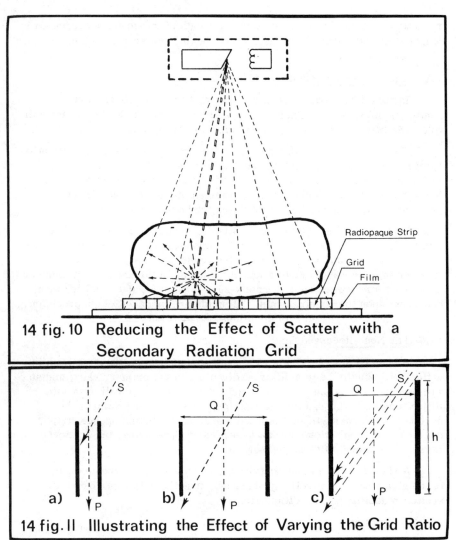

14 fig. 10 Reducing the Effect of Scatter with a Secondary Radiation Grid

Radiopaque Strip

Grid

Film

14 fig. 11 Illustrating the Effect of Varying the Grid Ratio

In 14 Fig. 11c, the height of the metal strip h is increased, and once again the scattered ray will be prevented from reaching the film.

It is thus possible to achieve a similar reduction in the transmission of scatter, by either having a thin grid in which the strip height h is small, but with a high number of lines per cm., or with a thicker grid in which the strip height h is increased, and the distance between adjacent metal strips is comparatively large.

14.7.2 The Problems of a Non-focussed Grid

In the description of the non-focussed grid, it was apparent referring to 14 Fig. 10 that the diverging primary beam will be absorbed towards the lateral edges of the irradiated area. Of course this primary beam is information carrying and not scatter. To absorb it within the grid structure means that information is being lost. The radiographic image will diminish towards these edges, and the reduction will become more apparent as the size of the image is increased, or as the F.F.D. is reduced.

In the manufacturer's search for a universally acceptable grid, early attempts were made to taper the height of the strips from the centre of the grid towards its lateral edges. Due to manufacturing difficulties, the ratio of the grid was already low and so was reduced almost to zero at the edges. An initial higher ratio at the centre was therefore required, but this higher ratio necessitated more accurate centring, as well as the manufacturing problem.

It has been seen that even the primary peripheral ray is attenuated by the grid towards the edges. In fact I.C.R.U. "International Commission on Radiological Units Measurements" recommendations specify that the focus-grid distance should be such that a variation in density between the centre and lateral edges of a 30 cm. square film does not exceed 50%. In practice, this is achieved by a focus-grid distance not less than the width of the image multiplied by the grid ratio.

The higher the ratio, the better the scatter absorption obtained. Assuming that a ratio of 10:1 is needed to achieve an optimum absorption, the minimum tube focus to grid distance for an area of 30 cm. square is equal to 30 x 10 cm. (300 cm.). A non-focussed grid of high ratio is thus impractical because of the large distances involved. If the F.F.D. is reduced, the lateral sides of the film will have the metal strips so closely projected, they will eventually overlap with total attenuation of the X-ray beam. This can be visualised by imagining a scene viewed through a venetian blind. As an example, for a 10:1 ratio grid at a F.F.D. of 100 cm, the usable data on a film of width of 30 cm., will be only about 11 cm.,wide.

14.8 The Focussed Grid

So far, only the parallel or non-focussed grid has been considered, but it is more general now to find focussed grids in use. In a focussed grid, the strips are inclined towards the tube focus as illustrated in 14 Fig. 12.

With a focussed grid, the metal strips form part of the radii of a circle, the centre of which is the focal point of the X-ray tube. The divergent beam of primary radiation is able to pass through the inter-strip spaces with little absorption,(see 14 Fig. 12).

A grid of this form can be used with quite a tolerable latitude in focus-grid distance and allows a reasonable latitude in the centring of the beam. A table of these limits is given in 14 Fig. 13.

It is apparent that the advantages of a focussed grid far outweigh

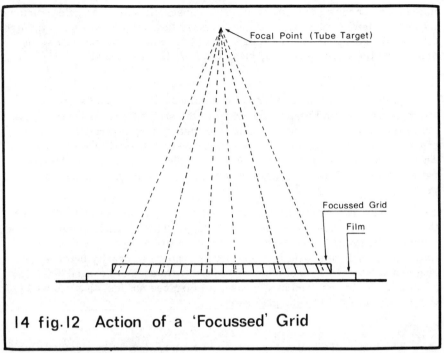

Focal Point (Tube Target)

Focussed Grid

Film

14 fig.12   Action of a 'Focussed' Grid

those of a non-focussed type.

· Obviously, when a non-focussed grid is employed, it is irrelevant
which face of the grid is opposite the tube, but it is essential the correct
side of a focussed grid faces the tube. The appropriate side and the
specification of the grid is normally indicated on the grid itself.

In the general explanation of Compton scatter, it was seen in 14 Fig. 4
that the scattered quantum was a vector BD at an angle ϕ to the incident
beam, and the recoil electron acting along the vector BC at an angle θ
As the X-ray tube voltage is increased, these two angles diminish, resulting
in scatter at a narrower angle. For this reason, high ratio grids are
selected to counteract the high energy level scatter at comparatively narrow
angles.

14.9   The Scatter Problem in Bi-plane Radiography

There is quite a problem to be solved in reducing scatter in bi-plane
techniques. The actual technique of bi-plane working is covered in
Chapter 19, the problem of scatter reduction will be dealt with here.

So far, the scatter problem, and the grid has been considered in a
two dimensional aspect only. In bi-plane techniques as depicted in 14 Fig 14,
scatter radiation is produced by both tubes in all directions and therefore
efficient selective absorption is important. As the grid described so far is

Ratio	Lateral Decentralising possible	F.F.D. Range			
		80 cm*	100 cm*	150 cm*	200 cm*
		cm	cm	cm	cm
1:4	0 cm	50 – 240	55 – ∞	70 – ∞	85 – ∞
	1 cm	50 – 230	60 – ∞	75 – ∞	90 – ∞
	2 cm	55 – 210	65 – ∞	80 – ∞	95 – ∞
1:7	0 cm	60 – 130	70 – 195	90 – ∞	100 – ∞
	1 cm	65 – 120	75 – 180	95 – ∞	110 – ∞
	2 cm	70 – 115	80 – 170	100 – ∞	115 – ∞
1:10	0 cm	65 – 110	75 – 150	100 – 300	120 – ∞
	1 cm	70 – 100	80 – 140	110 – 290	130 – ∞
	2 cm	75 – 95	85 – 130	115 – 280	135 – ∞
1:12 or 1:13	0 cm	63 – 100	80 – 135	110 – 250	130 – 350
	1 cm	70 – 95	85 – 130	115 – 240	140 – 340
	2 cm	75 – 90	90 – 120	120 – 220	150 – 330
1:15	0 cm	70 – 95	80 – 130	110 – 225	140 – 300
	1 cm	75 – 90	90 – 120	120 – 210	150 – 290
	2 cm	80 – 85	95 – 110	125 – 200	160 – 280

* F.F.D. specified for the grid

Table for the selection of the
most suitable grid for varying
F.F.D.(based on a width of 30cm).

14 fig. 13 Selection Table

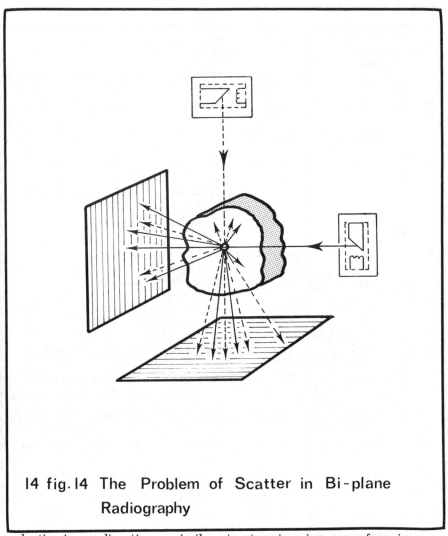

14 fig. 14 The Problem of Scatter in Bi-plane
Radiography

selective in one direction, a similar structure in criss-cross form is
employed.

The cross-grid combines the elements of two grids superimposed one
on the other, with the strips intersecting at an angle, usually at 90° to each
other.

The cross-grid can be either of the focussed or non-focussed type,
but in any event, the centring of the beam is more critical than with a single
grid. Combining the elements in two planes, will reduce by half, the ratio
of a comparable single grid.

14.10 The Metal Plate Technique

By virtue of the construction of all types of grid, no matter how finely made are the strips, the presence of the grid lines on the finished radiograph will always be discernible if the grid remains stationary throughout the exposure. The presence of fine grid lines may not detract from the diagnostic value of the film except when fine detail is required, such as in skull examinations.

An interesting technique of particular use in skull examinations and work with portable apparatus utilises a suitably dimensioned thin plate of tinned iron, interposed between patient and film in a similar manner to that when using a stationary grid. When the applied X-ray tube voltage is reduced by approximately 10 kV, from that normally used, the resultant radiographs show great clarity, with a complete freedom from grid lines.

Of course, this technique has limitations one of which is that as the applied kV rises, the increased energy level scatter is not sufficiently absorbed by the plate.

14.11 The Potter-Bucky Diaphragm

Doctors Potter and Bucky invented a device which overcomes to a great extent the problem of grid lines showing on the film.

A grid of a construction similar to the stationary focussed grid already described is mounted in a frame, the difference in the operation being that during the exposure, the grid is made to move across the X-ray beam in a direction at right angles to the long axis of the grid strips. In moving, the image of the individual strips is blurred out and so the presence of grid lines will no longer be apparent on the film.

The device which achieves this is known as a Potter-bucky, or simply Bucky. The grid is often called the bucky diaphragm, but to avoid confusion with the light beam diaphragm, it can be simply called the grid.

There are various methods of moving the grid, but all buckys include certain common design features which are :-

a) The exposure sequence of the X-ray apparatus is initiated at some pre-determined point during the grid movement cycle.

b) The velocity and distance moved by the grid during the exposure must be sufficient to effectively blur out the shadow of the grid line.

c) The unit is fitted with a framework which secures the grid and allows the grid to be simply and easily exchanged.

d) A mechanism, similar to one of the types described later in this Chapter, to move the grid and control exposure initiation.

e) A facility to hold the cassette, usually a metal tray with automatically centring jaws.

Bucky units fitted to diagnostic tables and vertical stands for general work, are held in a framework supported on bearings, effectively counter-balanced so it is possible to secure the bucky with a mechanical or electro-mechanical brake.

For serial changer operation, the bucky grid is supported by bearings or guide rails, and forms an integral part of the serial changer. The grid can be slid in and out of the irradiated area, as for some examinations it may not be required, for example, in a fluoroscopy examination of a child where the scatter problem is less pronounced.

Mention has been made of the effect of decentralising the grid with respect to the central ray of the X-ray beam. Obviously, during the movement of a bucky grid, decentralisation must occur, the degree of movement being 2.5 - 5.0 cm.

The centre line of the examination table is referred to as a datum line, and the grid should be mid-way in its travel when the centre of the grid is co-incident with this datum.

It is normal to orientate the grid so that the strips lie parallel to the centre line of the table. This is owing to the fact that the angulation of the X-ray beam for most examinations is in this direction. Should the axis of the grid be at 90° to the direction of beam angulation, excessive absorption of the primary beam will occur.

14.12 The Single Action Hydraulic Bucky

The manner in which the movement is transmitted to the grid varies between manufacturers. Early models utilised tension springs working against a hydraulic damper as is shown in 14 Fig. 15a. The mechanism is loaded by the operator pulling the handle, moving the grid against the tension of the springs. A mechanical catch locks the grid in the cocked position. The catch can either be electrically released, by energising the solenoid (the plunger of which strikes the catch and releases the grid), or mechanically released by pulling a cord attached to the catch. The springs draw the grid across the film which is positioned in a cassette tray immediately below the grid.

The grid, coupled to the hydraulic damper piston will move against the resistance of an oil flow between the two chambers A - A' . The oil, displaced from chamber A passes through an expansion bellows to an adjustable orifice. According to the orifice size, more or less oil can pass through in unit time. The orifice size is adjusted by the rod and knob calibrated in the time of grid travel.

During the movement of the grid, electrical contacts in the bucky initiate the exposure, these contacts shown at "x" in 14 Fig. 15. Just prior to the grid coming to rest, these contacts are opened. An exposure is thus only possible during the period of time that the grid is moving.

In 14 Fig.15b the handswitch will complete the release solenoid circuit when contacts 'Y' are closed. These are only closed when the bucky grid is loaded, thus forming an interlock to prevent the solenoid being energised when the grid is not loaded.

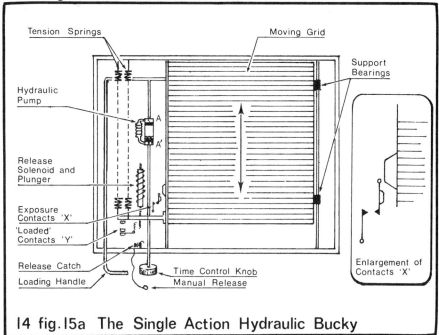

14 fig.15a The Single Action Hydraulic Bucky

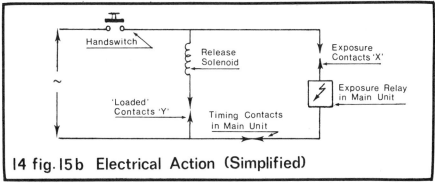

14 fig.15b Electrical Action (Simplified)

It is always necessary with this type of unit to set the time on the hydraulic control slightly longer than that selected on the exposure timer, so the exposure sequence is initiated by the contacts in the bucky, and terminated by the exposure timer which has a far greater accuracy.

There are of course other disadvantages to using this type of control; for example, it requires manual loading prior to each exposure. This is inconvenient and may be forgotten.

The single action type, as described, has another disadvantage when using short exposure times available with high output X-ray generators. The velocity of the grid is constant for practically the whole of the movement, (it will initially accelerate and close the contacts for the exposure to begin). If this velocity, which can be established **as** a rate of x lines per second, is the same as, or a harmonic of, the rate at which the X-ray pulses emanate from the tube, then stroboscopic grid lines will be recorded on the film and give the appearance that the grid has not moved. It will be necessary to avoid the bucky time settings at which this occurs.

14.13 Oscillating Buckys

In order to eliminate the need to load the mechanism manually prior to each exposure, some form of electro-mechanical actuator is now incorporated. By using an electric motor, coupled to the grid by a crankarm, the reciprocating bucky was introduced.

The grid drive motor is normally energised during "Preparation". The cyclic nature of the grid movement means that at either end of the grid stroke, it is almost stationary. This type of bucky is provided with phasing contacts to ensure that the X-ray exposure is initiated at or near maximum grid velocity, which is of a sinusoidal nature. The contacts can be adjusted to close at any moment in the grid cycle, so providing a means of correction for the zero time of the X-ray apparatus as referred to in Chapter 10. The contacts close twice in each revolution of the cam, so exposures always start at the same relative point in the cycle. Short exposure times occur at peak grid velocity, and the long exposure times commence at this point, and extend over the period when the grid is reversing. Should an exposure be terminated when the grid makes its first reversal, and an X-ray pulse occurs when the grid is stationary, the image produced by that pulse would have a contrast inversely proportional to the number of X-ray pulses contained in the total exposure. In order to compromise between the requirements of short and long exposure times, the exposure is initiated at a point 50° from either end of the grid stroke, the centre point of the grid position being 90° (See 14 Fig. 16).

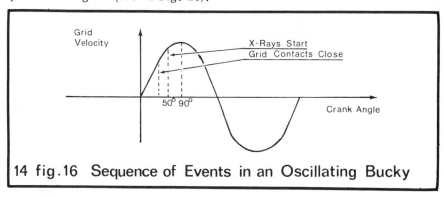

14 fig.16 Sequence of Events in an Oscillating Bucky

In order to reduce the effect of the grid reversal producing grid lines the sprung or "Trill" bucky was developed and introduced, this being explained later in this Chapter.

The type of grid drive explained in Section 14.13 is often found in a serial changer. The following brief explanation of the electrical functioning refers to 14 Fig. 17.

On "Preparation", the motor is energised, driving the grid and adjustable cam. The exposure circuit of the X-ray generator will be initiated by the phasing contacts closed by the cam. These complete the circuit for the self holding relay, closing contacts 'a ' and "b'. Contacts "a" by-pass the phasing contacts, and 'b' start the main exposure sequence. The exposure will be terminated by the main timer in the general control, and on release of the operators switch, the circuit will revert to its rest condition.

14 fig. 17 Simplified Electrical Functioning of a Motor - Driven Bucky

14.14 Two Speed Reciprocating Bucky

The motor driven reciprocating bucky described in Section 14.13 has a grid velocity which is sinusoidal, and a crankarm drive of a constant angular velocity. An optimum setting was given to the instant at which the exposure is initiated to compensate for both short and long exposure times.

A bucky drive having two speeds; an initial fast movement across the face of the film to the limits of the stroke, and a slower return movement, will compensate for a considerable variation in exposure time.

The cyclic grid movement is shown graphically in 14 Fig. 18.

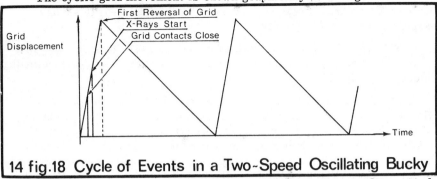

14 fig.18 Cycle of Events in a Two-Speed Oscillating Bucky

A simple way of achieving the two speeds, which are pre-determined and not adjustable, is with a combination of springs, hydraulic damper, and solenoid actuator. An illustration of a simple arrangement is shown in 14 Fig. 19.

At rest, the actuating solenoid is not energised and the springs are relieved of tension. When an exposure sequence is commenced, the solenoid is energised, rapidly drawing the grid across the X-ray beam. Soon after the grid starts to move, the exposure contacts close, initiating the actual exposure.

At the limit of grid travel, the solenoid supply is switched off, allowing the grid to be drawn in the opposite direction under the tension of the springs against the action of the hydraulic damper.

The solenoid circuit is remade when the grid reaches its starting point, the cycle of events being repeated until the exposure time has elapsed.

Although the two types of reciprocating bucky already described are a great improvement over the single action type, there is still a possibility that when a pulse of X-rays occurs at the instant of grid reversal an image of the grid lines will be recorded. During a lengthy exposure, there could be several of these reversals. With the types of reciprocating buckys, dealt with in this chapter so far, the displacement of the grid to its limits of travel is equidistant either side of the mid-point. This means that the grid reversal will occur at the same positions each time, with a cumulative effect of grid line recording.

14.15 The Trill Oscillating Bucky

By ensuring that the movement of the grid is in the form of a damped oscillation as shown in 14 Fig. 20, the reversal point will occur at different positions during a lengthy exposure.

The bucky grid is supported at four points by flat springs, and is free to swing over its limits of travel. The total time of oscillation is designed to be at least 15 seconds which is far in excess of maximum expected exposure time.

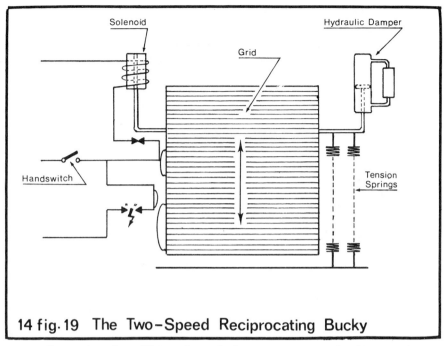

14 fig. 19 The Two-Speed Reciprocating Bucky

The period of oscillation is such that an exposure of 0.12 seconds can be made before the first grid reversal. As can be seen in 14 Fig. 20, the subsequent reversals will occur at different displacements of the grid.

An illustration of a Trill oscillating bucky is shown in 14 Fig. 21 and an electrical circuit in 14 Fig. 22.

14.16 Electrical Operation of a Trill Oscillating Bucky

At the start of the exposure sequence, the solenoid S1 is energised via a contact S2A of relay S2. The core of solenoid S1, attached to the grid, is thus drawn into the coil of the solenoid and the grid moved to the extreme position. In so doing the following actions result.

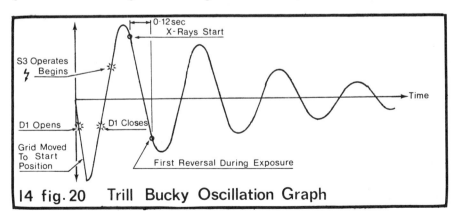

14 fig. 20   Trill Bucky Oscillation Graph

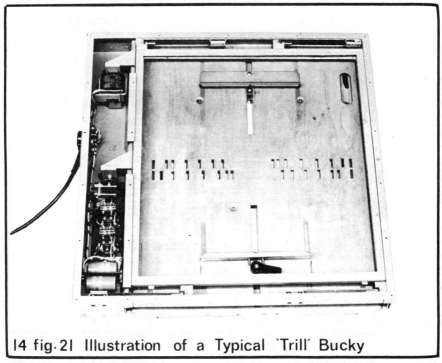

14 fig. 21 Illustration of a Typical `Trill´ Bucky

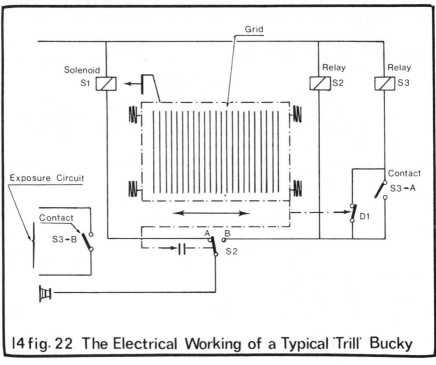

14 fig. 22 The Electrical Working of a Typical `Trill´ Bucky

a) The contact D1 is opened preventing the exposure start relay S3, being energised whilst the grid is stationary.

b) Contact S2A is changed over mechanically, completing the circuit for relay S2, which holds itself on.

c) The tripping of S2A will open the circuit for the actuator solenoid S1, so allowing the grid to oscillate freely.

Soon after the grid is released and starts to move the contact D1 is closed by the grid action. Relay S3 is then energised closing its contacts S3A and B. Contact S3A is a hold on contact, maintaining S3 in the on position irrespective of the subsequent opening of the contact D1. Contact S3B initiates the exposure.

14.17 Effect of Grid Ratio on Exposure Factors

It is necessary, when using a stationary or moving grid, to increase the exposure factors, because as well as absorbing scatter, some of the primary radiation is attenuated. The effectiveness of the grid is determined by several parameters, the attenuation of scatter being the most important. This attenuation should be high. It is also important that the primary beam attenuation is low, as this affects the exposure time, and the consequent dose of radiation to the patient.

In absorbing the scatter radiation, some primary attenuation is inevitable, the factors affecting the overall attenuation being a function of the grid ratio, the thickness of the radiopaque strips, and the number of strips per centimetre (line density).

The amount by which an exposure has to be increased, compared to that needed for non-grid working is shown in 14 Fig. 23 for various grid ratios, all other conditions being equal.

Ratio	70 kV	95 kV	120 kV
No grid	1	1	1
5:1	3	3	3
8:1	3.75	4	4.2
12:1	4.75	5	6
16:1	5.75	6.75	8

14 fig. 23   Table Showing How the Exposure Factor is Influenced by Varying Grid Ratios

14.18 Effect of Grid Line Density on Exposure Factors

For a given thickness of absorbent strip, the primary beam attenuation rises with an increase in line density. An increase in the line density results in a decrease in the thickness of the radioluscent spacers, between the absorbent strips. It follows that as there is an increase in percentage of radio-absorbent material, there will be an overall increase in absorption. An increase in the line density calls for greater accuracy in centring the X-ray beam to the grid centre, and the focus - grid distance becomes more critical.

14.19 Selection of Grids and Their Use

The table shown in 14 Fig. 24 may be of value in the selection of a suitable grid. It must be used only as a guide, because it has already been established that there are many variables in techniques which will affect the ultimate choice.

In general cross grids will be superior to the single axis grid, but are unsuitable for any angled beam techniques.

14.20 Air Gap Technique

A suggested technique for the reduction of scatter effect, applied mainly to chest radiography, utilises an air gap of about 15 cm., between subject and film. This gives comparable results to the scatter reduction obtained by the use of a stationary grid, as the scatter produced is prevented from arriving at the film.

The focus - film distance required has to be increased to about 4 m. to produce the same magnification as that found in conventional techniques. This increased F.F.D. requires much higher kV's than that normally employed.

Kilovoltages up to 190 kV have been used utilising this method with excellent results, the final radiographs showing the area of the lung fields without the rib cage.

In an installation of this kind, it is recommended that the tube be permanently fixed, and a suitable patient support provided. The tube has to be fitted with a specially shaped diaphragm and cone to accurately collimate the beam, and reduce the effect of "off focus" radiation.

The 15 cm. air gap is maintained by interposing a suitably dimensioned lead lined box between the subject and film. The front of the box is covered by a sheet of 0.5 mm Aluminium, the rear being open.

The results obtained give films of high quality, with absence of grid lines, as well as the important factor, a reduced patient dosage compared to that received using a stationary or moving grid.

226

Ratio	Line density	Performance	Suggested use
4:1	up to 28 per cm.	Adequate absorption for small areas, and low dosage.	Moving grid, useful for image intensification and spot film work.
5:1	up to 28 per cm.	Reasonable efficiency up to 85 kV with wide latitudes in centring and F.F.D.	Moving grid, general purpose.
7:1	up to 28 per cm.	Reasonable efficiency up to 85 kV with good latitude in centring and F.F.D.	Moving grid, general purpose.
8:1	up to 28 per cm.	Moderate efficiency, medium tolerance in positioning. Up to 100 kV working.	Moving grid, general purpose, but centring now fairly critical.
12:1 13·1	23 to 40 per cm.	Better efficiency than lower ratio grids but little positioning latitude. Up to 110 kV.	Moving or stationary role – great care needed in alignment.
15:1 16:1	35 to 42 per cm.	Very high scatter absorption. No positioning latitude. For use above 100 kV.	Moving, but more often stationary. Useful in tomography of dense regions.
10:1	greater than 50 per cm.	Minimal line visibility. Very little positional latitude.	Ultrafine stationary grid working.

N.B. Due to standardisation, not all combinations of grid ratio/line density may necessarily be available.

14 fig. 24 Guide to the Selection of Suitable Grid Parameters

Chapter 15

Fluoroscopic Equipment

15.1 Fluoroscopy

Fluoroscopy, sometimes incorrectly termed screening, is the dynamic radiological study of the human anatomy. In these examinations, X-rays are converted into a visual image on a fluorescent screen. Sometimes the fluorescent screen forms part of an image intensifier and this is discussed in Chapter 16.

As these procedures can last several minutes every effort must be made to limit the radiation dose to a low level. It therefore follows that the fluorescent screen should convert as much radiation energy into light as possible. The essential requirements are an X-ray source, a patient and a fluorescent screen. The patient is usually supported on a table which has various movement facilities. This is to ensure that the examination may be carried out with the patient in any desired position. We will now look at each item in some detail.

15.2 The Fluorescent Screen

All materials which change radiation into light are known as phosphors. The substance most widely used in the manufacture of fluoroscopic screens is a mixture of zinc sulphide and cadmium sulphide. This has the advantage, when subjected to X-ray bombardment, of emitting a green/yellow light to which the human eye is most sensitive. The phosphor also contains minute traces of an actuator such as copper, which increases green/yellow light emission.

Commensurate with the production of light, the screen must be thick enough to absorb the maximum amount of X-radiation to which it is exposed. Increasing the thickness, will always increase the absorption; but the human eye would be incapable of viewing the light produced from the depths of the screen. For this reason, and subsequent considerations to be discussed, an optimum thickness exists for each type of fluorescent screen. A typical screen is depicted in 15 Fig. 1.

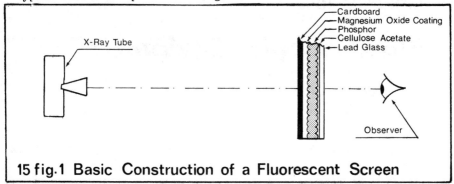

15 fig.1 Basic Construction of a Fluorescent Screen

A white undercoat of magnesium oxide is incorporated to create a smooth reflecting layer which will direct most of the light towards the surface viewed. The phosphor itself is given a very thin coat of cellulose acetate to protect it and also to prevent optical contact between the screen and the lead glass. Optical contact manifests itself in the appearances of dark patches on the screen when subjected to X-rays. The cellulose acetate coat will also afford a certain amount of protection to the phosphor against exposure to ultra violet and blue light, since the emission of an unprotected screen would rapidly deteriorate when exposed to daylight. Since the fluorescent screen does not absorb all the X-rays falling on it, the observer must be protected by a sheet of lead glass through which he views image. This glass has an absorption factor known as the lead equivalent. This is the thickness of lead that would be required in place of the glass to obtain the same absorption. The regulations vary from country to country; but generally call for a glass with lead equivalent of 2.0 mm of lead for examinations conducted between 50 kV and 100 kV and 2.5 mm of lead for examinations up to 150 kV. Relevant codes of practice should be consulted.

15.2.1 Intrinsic Unsharpness

The fairly large thickness of fluorescent screens, varying in practice from 0.5 mm to 1.0 mm, causes what is known as intrinsic unsharpness of the resultant image. The phosphor material is made up of crystals, the size of which can be predetermined during manufacture. For example, should the crystals be small the eye is able to integrate over a smaller area, so observing greater detail. The drawback is that this results in a lower brightness level.

15.2.2 Fluoroscopic Image Brightness and Contrast

As the brightness of a typical phosphor is very low, the best way to view is in darkness. The observer requires time for his eyes to adapt to see in a darkened room. If this is not done, it will not be possible to perceive sufficient detail on the screen. The situation may then only be improved by increasing the input X-ray dose or replacing the screen by an image intensifying system. Contrast is low when using a combination of high kV and low mA, because the differential absorption resulting from the beam passing through the various organs of the patient is minimal. This also leads to lower detail perceptibility.

15.2.3 Geometric Unsharpness

Geometric unsharpness in fluoroscopy generally results from the fact that the screen to focus distance is less than that used for general radiography. The patient to screen distance will also be greater than in radiography. Both these factors contribute to image unsharpness. The focal size of the X-ray tube is significant and a small focus is generally chosen for fluoroscopy to minimise geometric unsharpness.

15.3 Fluoroscopic Tables

The design of modern tables has been greatly influenced by the universal acceptance of image intensification and television in place of the fluorescent screen.

There are two broad approaches; tube below the table and image intensifier above, as shown in 15 Fig. 2, or with the tube above the table and image intensifier below.

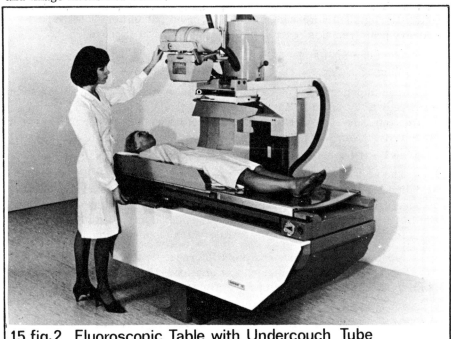

15 fig. 2   Fluoroscopic Table with Undercouch Tube

Both types of table are manufactured in a variety of versions but include the following features:-

In all cases the table base must be of a robust construction as it has to bear the weight of the table, tube assembly, serial changer, bucky assembly and all the counterweight devices required to enable their balanced movement. It is usual to incorporate a table tilt drive which enables examination of the patient to be carried out in the horizontal, vertical or any intermediate position. The modern drive is usually powered by a d.c. motor which enables infinite speed variation from zero to maximum. A present day unit would be expected to tilt from 0° to 90° in approximately 25 seconds at maximum speed. An alternative method of tilting is the hydraulic drive which also gives a smooth, infinitely variable drive characteristic.

Nearly all tables have the Trendelenberg,or adverse tilt,facility which varies up to 90° according to design. A popular application of this feature is in myelography. Most tables can be made to stop automatically in the horizontal position. On some tables automatic speed reduction operates prior to stopping.

Power driven table top drives were introduced to facilitate patient positioning. Automatic centring is often provided on both longitudinal and lateral drives.

On the majority of present day tables the X-ray tube is mounted beneath the table top. It must be mechanically coupled to the serial changer which carries the fluorescent screen (or Image Intensifier) so that the primary beam remains centred to the screen when it is moved.

The table top to tube focus distance is usually fixed in the range of 40 - 50 cm.

It is important to protect the radiologist and his assistants against any stray radiation caused by scatter or misalignment of the primary beam. Scatter radiation is dealt with by fitting protective lead rubber slide flaps on the serial changer and table top, plus closure of the bucky slit when the bucky is parked.

The area of radiation is restricted by fitting a motorized diaphragm, or delineator, to the tube. The lead shutters within the diaphragm automatically compensate for a change in the field-focus distance. In addition filters of aluminium or copper are placed in the path of the primary beam to reduce the low energy radiation which performs no useful function.

Most control units incorporate a fluoroscopic timer to measure the time that each patient is subjected to radiation. Usually an audible warning is given at the end of a predetermined time (generally 5 minutes).

When radiographic films are taken by the serial changer, many diaphragms are now designed to sense the cassette size and adjust the shutter aperture accordingly.

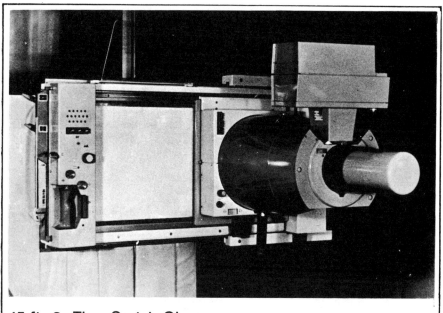

15 fig.3 The Serial Changer

15.4 Serial Changer and Image Intensifier Carriage

The serial changer, sometimes known as a spot film device (typical example shown in 15 Fig. 3), is designed for a sequence of radiographic exposures during a fluoroscopic examination. Basically, a cassette is inserted into the serial changer and by either a manual or automatic system a series of exposures are made on the one film, the film being exposed in sections. The area of the sections is determined by a shutter, or cap which is also used to compress the patient in the region of interest.

To obtain additional views, it is necessary to move the patient on the tables so far described which have a fixed undertable tube. For example, to obtain a lateral view, the patient must be turned on his side. Should a lateral view be required without turning the patient, a second X-ray tube may be attached to the side of the table (see 15 Fig. 4).

As mentioned in Section 15.3 the serial changer carriage is coupled to the X-ray tube. Provision is made so that the serial changer can be parked out of the way so that radiography, with an overtable tube, or techniques not utilising fluoroscopy, can be carried out.

Image intensification and television has influenced the grouping of controls on the serial changer and certain manipulations, which had to be done separately in former times, are now performed concurrently. Controls are now generally found on the lefthand side of the serial changer, as is the facility for lefthand loading of the cassettes. Automatic diaphragms, operated by the programme selector on the serial changer, are a general feature of modern examination tables. Programme selection itself has been simplified since the programme is now determined by the size of the cassette placed in the serial changer and by the size of compression cap used.

The serial device moves in three planes relative to the table top; longitudinally, laterally and vertically (sometimes known, incorrectly, as compression). It must be possible, with one switch, to energise the brake system which locks the serial changer at any instant. They must operate automatically under certain circumstances, for example, whilst tilting the table or moving the table top. A vibration free serial changer carriage is essential for radiography.

Radiological tables follow a common pattern as a result of standardisation in examination techniques.

With a second image intensifier for the horizontal beam, fluoroscopy in two planes becomes possible with rapid alternation from one plane to the other.

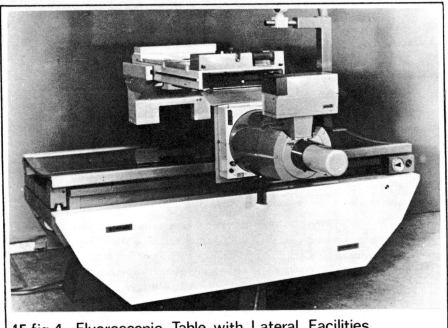

15 fig.4   Fluoroscopic Table with Lateral Facilities

15.4.1 The Cassette Transport

A mechanism is included in the serial changer to transport the cassette into the X-ray field so that phenomena, viewed on the fluoroscopic screen or television monitor, may be recorded on film. It is important that the delay between cessation of fluoroscopy and radiographic film exposure is minimal, as many observed phenomena are purely transient in nature. Several exposures are possible on one film, by exposing different areas successively. For example, four exposures can be made on an 18 x 24 cm film; two, four or six exposures on a 24 x 30 cm film or three exposures on a 35 x 35 cm film. Obviously other sub-divisions are possible and vary according to the manufacturer's design.

Spot films can now be taken via the image intensifier and this is discussed in the next chapter. The serial changer described employs film in cassettes, but future trends suggest that a method of film transportation without cassettes is desirable.

In modern, sophisticated units the sub-division and correct positioning of the cassette for successive exposures is automated. Thus the operator has only to select a given exposure series on the programme selector. The serial changer then looks after everything else, even setting the diaphragm to the required aperture in certain cases, as described in 15.3.

To obtain radiographs during a fluoroscopic session, a certain sequence of events must take place :-

a) Fluoroscopy must be switched off as the cassette carriage starts to move.

b) The X-ray tube anode must be accelerated to the required speed and the filament heat boosted for radiography.

c) The cassette carriage must be brought into the exposure field and held in the correct place.

d) The grid, when fitted, must be set in motion (unless a stationary fine line grid is used.

e) An exposure can then be initiated having previously selected the required kV and mAs values.

All the above operations on modern units are executed automatically by depressing one button. After the exposure the cassette is returned to the parked position. Fluoroscopy can only then be resumed after a short delay to allow cooling of the X-ray tube filaments. On the second and subsequent exposures the cassette takes up a different position in relation to the exposure area and the above procedure repeated. On simple changers these operations are still hand-operated.

15.5 Remote Control Tables

Remotely controlled tables are now rapidly gaining general acceptance. A typical example is illustrated in 15 Fig. 5. This shows the overtable tube configuration. As the radiation protection presents a greater problem, nearly all of these types are remote controlled. The reason for continuation and perfection of this type of table was that there are certain advantages in comparison with conventional methods, amongst which the following should be mentioned:-

a) It is easier to carry out many examinations with this type of table.

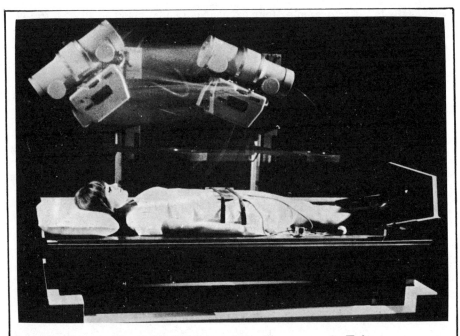

15 fig.5 Fluoroscopic Table with Overcouch Tube

Considering for instance, gastro-intestinal work, it is certainly more convenient to do this by remote control than by manipulating a large spot-film device with an image intensifier and its accessories. Remote control reduces the physical effort required and allows a greater number of examinations to be carried out.

b) The protection screen between the control desk and examination table ensures that the radiologist is fully protected from the hazards of ionising radiation.

c) The necessity for wearing heavy protective clothing is now removed. The radiologist is not obliged to wear heavy rubber gloves.

d) Most remotely controlled tables have the X-ray tube above, so providing a better view of the patient.

It must be said that a few disadvantages also exist so provision is often made to operate the control desk adjacent to the table. Palpation of the patient is then possible during the examination.

A remotely controlled table is a rather complicated device with intricate circuitry and many moving parts. Consequently, the complete set-up may be expensive, but viewed overall the concept of remote tables is gaining universal favour.

15.6 Compression Devices

It is necessary to compress and reduce the thickness of patient in the

236

field of view in order to minimise the scatter.

A common device is known as the distinctor, or palpation spoon (15 Fig. 6) which enables the radiologist to compress the patient without having to expose his hands to radiation.

Conventional serial changers are fitted with manually operated compressors.

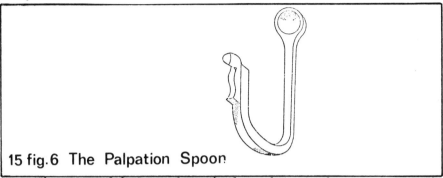

15 fig.6 The Palpation Spoon

These manual devices rely on the doctor being in close proximity to the patient and so are not applicable to remote controlled units. As can be seen in 15 Fig. 5, a motorized compression arm is mounted beneath the tube. This arm stops when contact is made with the patient, after which additional compression can be applied.

15.7 Specialised Tables

Many tables have evolved over the years with varying degrees of success. Some were so specialised that they spent much of their time out of use, whilst others, because they were designed for many techniques, had severe limitations placed on their specialised facility. A unit suitable for conventional fluoroscopy and also specialised techniques is shown in 15 Fig.7. As well as providing all the standard projections this table has facilities for the following additional projections.

Longitudinal oblique projections can be made by angulation of the X-ray beam in the cranio-caudal or caudal-cranial direction. This facility, giving about 30° to either side of centre, is helpful in colon examinations and many types of skeletal work and enables visual separation of overlying structures. Rotation of the beam around the longitudinal axis of the table enables a lateral oblique beam to be passed through a patient, who may be in a supine, lateral or prone position. The patient can be turned about his longitudinal axis in a cradle. This, in combination with all the other movements, makes it a truly comprehensive table.

A pneumatically inflatable compressor diaphragm mounted on the patient side of the serial changer is also included. When deflated, the compressor is not visible in the field.

Chapter 16

Image Intensifier and Television Technique

16.1 Introduction to Image Intensification

From Roentgen's first experiment until about 1950, the only
satisfactory method of viewing the X-ray image was with a fluorescent
screen which emits light when X-ray quanta are absorbed. The intensity
of the light emitted by the fluorescent screen is proportional to the rate
of absorption of the X-ray quanta. The energy is transformed into
heat and light; very little heat but a relatively large amount of light.

To appreciate why it was necessary to depart from this method of
viewing the image, the characteristics of the eye must be understood.
(See 16 Fig. 1).

Two kinds of light sensitive cells are present in the eye, namely
rods and cones. These cells form the layer in the eye called the retina.
The rods are highly sensitive to light, but cannot differentiate colour. The
cones are concentrated in the area of the fovea centralis and these are less
sensitive but able to differentiate colours. The combination of the two
accommodate a brightness range of about 10^9. (A normal camera will
cover a brightness range of 5×10^3).

Since there is an increase in the number of cones at the centre of the
fovea centralis, this is the area of greatest visual acuity, although it is
rod free.

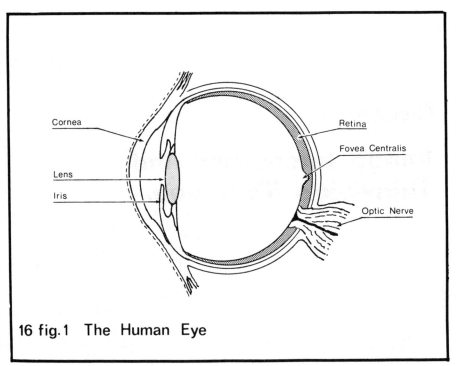

16 fig. 1 The Human Eye

As the level of light is reduced the cones cease to function whereas the sensitivity of the rods increases, giving a gradual improvement in vision due to the ability of the rods to adapt to low levels of illumination.

Since the fovea centralis does not contain rods the area of keenest vision is now just off the centre where the rods are most numerous. The density of the rods is, however, not as great as that of the cones in the fovea centralis, so that the visual acuity is not as great. Vision depends upon cones down to about 0.1 millilamberts (an average daylight scene is about 1 lambert) and below this depends on the rods, although there is no sharp transition.

The amount of light available for X-ray film reading is about 10 millilamberts, which is in the range of cone vision giving extremely good acuity. The amount of light emitted from a fluorescent screen during fluoroscopy is about 0.001 millilamberts which is in the range of rod vision.

In order to increase the amount of light available to the amount required to give cone vision, it is advisable to effect an improvement of about 5000 times. This could be achieved by a 5000 fold increase in radiation, but since this is not acceptable, other means have to be sought to bring about the required increase in light.

Over the years, a number of devices have been proposed having light gains ranging from 10 to 100 times. Although it may seem worthwhile to

240

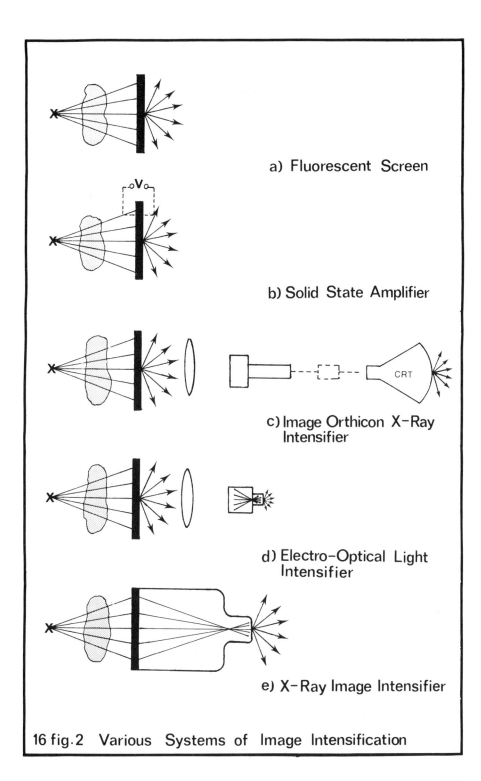

a) Fluorescent Screen

b) Solid State Amplifier

c) Image Orthicon X-Ray Intensifier

d) Electro-Optical Light Intensifier

e) X-Ray Image Intensifier

16 fig. 2 Various Systems of Image Intensification

effect a reduction in dose rate of this order, it is not the principle reason for adopting image intensification. The main reason for using intensification is to raise the light level to a point where cone vision takes over, giving both an increase in visual acuity and contrast perception.

Many ways of increasing the amount of light have been tried (See 16 Fig. 2), but only the X-ray image intensifier system has been widely adopted.

16.2 The Image Intensifier

An X-ray image intensifier consists of an evacuated glass envelope with a fluorescent screen on the inside front surface as shown in 16 Fig. 3. A photo-cathode is deposited on this, using a chemically inert adhesive.

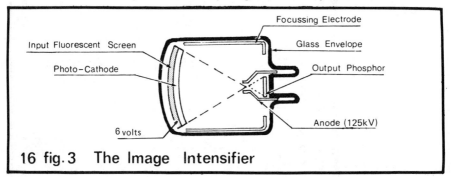

16 fig. 3   The Image   Intensifier

Stokes' law states that a phosphor may be excited by a radiation having an energy equal to, or greater than, the photons to be emitted. In order that the principle of conservation of energy may be preserved, the absorption of one high energy photon of X-radiation must release a larger number of photons of lower energy. For example, with a zinc cadmium sulphide screen, one X-ray photon yields 5000 light photons.

The photocathode is a thin layer of caesium to which a small amount of silver is added. This layer emits electrons under the influence of light, giving off one electron for every five light photons absorbed. In fact the photocathode also gives off electrons under the influence of X-rays, but since the absorption of the photocathode is low, the effect is negligible.

It should be noted that two factors are concerned in the efficiency of the input screen :-

    a) the number of light photons emitted for each X-ray photon absorbed,

    b) the number of X-ray photons absorbed against the number of X-ray photons transmitted,

The first factor mentioned is a function of the composition of the phosphor, whilst the second factor is a function of the density and the thickness of the phosphor.

242

The gain of an intensifier is also dependent on two factors :-

a) the acceleration of the electrons across the gap between cathode and anode,

b) the geometric reduction in image size, which results in a smaller and brighter image on the output phosphor.

The input screen converts the X-rays into visible light which is readily absorbed by the photocathode,which then gives off electrons and these are accelerated by a potential difference of about 25 kV towards the cylindrical anode. The electron pattern is reduced in size and focussed by an electro-static field onto the output screen. This electro-static field is produced by the potential difference between the anode, cathode and the focussing electrode. The output screen then emits light in proportion to the number of electrons absorbed.

Using a linear reduction of about 10 times (ratio of input to output screen diameters), the area within which the electron energy is concentrated is reduced by a factor of 10^2 . Thus the luminous flux is emitted from an area about 100 times smaller than it would be with a reproduction scale of 1:1. An increase in luminance by a factor of 100 due to the electro-optical reduction is therefore achieved.

It may be felt that the gain in light due to the minification is not a true gain and so should be disregarded. This is in fact not the case where electron-optics are concerned, as can be seen from 16 Fig. 4.

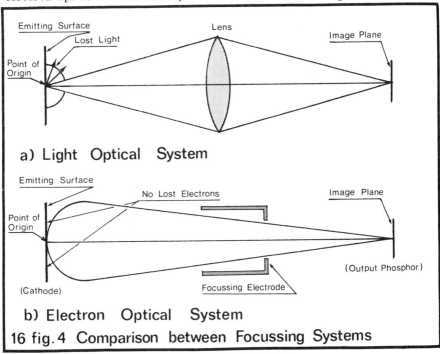

a) Light Optical System

b) Electron Optical System

16 fig. 4 Comparison between Focussing Systems

In the case of the lens system, only those rays of light from the point of origin which travel at the correct angle are refracted by the lens to come to focus on the output screen. However with the electron-optical system, all electrons, including those travelling almost parallel with the photocathode, will be turned to focus on the output screen.

16.3 Conversion Factor (or Gain)

It is essential to have a measure of the efficiency of an intensifier and until recently a figure of gain or amplification was often quoted.

The gain of an image intensifier is expressed as the ratio of illumination from a standard Levy West fluorescent screen to the illumination from the output phosphor of an intensifier when both are irradiated under identical conditions. This is a very difficult measurement to undertake because the quality of the incident radiation is, in part, dependent on the waveform of the X-ray generator and will influence the result. Also the low level of illumination raises further problems.

The International Committee on Radiological Units has now recommended that the conversion factor would be a more realistic measure of intensifier efficiency. The conversion factor is expressed as the ratio of luminance of the output phosphor to the dose rate at the input phosphor.

$$\text{Conversion Factor} = \frac{L}{R}$$

where L is light output in Candela per square metre (cd/m^2)

R is radiation at input screen (mR/sec.)

A comparison between the two methods of measurement is possible since a gain of 5000 times approximates to a conversion factor of 70.

16.4 Information Content

The resolution in the centre of a modern 23 cm (9") image intensifier is better than 20 line-pairs per cm. (Each line-pair is one black and one white bar spaced by their own width). If there is provision for enlarging the image to cover a 12 cm (5") field, the central resolution will have increased to about 28 line-pairs per cm.

It must be noted that when the 12 cm field of a dual field intensifier is in use, the image forming area of the input phosphor is reduced to about ¼ that of the 23 cm field. Thus a corresponding increase in dose rate is required to produce the same number of electrons per unit area at the output phosphor. It is usual to increase the X-ray tube voltage by about 15 kV when using the 12 cm field to compensate for this loss of gain (decrease in conversion factor).

It is possible to see variations in contrast of about 4% with a typical intensifier, providing an adequate dose rate is used to produce enough X-ray quanta per unit area on the input screen.

If the dose rate reaching the input phosphor of the image intensifier is too low, there is insufficient quanta per unit area to visualise all the information. In order to obtain a relatively "grain free" image, a minimum dose rate of about 50 μR per second at the input phosphor is required.

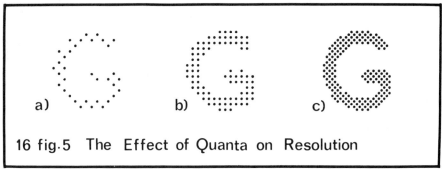

16 fig. 5   The   Effect of Quanta on Resolution

As the number of X-ray photons falls, the effect of each one becomes more noticeable.

An example of this is shown in 16 Fig. 5 where (a) shows a small number dots representing the image produced with a low dose rate on a intensifier. Figs. (b) and (c) show the improvement in detail by increasing the dose rate (increase in the number of dots per unit area).

16.5   Viewing Systems

The output phosphor can be directly viewed, but is too small to be conveniently observed in this way. If viewed via a single lens (magnifying glass), then providing that the diameter of the lens is greater than the diameter of the pupil of the eye, there will be no detectable loss in brightness even though the lens enlarges the image up to the apparent diameter of the input screen. The image so viewed is called the aerial image (16 Fig. 6a). If however a second screen is introduced and a real sized image projected onto this then the advantage of the small bright image will be lost.

This is shown in 16 Fig. 6b where it can be seen that the translucent screen once again diffuses the incident light to cover all angles so the eye is able to make use of only a small fraction of the light from each point.

There are clear advantages in viewing the aerial image. The disadvantage is that the exit beam is about the same diameter as the lens and in order to see the output phosphor the eye must remain within the beam. For economic reasons it is necessary to use a comparatively small lens, which then causes difficulty in viewing. For binocular viewing, the exit beam needs to be large enough to cover both eyes simultaneously which involves the use of a lens of about $2\frac{1}{2}$" in diameter. As those who are interested in photography will appreciate, a fully corrected lens having a diameter of 2½" is very expensive.

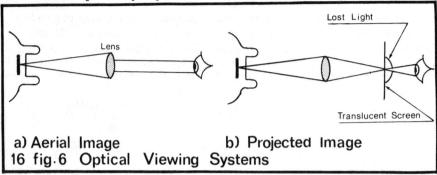

a) Aerial Image   b) Projected Image
16 fig.6 Optical Viewing Systems

There are a few people who still use an optical viewer although nowadays television is more or less universal. However, the large diameter lens is still retained but for a different reason. If the intensifier is to be used only for television,then in theory, a single lens system as shown in 16 Fig. 7 is sufficient. The diameters of the intensifier output phosphor and the standard camera tube are the same. For an image size equal to that of the object size, the nodal point (centre) of the lens is 2 times the focal length of the lens from the focal plane. Also the distance from lens to object must be the same as the distance from lens to the plane of focus. However, under these conditions problems may be encountered if the lens is not designed for this short distance.

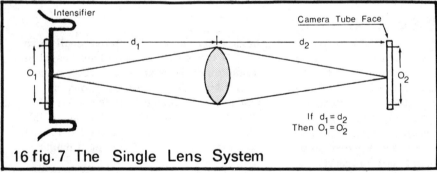

16 fig. 7 The Single Lens System

Under close-up conditions such as these, the normal method of calculating lens efficiency ('f' number) does not apply. For a 1:1 ratio the 'f' number must be multiplied by 2 (thus an f8 lens is equivalent to f16) so that the amount of light is now $\div$ 4. In addition to this, at short distances the depth of focus is very small, so that unless the lens is rigidly mounted, variations in the defintion of the picture will occur. This is due to slight changes in the position of either phosphor, lens or camera tube.

Where the output from the intensifier is required to supply a number of different optical devices some other method must be used. The Tandem lens system,shown in 16 Fig. 8,is the one generally adopted.

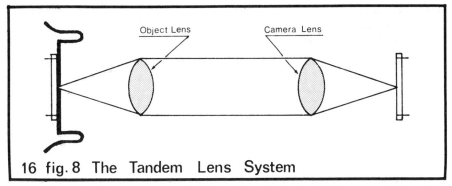

16 fig. 8 The Tandem Lens System

Here two lenses are used. The object lens is rigidly mounted on the intensifier and is adjusted to bring the image of the output phosphor to focus at infinity. The light output from this lens is therefore a parallel beam of light. The camera lens is adjusted to bring to focus an object at infinity (that is, it will focus a parallel beam of light).

The size of the image will be determined by the relative focal lengths of the two lenses –

$$\frac{\text{output phosphor diameter}}{\text{object lens focal length}} = \frac{\text{image diameter}}{\text{camera lens focal length}}$$

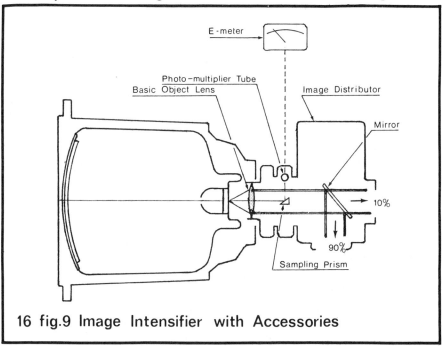

16 fig.9 Image Intensifier with Accessories

The camera lens is rigidly mounted on the camera and the focus set to infinity. Where the two lens systems are mounted as shown in

247

16 Fig. 8, the focus is independent of distance between the lenses, although too great a distance will produce vignetting (the image will be brighter at the centre than at the edge).

Since there is now considerable flexibility in the relative positions of the two lenses, it is a simple matter to exchange cameras, etc. The operation of the equipment can be further simplified by inserting a surface silvered mirror into the light beam (16 Fig. 9) so that by rotating the mirror the light beam may be directed into the appropriate lens. A specially made mirror having a very thin coating may be used so that only 90% of the light is reflected. The other 10% of the light passes through the mirror so that two devices may be used simultaneously (TV and Cine).

16.6 Television

Television is the transmission and reception of moving pictures over a distance. The use of television in X-ray diagnosis overcomes several of the limitations of the previously discussed systems, namely :-

(a) Since a number of moveable monitors can be used to display the image, the operator's freedom of movement and angle of viewing is not limited as it was with the optical viewer.

(b) Any X-ray image is essentially of low contrast, (in fact X-ray films compensate for this by an inherent contrast increase of about 1.5 times), but with T.V. systems the operator has control of image contrast and brightness, allowing daylight viewing.

A simplified block diagram of the closed circuit T.V. system used in medical diagnosis is shown in 16 Fig. 10. The following sections will discuss each part in detail.

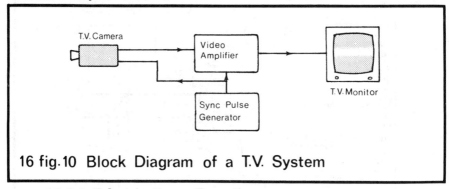

16 fig. 10 Block Diagram of a T.V. System

16.6.1 Television Image Formation

Like the cinema, television makes use of the persistence of vision: if the information can be assembled sufficiently rapidly on the screen, the viewer will see a complete picture. The picture is formed by moving a spot of light over the screen area in a regular system of lines (called scanning) and by increasing or reducing the spot intensity to make light

248

and dark areas (See 16 Fig. 11). The picture is scanned by starting the spot at point 'A', moving it to 'B' by electromagnetic deflection (see section 7.8), then returning it instantly to 'C'. From there it is moved to 'D' and the process repeated until point 'X' is reached; from there it is quickly returned to 'A' to begin the cycle again. This system of lines is called the raster or frame.

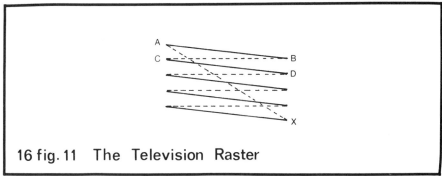

16 fig. 11   The Television Raster

Most television systems in Europe use 625 lines per frame to give good vertical resolution and require 50 images per second to give a flicker-free picture. For the picture to have sufficient horizontal resolution, each line must contain about 300 pieces of information and this represents a frequency of over 10 million cycles per second (10 MHz). Since a frequency of this order is difficult to process, a system known as double

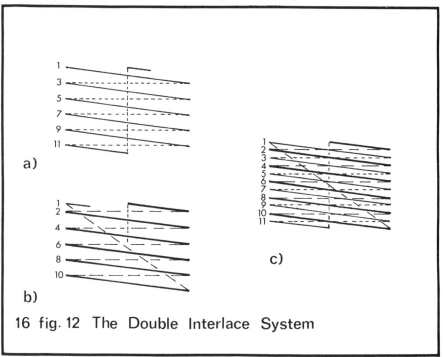

16 fig. 12   The Double Interlace System

interlace is employed to give the same resolution, but using only half the frequency.

In this system, the first vertical scan only covers the "odd" lines (see 16 Fig. 12a). The next time, only the "even" lines are scanned (see 16 Fig. 12b). A complete picture scan is termed a frame and consists of 2 fields as shown in 16 Fig. 12c. Thus there are 50 fields (images) each of $312\frac{1}{2}$ lines.

In order to obtain the full benefit of the double interlace system it is obvious that the lines must be equally spaced. To achieve this, the monitor uses time base circuits (described in section 7.19.2) which are controlled by synchronising pulses incorporated in the complete television signal from the video amplifier.

16.6.2 The T.V. Camera

The T.V. camera converts the optical image appearing at the output phosphor of the image intensifier into a series of electrical signals. Inside the camera housing there is a set of deflection coils (explained in section 7.8), a camera tube and a video pre-amplifier.

Several different types of camera tubes are available, the most common of which is the "vidicon" tube shown schematically in 16 Fig. 13. It may be assumed to consist of three sections; the electron gun, the scanning section and the target.

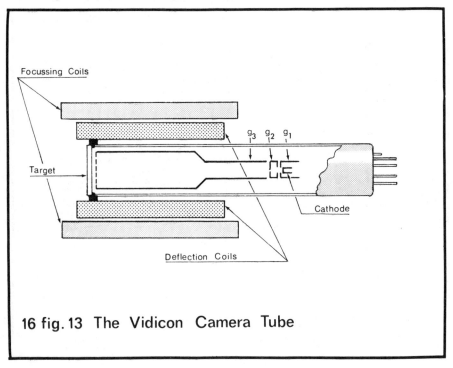

16 fig. 13 The Vidicon Camera Tube

The electron gun consists of a heated cathode which emits electrons, a grid (g_1) controlling the electron beam current, and a second grid (g_2) which accelerates the electrons and focusses them into a fine beam.

The electron beam released by the second grid enters the space enclosed by the cylindrical electrode (g_3). This is the scanning section where, by means of the adjustable electrostatic field of g_3 and the axial electro-magnetic field of an external coil, the electrons are focussed onto the target.

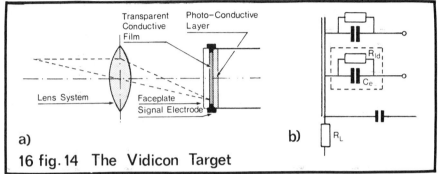

a)   b)

16 fig. 14   The Vidicon Target

The target section is illustrated in 16 Fig. 14a where it can be seen that a conductive transparent layer is laid down on the glass faceplate upon which is formed a layer of photo-conductive material. The optical image to be televised is focussed onto the conductive film by means of a lens system. The target can be considered to consist of a very large number of "target elements" (see 16 Fig. 14b), each element acting as a small capacitor (C_e), with one end connected to the signal electrode and in parallel with a light dependent resistor (R_{ld}). If the electron beam is now made to scan the face of the target in exactly the same way as described for the monitor, each capacitor will be charged to nearly the same potential, provided the faceplate is not illuminated. The photo-conductive material is a fairly good insulator so that only a very small part of this charge will leak away between scans. This means that very little beam current will flow and there will be hardly any voltage drop across the load resistor R_L. (The small current which does flow is called "dark current"). If however an optical image is focussed on the faceplate, those target elements that are illuminated will become more conductive and the capacitors concerned will be partially discharged to an amount proportional to the illumination. As a consequence the electron beam, while scanning the charge pattern, will re-charge depleted elements to their original state. This current also flows through R_L and produces a varying voltage drop across it. The voltage, negative going for highlights, is the video signal and is fed to the pre-amplifier stage. An example of the type of voltage waveform produced during this process is shown for one line in 16 Fig. 15.

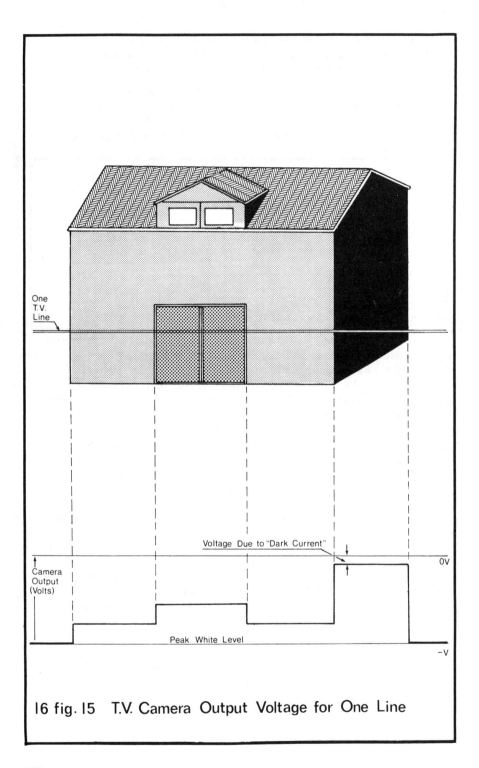

One
T.V.
Line

Voltage Due to "Dark Current"

0V

Camera
Output
(Volts)

Peak White Level

−V

16 fig. 15   T.V. Camera Output Voltage for One Line

Another type of camera tube now available is known as the "Plumbicon". The construction of this device is very similar to a vidicon, except for the target which is shown schematically in 16 Fig. 16.

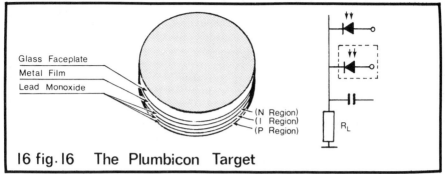

Glass Faceplate
Metal Film
Lead Monoxide

(N Region)
(I Region)
(P Region)

R_L

16 fig. 16   The Plumbicon Target

The target structure can be considered as being formed of a large number of tiny photo-diodes, reverse biased by the electron beam. Incident light focussed onto the face of the plumbicon falls on the junction of these diodes and generates current carriers. This means that when the electron beam scans the target, current will flow through those diodes whose junctions are illuminated and in doing so will also pass through the load resistor R_L. The voltage drop thus produced across R_L will be proportional to the illumination of the diode being scanned.

The main advantages of the Plumbicon are :-

(a) As the diodes are reverse biased, virtually no "dark current" will flow. This is important because the "dark current" is not constant across the face of the tube and is temperature dependent.

(b) The Plumbicon has a much faster response (shorter lag) than the vidicon, since the photo-diodes react more quickly than the light dependent resistors of the vidicon.

The Plumbicon can thus be used to advantage to televise fast moving phenomena.

16.6.3 The Synchronising Pulse Generator

Having seen how the picture is traced out line by line and frame by frame in both the T.V. monitor and camera, it is fairly obvious that the electron beam in the monitor must move in exact synchronism with the beam in the camera. Not only must the beams move at exactly the same speed, but in addition, they must always be at the same relative positions in their scan. This result is achieved by sending suitable synchronising pulses (sync pulses) to the T.V. camera and combining the same pulses into the complete television signal leaving the video amplifier. At the monitor, the sync pulses are separated from the picture signal, and are used to control the time base circuits.

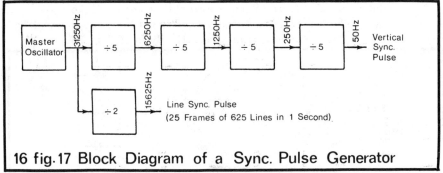

16 fig. 17 Block Diagram of a Sync. Pulse Generator

The sync pulse generator is shown in block diagram form in 16 Fig. 17. The master oscillator runs at a very accurate fixed frequency which is fed to two sets of electronic frequency dividers. The upper divider chain counts the number of lines for each field and generates a vertical sync pulse (50 Hz) whilst the lower divider generates the line sync pulse (15625 Hz). 625 lines were chosen because it is easy to make an electronic divider for this number.

16.6.4 The Video Amplifier

The video amplifier is used to amplify the small voltage variations from the camera to a suitable level to drive the monitor. At the same time as amplifying the camera signal, it must also mix in the sync pulses to form the complete television signal which is fed to the monitor via a single co-axial cable.

The main point to be remembered about this circuit is that compared with say, an audio amplifier which may have a frequency range (bandwidth) of 50 Hz to 18 KHz, the video amplifier must be capable of handling frequencies from 0 Hz (D.C.) up to 5 MHz without distortion. Also, any spurious signals must be eliminated to avoid degradation of the T.V. image.

16.7 Automatic Gain Control (A.G.C.) Circuits

During T.V. fluoroscopy, the amount of radiation absorbed by a subject will vary over wide limits, so that unless an automatic system of control is used, the setting of kV and mA will have to be continually varied in order to bring the video output voltage to the desired value.

Because of this, the earliest types of X-ray television used a system of automatic gain control. The system worked by measuring the amplitude of the output signal from the camera and comparing the result against a reference voltage. This generated a control voltage which altered the gain of the video amplifier and so maintained the brightest part of the picture at 1.4V, this being the voltage selected as an international standard.

Although the system can be made to work very satisfactorily it must be remembered that it can only operate by reducing the gain. The dose rate must be set to give an input to the face of the intensifier which is sufficient to produce an acceptable picture of the thickest part of the patient. When a less dense area is under examination, the gain of the video amplifier will be reduced, so that an acceptable picture will still be obtained, but still at the original dose rate.

A better system maintains a constant gain but automatically varies the kV, mA or both to give sufficient dose rate to produce an acceptable picture.

16.8 Automatic Dose Rate Control

The first development in dose rate control took the form of an add-on unit which used a small mirror to direct a percentage of the light out of the intensifier into a photomultiplier tube (see 16 Fig. 9). This in turn controlled the X-ray tube filament current, and so stabilised the brightness of the image on the intensifier output phosphor. The same photomultiplier tube is often switched between the brightness stabiliser circuit and a phototimer. The same tube can thus be used to control radiographic exposure times as well.

The main disadvantage of this system is that it is area sensitive. If the collimating diaphragm is set to give a square and the dose rate noted and then the diaphragm closed to reduce the irradiated area by half, then the dose rate will approximately double. The problem may be overcome by using some system which detects the level of the brightest part of the picture rather than the average brightness, but to do this one would have to scan the picture in some way. Since the television camera does just this, a peak level sensing circuit can be built in to the television unit. There will still be some increase in dose rate when the irradiated area is reduced, but this is due mainly to the reduction of scatter.

To be effective, the automatic dose rate control circuit must operate on only a small area, so that under normal conditions it is not area sensitive. This in turn can produce problems if, for example, one is examining the stomach in the lateral position where the area of interest is close to the surface of body. The area of peak white due to direct radiation falling on the input screen may easily be 100 times brighter than the average brightness. This can be minimized by arranging that the sensing circuit looks at an area less than the whole picture area. This causes problems if the entire sensing area is covered by a bolus of contrast medium.

These difficulties are best resolved by having a switch which permits selection of the most appropriate area for the examination. This is normally preset to operate on, for example, 40% and 80% of the screen area.

Advances in the field of semiconductors have given improved signal to noise ratios, increased bandwidths, and reduction in the number of breakdowns. Camera tubes have undergone similar improvements to give greater output, shorter lag, more even sensitivity across the face of the target and a lower "spot count" (blemishes on the target).

One would expect there to have been a similar improvement in the gain of intensifiers, but although intensifiers have indeed improved in a number of ways there has not been any significant reduction in the dose rate required for the following reason. As has already been stated, the X-ray input to the intensifier consists of a relatively small number of high energy X-ray photons which strike the input phosphor to produce a larger number of lower energy light photons. A reduction in dose rate causes a fall in the number of X-ray photons striking the input phosphor per unit time. An increase in the intensifier gain raises the number of light photons produced by each X-ray photon, but cannot make up for a shortage of X-ray photons which are the only information carriers. Thus a low dose rate gives rise to a granular image due to what is called quanta noise.

Particularly where only television is in use, the noise is often blamed on the T.V. system itself, although exactly the same effect can be demonstrated on cine and photofluorographic films. The only way in which this noise may be reduced is by increasing the number of X-ray quanta available, in other words, increasing the dose rate.

The combination of a high gain intensifier and camera tube produces sufficient light to operate the T.V. system, but the dose rate is too low to give an image with an acceptable amount of quantum noise. The solution is to stop down the lens which allows the dose rate to be set to an acceptable level. This also improves the performance of the lens system, giving an overall increase in picture quality.

An alternative approach is to use a different type of material for the input phosphor of the image intensifier. A new type of phosphor (caesium iodide) is now available which has a greater absorption thus converting a greater proportion of the input dose rate into light. This also makes possible the use of a thinner phosphor layer which, by reducing the lateral spread of light, gives improved resolution.

16.9 Kinescopy

When X-ray television first became available it was obvious that it would be advantageous to be able to record the T.V. monitor image on film. Even the introduction of the video recorder has not totally replaced this method of recording, since video tape cannot easily be edited or spliced.

When a cine film is recorded from a T.V. monitor the procedure is known as Kinescopy.

A study of the make-up of the T.V. image has revealed that it is composed of a spot of light tracing $312\frac{1}{2}$ evenly spaced lines across the monitor screen in $\frac{1}{50}$ of a second. The spot then returns to the top of the monitor and repeats the operation, the second set of scanning lines being interlaced with the first. This makes one 625 line interlaced picture in $\frac{1}{25}$ of a second.

The cine camera shutter should be opened when the spot is at the top of the monitor (start of the picture field) and closed when the spot is at the bottom of the monitor (end of the picture field). Since the television image frequency is synchronous with the mains cycle, the camera shutter must be driven by a special motor. This is a synchronous motor which may be locked to a certain part of the mains cycle, thus keeping the T.V. image and camera shutter in phase. A table to indicate the shutter openings and frame speed combinations which can be used for Kinescopy is shown below.

Frames per Second	Shutter Opening Angle	Information Recorded per Cine Frame	Information Lost per Pull Down
$12\frac{1}{2}$	180°	2 Monitor Fields	2 Monitor Fields
$8\frac{1}{3}$	180°	3 Monitor Fields	3 Monitor Fields
$6\frac{1}{4}$	180°	4 Monitor Fields	4 Monitor Fields
$16\frac{2}{3}$	240°	2 Monitor Fields	1 Monitor Field
$8\frac{1}{3}$	240°	4 Monitor Fields	2 Monitor Fields
25	180°	1 Monitor Field	1 Monitor Field

The most satisfactory system for medical use has proved to be a shutter opening of 240° and a speed of $16\frac{2}{3}$ frames per second. Using this system, the shutter is closed and the film moved through the camera gate during a T.V. field ($\frac{1}{50}$ second). The film is then held stationary and the shutter opened for 2 T.V. fields ($\frac{1}{25}$ second) whilst the image is recorded. It can be seen that there is a loss of $\frac{1}{3}$ of the information during the film pull down time. (Shutter opening angle is discussed in section 16.11).

The dose rate at the face of the image intensifier during fluoroscopy is normally about 50 μR per second and as Kinescopy is recorded at these factors it can be seen that the amount of radiation for each cine frame is only about $\frac{50}{25}\mu$R/frame = 2 μR per frame.

When the film is being projected the eye integrates the individual frames, and the grain caused by the X-ray quanta, into one continuous moving image. However, if the film is analysed frame by frame there is then insufficient quanta per unit area in $\frac{1}{25}$ of a second to convey all the available information and the result is a grainy low resolution image. This can be rectified by increasing the fluoroscopic current during recording and a factor of 1.5 or 2 gives a noticeable increase in picture quality.

In finite terms it is possible to resolve about 20 line-pairs per cm. in the centre of the field of a 9″ image intensifier, but when this has been passed through the optical and video system less than 10 line-pairs per cm. can be seen on the film. This determines smallest detail which can be isolated by its own diameter from surrounding objects but it does not tell us much about the diagnostic quality of the image which is dependent upon blackening (gamma) and contrast (grey scale). These two factors can be adjusted by means of the brilliance and contrast controls on the T.V. monitor built into the kinescope. The success of this system is dependent upon the ability of the equipment to provide adjustment to both gamma and grey scale and the ease with which they can be matched to the characteristics of the recording film.

Kinescopy thus provides a method of recording with the advantage of low dose rate, but with the disadvantage of some loss of information.

16.10 Video Tape Recording

The basic principles of magnetic tape recording are not difficult to understand. A plastic tape coated or impregnated with a ferrous oxide is passed in front of a small electromagnet (the recording head). The coil of the recording head is fed by the input signal and as the tape passes across the gap in the head the oxide coating becomes magnetised in proportion to the strength and frequency of the signal (see 16 Fig. 18).

Playback is achieved by passing the tape in front of a similar coil (replay head) and the variable magnetic flux from the tape induces a signal, similar to the original, in the replay head winding. The range of frequencies which can be recorded is dependent on the speed of the tape and the width of the gap across which the magnetic flux is developed.

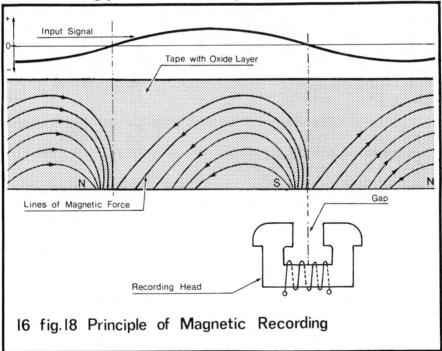

16 fig. 18 Principle of Magnetic Recording

A modern domestic audio tape recorder with a tape speed of 19 cms/ sec. ($7\frac{1}{2}$ins. per sec.) will record frequencies up to 15 KHz. The range of the recorded frequencies is termed the bandwidth of the instrument.

To record a video signal of reasonable quality, a bandwidth of at least 3 MHz is required. This frequency range is 200 times that of the audio recorder and requires a tape speed across the head in excess of 96 km/h (60 m.p.h.) assuming that a simple recording head is used. The mechanical problem of this high tape speed is overcome by passing the tape in a helical configuration around a drum inside which the recording head or heads rotate at 3000 r.p.m. as shown in 16 Fig. 19. Consequently the actual tape speed can now be reduced to 19 cms/sec. since the recording head is made to rotate in the opposite direction to tape movement, giving the same relative tape to head speed. It is normal practice to use the same heads for recording and playback. Several geometrical arrangements are available for forming the helix around the drum, the most popular being the Ω and α wrap format. The drum is 15.25 cm (6") in diameter and the tape starts at the top and comes off at the bottom, passing round the drum in a helix of almost one loop. There is a slit all the way round the circumference of the drum through which the head protrudes to wipe the tape. If the head is rotated at 3000 r.p.m. then the peripheral speed of the head is π15.25 x 3000 which is approximately 85 km/h (53 m.p.h). Added to this there is the linear tape speed of approximately 1 km/h.

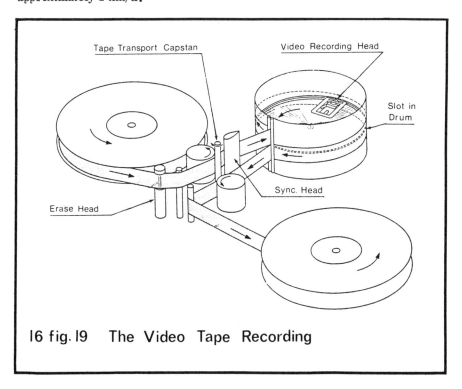

Tape Transport Capstan

Video Recording Head

Slot in Drum

Sync. Head

Erase Head

16 fig. 19   The Video Tape Recording

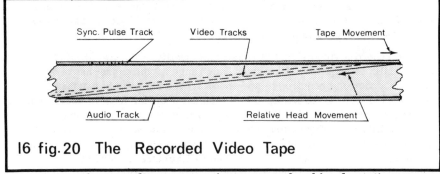

Sync. Pulse Track   Video Tracks   Tape Movement

Audio Track   Relative Head Movement

16 fig. 20   The   Recorded   Video   Tape

During the recording process the tape speed and head rotation are synchronised to the mains frequency. The vertical synchronising pulses are recorded separately on the tape to mark the start of each T.V. field (see 16 Fig. 20). During replay these pulses are compared with the mains frequency and any difference signal converted into a control voltage used to keep the speed and angular rotation of the head such that the start of each T.V. field coincides with the start of a recorded magnetic track.

It is not always possible to replay a video tape on a machine other than the one on which it was recorded because the drum diameter determines the length of the magnetic track. If compatability is required, the drum has to be manufactured to very close tolerances. The geometry of a helix of tape around a 15.25 cm drum records a 45 cm magnetic track at an angle of approximately 10° for each head revolution. As the tape moves forward at about 19 cm/s, a series of parallel diagonal magnetic tracks are recorded very close together. Each sloping magnetic track on the tape contains all the information for one T.V. field (2 interlaced fields are required for one complete frame).

Stationary images are obtained by stopping the tape and allowing the head to continue to revolve, playing back only one magnetic track continuously. With a single head recorder only half the picture (312½ lines) is played back, and a considerable amount of information is lost. A slight amount of information is also lost at the top and bottom of the field because the tape is now stationary and the path of the head and the recorded magnetic track do not have the same geometry.

X-ray television installations require the video recorder to be connected in the monitor circuit such that it is available for immediate use during the examination. The video signal to the recorder is fed by a matched co-axial cable, thus the recorder can be located at any reasonable distance from the examination room, provided remote switching facilities are available. Several monitors can be used with a recorder or T.V. installation and may be located at any convenient point in the hospital. A simultaneous sound track can be recorded on the edge of the tape for commentary.

If the tape is kept clean, it can be passed across the head about 200 times but just a small amount of dust or dirt will reduce this very drastically and also degrade the quality of the picture.

The signal on the tape is in the form of a variable magnetic flux and, if the tape is stored too long without being replayed, an increase in signal to noise ratio is noticeable due to the "print through" from one track to another. It is recommended that the tape should be rewound backwards and forwards on the fast rewind position of the recorder every six months to reduce this degradation.

16.11 Cinefluorography

In its simplest form cinefluorography consists of filming the images on the output phosphor of the image intensifier.

Cinefluorography has many useful applications where dynamic studies of physiological phenomena are undertaken. Events may be speeded up or slowed down by varying the speed of the camera or projector. Film loops may be made to study repetitively a single event. Editing and splicing can easily be undertaken for teaching or storage purposes. Conventional photographic optical systems are unsuitable for filming from the image intensifier where the object to image ratio is in the region of 1:1 or less (see section 16.5).

This problem was solved with the early intensifiers by using two ordinary photographic lens systems in tandem so that the image produced at infinity by one is focussed by the other onto the film (see 16 Fig. 8).

This system uses each lens in a manner best suited to its optical design; the optical efficiency, is twice that of a single optical system forming an image in the ratio of 1:1. Modern image intensifier installations already have part of this tandem lens system in the form of the basic objective (See 16 Fig. 9) so that it is only necessary for the cine camera to be mounted in a manner which accurately aligns the two optical axes.

The focal length of the camera lens can then be chosen to produce the required image size and the focussing mechanism adjusted to infinity to produce a sharp image. This point was discussed in section 16.5 and the method of calculation follows:-

To calculate final image size

Let D_1 = diameter of image on output phosphor of intensifier
D_2 = diameter of final image on film
F_1 = focal length of basic objective
F_2 = focal length of camera lens

then

$$D_2 = D_1 \times \frac{F_2}{F_1}$$

Example for 16 mm cine camera

D_1 = 20 mm
F_1 = 65 mm
F_2 = 25 mm
D_2 = 20 x $\frac{25}{65}$ = 7.6 mm (diameter of image on film)

Example for 70 mm camera

D_1 = 20 mm
F_1 = 65 mm
F_2 = 220 mm
D_2 = 20 x $\frac{220}{65}$ = 68 mm (diameter of image on film)

Example to find lens focal length for a 70 mm camera

D_1 = 20 mm
D_2 = 70 mm
F_1 = 65 mm
$F_2 = \frac{F_1 \times D_2}{D_1} = \frac{65 \times 70}{20} = \frac{4550}{20} = 227.5$ mm

Cameras used for cinefluorography have an intermittent film movement, the film being stationary while the shutter is open and pulled down through the gate while the shutter is closed. It is usual to locate the film in register with a pin through the perforations while the shutter is open, so that it cannot move causing the image to be blurred.

The shutter is in the form of a rotating disc with a segment removed, and is situated between the lens and the film as shown in 16 Fig. 21.

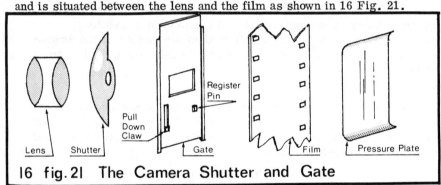

Lens   Shutter   Pull Down Claw   Gate   Register Pin   Film   Pressure Plate

16 fig. 21   The Camera Shutter and Gate

If, in a complete cycle, film pulldown and exposure occupies 360° and the shutter is open for 50% of the cycle, the camera is then said to have a 180° shutter. Likewise if the shutter is only open for 25% of the cycle the camera is said to have a 90° shutter.

It can be seen that if a camera has a 180° shutter, rotating at 25 revolutions per second, the exposure time will be $\frac{1}{50}$ sec. (or 0.02 sec). If the radiation is continuous with an X-ray tube current of 20 mA, then the mAs per frame = 0.02 x 20 = 0.4 mAs. Only 50% of the patient dose contributes to the film blackening; the other 50% is wasted because the shutter is closed.

A disadvantage of this system is that the exposure time is determined by the camera speed and if it is required to analyse the frames individually there is often movement blurring, unless the camera is run at a high speed.

If the radiographic factors and camera film speed are constant,the film blackening will vary considerably due to variations in patient density and the amount of opaque medium used in the investigation. A small proportion of the light from the centre of the image on the output phosphor of the intensifier is therefore monitored by a photo-multiplier with a prism optical system (16 Fig. 9). The result is displayed on an exposure meter (E-meter) so that the X-ray tube current can be varied to keep the meter reading constant and hence the film correctly exposed. The signal from the photo-multiplier may also be amplified and used to vary the X-ray tube current so that the film blackening is automatically kept constant. The sensitivity of the exposure meter can be varied to suit different film speeds.

16.12 Pulsed Cinefluorography

A considerable increase in efficiency, image quality and reduction in patient dose can be obtained by synchronising the X-ray exposure with the camera shutter such that there is no radiation when the film is being pulled through the gate. If the X-ray exposures are pulsed for each frame and are relatively short, (between 1 - 10 ms.), each frame will have less movement blurring and will be suitable for individual analysis.

The mAs per frame is calculated by multiplying the pulse width by the tube current. For example, if the tube current is 120 mA and the pulse width 3 ms., then mAs per frame = 0.003 x 120 = 0.36 mAs.

Automatic control of density is again achieved by diverting a small proportion of the light from the centre of the field to a photo-multiplier, and the amplitude of the pulses integrated to give a meter reading proportional to film density. The signal from the integrator can also be amplified and used to control the X-ray tube current and thus the film blackening.

The pulse width must be shorter than the shutter-open time and thus the exposure time per frame is independent of camera speed. Various pulse widths may be selected to provide minimum film blurring, consistent with X-ray tube loading and film blackening.

16.13 Bi-plane Cinefluorography

It is advantageous in cardiac procedures for cine films to be taken in bi-plane so that lateral and AP (antero-posterior) views can be recorded at the same time.

In order to obtain satisfactory results in bi-plane operation, it is necessary for the cameras to be accurately phased such that the film is passed through the gate in one plane, while the exposure takes place in the other plane. If the two exposures are allowed to take place simultaneously, or overlapping one another, the cross scatter between the two channels will cause a noticeable loss of image quality and contrast (see section 14.9).

The need for more diagnostic information has produced a demand for higher camera frame speeds. It is possible to achieve up to 150 f.p.s. with 35 mm cameras, but 16 mm cameras are used for speeds above this due to mechanical and power considerations. The maximum speed currently in use is 200 f.p.s.

16.14 Cine Film Marking

It is possible to mark the cine film to coincide with the start of an event such as the injection of contrast medium or the R-wave of an E.C.G. Such a device is called an event marker and would consist of a small light emitter in the film gate. A more complex system,using computer principles,is available which records two physiological traces on the edge of the film (see 16 Fig. 22).

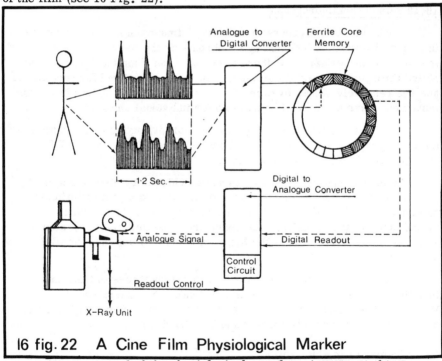

16 fig. 22   A Cine Film Physiological Marker

About a second of the physiological waveform is converted to a computer type signal consisting of 300 pieces of information. This is then stored in a ferrite core memory bank until it is required.

The contacts on the camera which initiate the X-ray pulse circuits also produce the signal to command the stored data readout. This data is fed to a small oscilloscope mounted on the side of the camera and focussed via a lens system onto the edge of the film.

The stored signal is renewed 300 times per second so even at the highest frame speeds, the patient's data recorded on film is always the latest information available.

16.15 Spot Film Fluorography

As we have seen, the image recorded on 16 mm or 35 mm film is best suited to dynamic examinations because individual cine frames do not record all the information available on the image intensifier output phosphor. In order that the high definition image on the output phosphor can be adequately recorded, a larger film format was necessary. Therefore, systems have been developed utilising 70 mm or 100 mm miniature film.

70 mm cameras are capable of operating up to 6 frames per second, and have a magazine which will hold up to 45 metres of polyester based film (approximately 600 shots). The camera operates without a conventional shutter, film exposure being controlled by the length of time X-rays are emitted from the tube. A mirror in the image distributor turns during the X-ray set preparation time to reflect the radiographic image onto the film. After exposure, the mirror is returned and light cannot therefore enter the spot film camera during fluoroscopy.

For consistent results a photo-timer is necessary, the exposure being about $\frac{1}{4}$ to $\frac{1}{6}$ of that required for a full size radiograph. Provision can also be made to record patient data in the space between frames.

Films are available for normal or rapid processing. It is usual to attach a large film as a leader to one end of the 70 mm film to feed it through the automatic processor.

100 mm cameras are now available but the maximum repetition frequency is 2 f.p.s. and there is a proportional increase in dose.

The magazines are loaded with cut film and although the storage and take-up cassettes are generally easier to load and unload, processing can be difficult unless specialised equipment is installed.

16.16 Films for X-ray Cinefluorography

The spectral response of the image intensifier output phosphor has a peak in the green region at about 5400Å and it is necessary to ascertain that any film used for recording this image also has a high sensitivity in this region.

Many manufacturers market film stock with a spectral sensitivity which matches this colour. The graph 16 Fig. 23 depicts the sensitivity of a film, used for cinefluorography, compared with the response of the intensifier output phosphor.

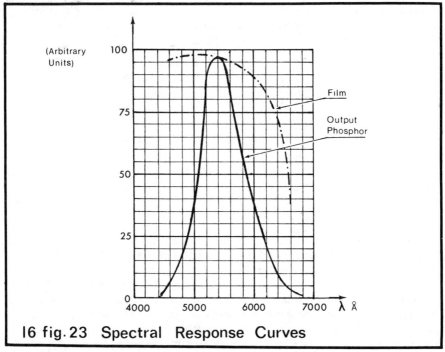

l6 fig. 23 Spectral Response Curves

It should be noted that the ASA or DIN standard ratings given to films by manufacturers refer to a polychromatic light source which includes all the colours found in daylight. As the response of the intensifier output phosphor is monochromatic, or mainly one colour, these ratings are not always an indication of relative film speed when used for cinefluorography. The only certain method of checking the compatability of a film for cinefluorography is to make a test run, process the film in the usual manner and then examine quality and blackening against an image of known quality.

16.17 Magnification Techniques

It is very difficult to record and visualise all the information from the image intensifier due to the limiting resolution of the lens, film, developer combinations which are available and the losses in the projection system.

The information obtained during analysis of films taken during cardiac investigations is often limited by the detail in the recorded image. This can be improved by enlarging or magnifying the image before it reaches the film.

The most satisfactory method of achieving this is by electron-optical enlargement within the construction of the intensifier. The inclusion

266

of a second anode at a potential of 17 kV, while keeping the first anode at 25 kV, still gives a 9" coverage. If the second anode is also connected to a potential of 25 kV, this alters the divergence of the electron beam within the glass envelope, and enables a 5" diameter circle in the centre of the 9" input phosphor to be enlarged to cover the whole of the output phosphor (16 Fig. 24).

The resolution is increased by this method from 20 line pairs per cm to approximately 28 line pairs per cm, but the input dose at the face of the intensifier has to be increased in proportion to the area enlargement in order that enough X-ray quanta per unit area are available to resolve the increased information (16 Fig. 5).

An alternative arrangement is to provide a long focus lens to project an enlarged image of the output phosphor onto the film as discussed in 16.11. This method provides an improved information content by enlarging the image and removing much of the limitations on resolution by the film—developer combination. In practice the irises of the two lenses have to be adjusted to give equal light transmission so that the film blackening is the same for each lens without adjustment to the control on the X-ray set.

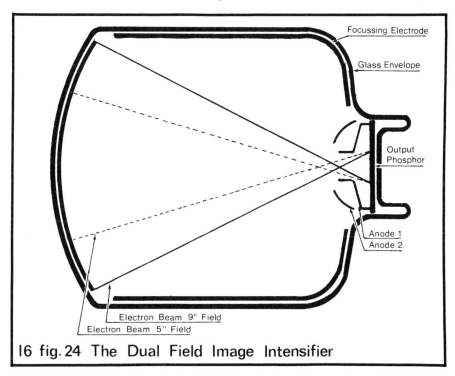

16 fig. 24 The Dual Field Image Intensifier

Chapter 17

Body Section Radiography

17.0 An Introduction to Tomography

A radiograph is simply a record of the shadow cast by the various structures through which the X-ray beam has passed. This means that the shadow of structures lying at differing levels within the subject will overlay each other making it very difficult to separate detail occurring at these various levels.

One may quote, for example, such cases as a kidney partially covered by an uneven intestinal gas shadow; or the fine structures of the inner ear which are obscured by other formations in the skull.

To separate the structures, use is made of a technique whereby objects in a selected plane are rendered sharp, whilst those above or below the plane cast blurred shadows. This technique is now known as "Tomography", but was previously known as Planigraphy.

Tomography involves a system of co-ordinated movement of film and focal spot about a fixed plane within a patient.

17.1 The Grossman Method

The "Grossman" method describes a system in which the tube and the cassette perform arc-shaped movements about a perpendicular plane during the exposure. (See 17 Fig. 1a). In 17 Fig. 1b it can be seen that objects lying on that plane will cast shadows which will always project

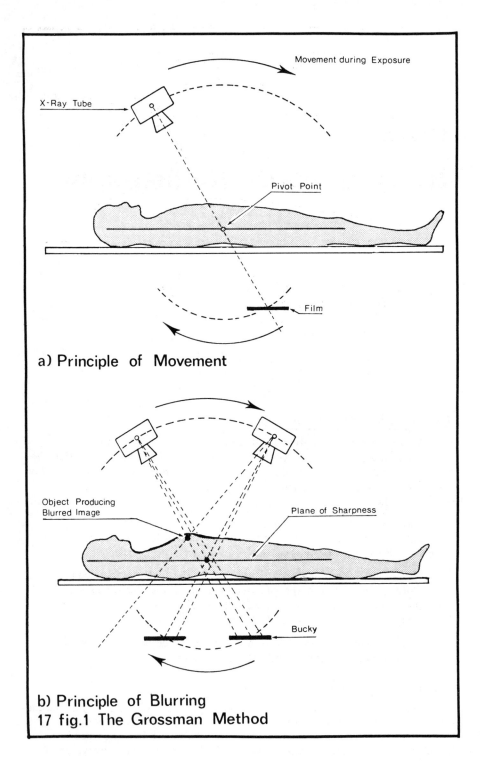

a) Principle of Movement

b) Principle of Blurring
17 fig.1 The Grossman Method

onto the same point on the film; whereas objects above or below the plane will cast shadows which will move across the film, and so be blurred out.

All forms of tomographic apparatus derive from this principle although a considerable number of variations are possible. Apparatus incorporating the full Grossman method is difficult to construct because the bucky has to execute an arc whilst remaining parallel to the plane of sharpness.

17.2 The Simplified Grossman System

The equipment may be simplified by eliminating the vertical movement of the bucky so that it now runs parallel with the table top.

A simplified system has certain limitations but, since the construction of the equipment is much cheaper, the shortcomings may be considered acceptable. Consideration of 17 Fig. 2 will show that the ratio of the distance from plane of sharpness to tube focus, and the distance from plane of sharpness to film is not constant. Since the magnification is a function of this ratio, the magnification will alter during the swing, the effect being more pronounced towards the edges of the film.

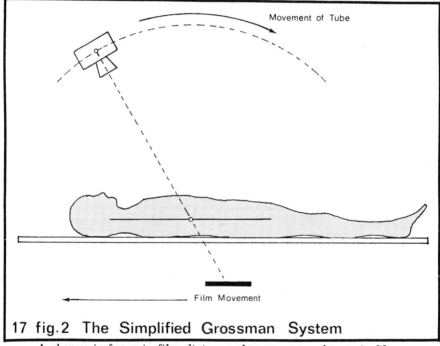

17 fig. 2 The Simplified Grossman System

A change in focus to film distance also causes a change in film blackening per unit time. Thus it follows that the amount of blackening which occurs at the centre of the swing is greater than that which occurs at the extremities. To counteract this the tube could be moved slowly at first, increasing in speed until the centre point is reached, and then slowing down towards the end of the swing, although in practice this is too difficult to achieve in simple apparatus.

17.3 The Jankers System

In the "Jankers" method both the tube and film move parallel to the plane of sharpness. Using the system shown in 17 Fig. 3 the magnification is constant over the entire swing. Although the distance between film and tube focus changes, the ratio of the distance from the tube focus to the plane of sharpness and film to plane of sharpness does not change.

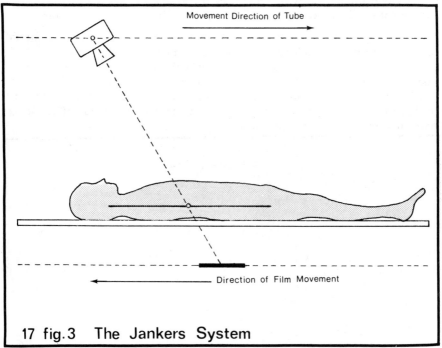

Movement Direction of Tube

Direction of Film Movement

17 fig. 3   The Jankers System

Since a change in tube to film distance throughout the swing will cause a change in dose rate to the film, one might expect that some means of varying the tube current would be needed. Fortunately this is not so, for if the tube support is moved down the table at a constant speed, the angular velocity changes; slow at the start and end of the arc, and fast in the centre, so giving constant blackening.

17.4 Alternative Tomographic Systems

In order to obtain tomograms the usual system is, as we have seen, to maintain the patient in one position and move the tube and film; but it is also possible to produce similar results by keeping the tube stationary and moving the patient and film, or by keeping the film stationary and moving the patient and tube. Examples of each of these systems are shown in 17 Fig. 4.

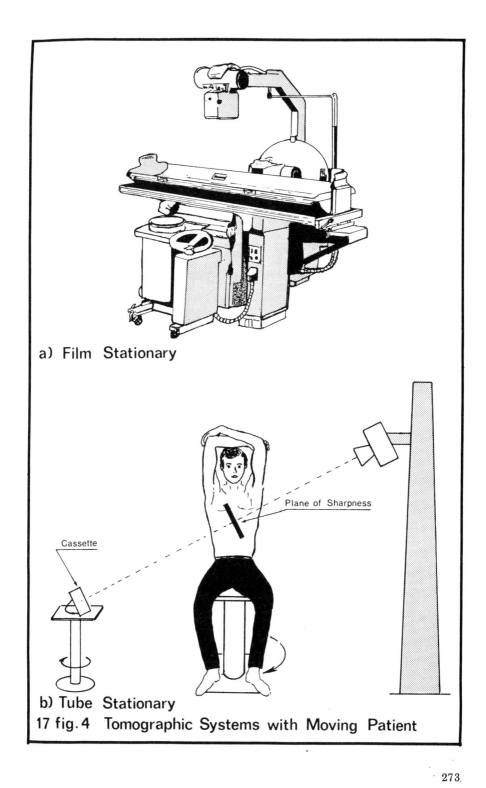

a) Film Stationary

Cassette

Plane of Sharpness

b) Tube Stationary
17 fig. 4 Tomographic Systems with Moving Patient

17.5 Layer Height

If one considers the Grossman system, it can be seen that the layer which is rendered sharp lies at the centre of the pivoting point of the tube arm. To alter the level of this layer (layer height adjustment), one can maintain fixed distances between tube, pivot, and film, and then raise and lower the patient. An example is shown in 17 Fig. 5. This system has the advantage that it gives a constant degree of magnification so that the size of structures lying at any level can be compared. It also has the advantage that the tube to film distance remains constant so that no variation in blackening will occur when the layer height is changed. The mechanism required to enable the patient to be raised and lowered simply but accurately is expensive to build and is only found on specialised tomographic units.

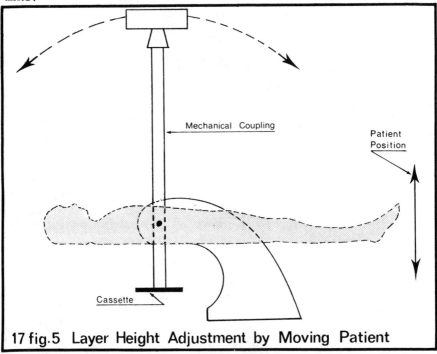

17 fig.5 Layer Height Adjustment by Moving Patient

The mechanical problem can be simplified by maintaining a fixed distance between tube, patient and film, but moving the pivot. In fact most simple tomographic units make use of this system. The main disadvantage of this method is that the magnification is a function of layer height so it is not possible to compare the size of structures at different levels. For example, one would not be able to compare structures of the middle ear on both sides of the skull.

The next method of altering layer height involves a fixed distance between tube, pivot, and patient, the layer height being changed by moving the level of the film. This is shown in 17 Fig. 6. The pivot point coincides

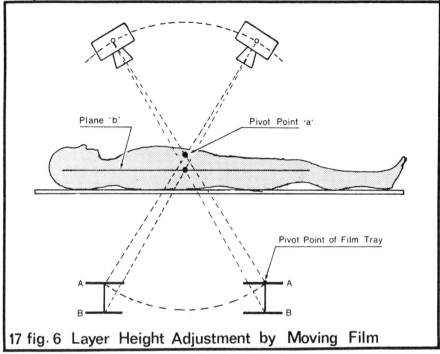

Plane 'b'

Pivot Point 'a'

Pivot Point of Film Tray

A

A

B

B

17 fig. 6 Layer Height Adjustment by Moving Film

with the plane of sharpness reproduced on film A. Film B, mounted
vertically below film A, and coupled to it by a rigid arm will reproduce
the plane of sharpness b. As can be seen the plane of sharpness only
coincides with the pivot point of the tube arm if the film is at the pivoting
point of the film tray.

If the film is dropped below the tray pivoting point, then the height of
cut will also fall by an amount related to the magnification of the system.
If the magnification is, for example, 1:1.3 then the film will have to be
lowered 1.3 cm to lower the layer height by 1 cm.

This principle is also used in a multi-section box where a number of
films are spaced at specified intervals,giving a series of films of different
heights for one exposure. It should be noted that,if a film is held above
the pivoting point of the tray,this film will show a plane above the normal
plane of sharpness.

17.6 Tomographic Attachments

The simplest type of tomographic unit is the attachment which can be
fitted to the side of most tables, an example is shown in 17 Fig. 7. In this
type of device the bucky travels parallel to the table top and,depending upon
the type of unit, the tube may either travel in an arc or parallel to the table
top. The height of cut is adjusted by moving the height of the pivot and as a
result the magnification will depend upon layer height.

275

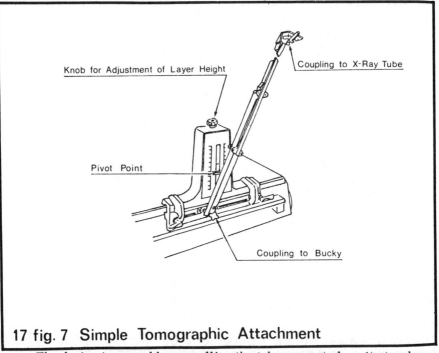

Knob for Adjustment of Layer Height

Coupling to X-Ray Tube

Pivot Point

Coupling to Bucky

17 fig. 7 Simple Tomographic Attachment

The device is moved by propelling the tube support along its track either by means of a spring or an electric motor (See 17 Fig. 8). The tube support may be either floor mounted, as shown, or ceiling mounted. The angle during which exposure occurs is determined by means of switches but the length of travel remains constant. The switches together with a screw mechanism to raise and lower the pivot are mounted in the assembly fitted to the accessory rail of the table. This device is often referred to as the "tombstone" because of its shape.

Although a great deal of routine work is done by means of such devices they are difficult to use, and the results tend to vary, making it hard to compare radiographs taken over a long period of time.

Since the exposure period is determined by the time taken for the tube to traverse a certain number of degrees of the arc, any variation in the duration of tube movement will cause an alteration in exposure time. This problem is particularly bad when a floor mounted tube support is used since dirt tends to accumulate in the floor track causing the time of travel to vary. In addition to causing variation in exposure time any roughness of the track will also tend to cause an increase in apparent thickness of cut. This comes about as a result of vibration of the tube – patient – film combination. There will also be a loss of definition, although this may not be so apparent.

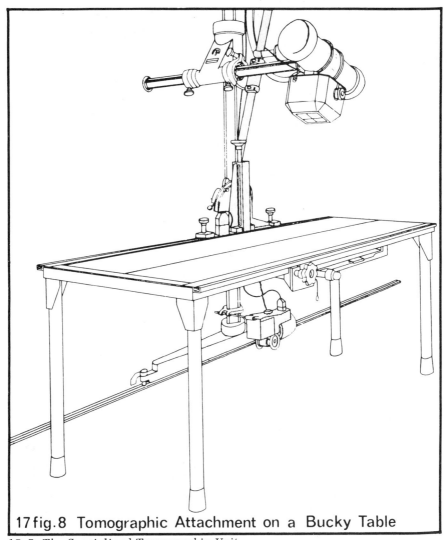

17 fig. 8 Tomographic Attachment on a Bucky Table

17.7   The Specialised Tomographic Unit

The above problems can be obviated by using a specially designed
unit in which the tube support does not have to travel on an exposed track.
Such a unit should include the following features:-

(a) Constant linear velocity of tube and film carriage.

(b) A means of controlling the time of travel independently of the
angle of movement.

(c) A drive system which does not cause the tube, table, or film to
vibrate.

The first condition can be met by making the tube support part of a flywheel system. This entails increasing the mass of the system, but brings with it the problem of accelerating the assembly up to speed. However, increasing the mass of the system will also help to reduce vibration providing the weight is rigidly mounted.

Points b and c are inter-related and so must be considered together. The travel time could be controlled quite simply by using a variable speed electric motor, but this may introduce too much vibration. The designer may be forced to use gravity or a spring, in conjunction with a speed regulator of the oil dashpot type, to meet both requirements.

As has already been mentioned, some means of switching the start and end of the exposure has to be incorporated, so that the tube swing can be longer than the exposure time. This permits the tube to accelerate up to speed before the exposure begins, and to decelerate after the exposure has ended.

Some method of selecting the angle of exposure is usually provided since the thickness of the plane of sharpness is dependent on (amongst other things) the length of the blurring path.

The amount to which the image of an object is blurred depends upon the angle through which the tube moves, and the distance of the object from the centre of the plane of sharpness. There is no sharp transition, the further away from centre of the plane of sharpness, the greater the blur. The thickness of cut is therefore defined as the range over which the amount of blur does not exceed 0.1 mm.

There is a practical limit to the angle which can be obtained using a linear movement, so that, in order to increase the length of the blurring path without further increasing the angle of swing, various complex movements are used. The one most frequently encountered is the circular movement in which the length of the blurring path is over three times that which could be obtained using the same angle with linear movement.

This movement gives thinner cuts and complete elimination of the familiar streaking which occurs with the linear movement, but can give rise to artefacts where a tomogram is to be made of a circular structure. Some tomographic units have provision for an elliptical movement, but linear structures outside the plane of sharpness can give rise to double edges. This is because the ellipse is really made up of two parallel linear movements displaced laterally by a small circular movement. (See 17 Fig. 9).

A fourth possibility is the spiral movement, which is a combination of a circular and a radial movement. This can eliminate many of the problems already mentioned, providing the speed of rotation is controlled so that the tube rotates more slowly at the outside of the spiral than at the centre. Unfortunately this is difficult to achieve and also means extending the exposure times.

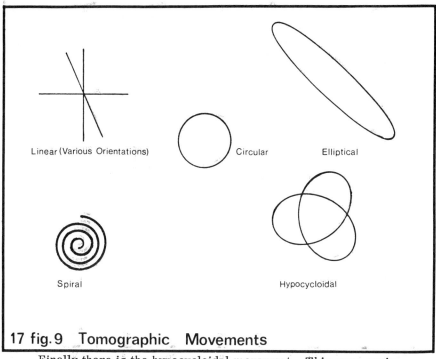

Linear (Various Orientations)   Circular   Elliptical

Spiral   Hypocycloidal

17 fig. 9   Tomographic   Movements

Finally there is the hypocycloidal movement. This once again consists of a circular and a radial movement – which gives about five times the blurring path that could be obtained using a linear system with the same angle of displacement.

The movement is a combination of two circular components and is brought about by the rotation of two gears of a certain ratio. The ratio required to produce a hypocycloid is 3:2 so that one could use, for example an outer gear having 96 teeth and an inner gear having 64 teeth. A fixed point on the inner gear will trace out a hypocycloid when the outer gear rotates. (See 17 Fig. 10).

A unit incorporating this technique consists of a heavy base supporting a parallelogram which is mounted in such a way as to be free to swing in any direction. The X-ray tube is fixed at one end of the parallelogram and the film holder at the other. The design of the system is such that the tube and film will always be correctly orientated no matter what the displacement of the parallelogram may be.

The driving mechanism to which the parallelogram is coupled is shown in 17 Fig. 11. The same basic system may be used to produce other figures, so that by a suitable choice of gearing, or by using a fixed coupling pin, linear, circular, or elliptical movements may also be obtained.

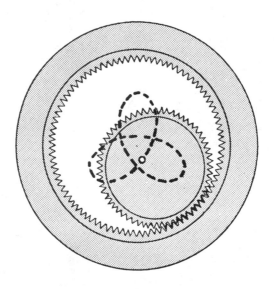

17 fig.10 Production of a Hypocycloid

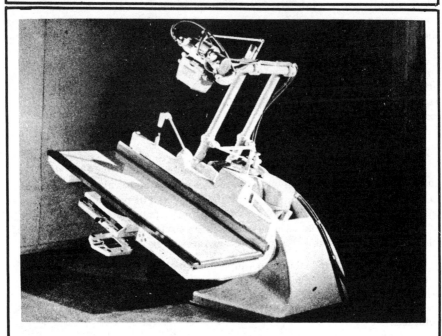

17 fig.11 Unit for Complex Tomography

The elliptical movement is obtained by means of a gear ratio of 2:1, the circular movement by coupling to the fixed position on the large disc, and linear by using an arm to convert the circular movement to a linear one.

The hypocycloidal movement gives extremely thin sections. In fact the thickness of cut is really determined more by the thickness of the two intensifying screens and the film, rather than the length of the blurring path. The screens and film combination act rather as a multi-section cassette box and detail occurring anywhere within the thickness of this pack will be displayed on the film. The top screen will project the image of a layer slightly above the plane of sharpness depicted by the film itself, whereas the lower screen will project the image of a lower layer. Since one cannot encounter a naturally occurring hypocycloidally shaped structure no artefacts should be introduced. Initially many users are disappointed at the results that they are able to obtain from this type of unit. The first impression that one has is that the films are lacking in both contrast and definition. It is inevitable that the contrast will be low, but in practice definition should be good. However, the lack of contrast gives the impression of poor definition. (A high contrast film always looks sharper than a low contrast film.) The lack of contrast is closely related to the thickness of cut. Although structures above and below do not add any detail to the film, the X-ray beam still has to traverse the full thickness of the object. The results are the same as one would obtain by taking a radiograph of an object having a thickness of about 1 mm, sandwiched between plates of homogeneous filter material having approximately the same density but a thickness of about 10 cm - 20 cm or more. This is shown in 17 Fig. 12.

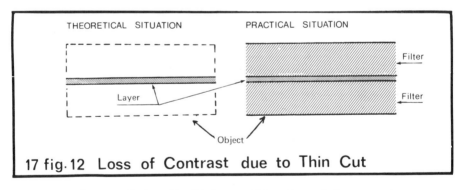

THEORETICAL SITUATION   PRACTICAL SITUATION

Filter

Layer

Filter

Object

17 fig. 12   Loss of Contrast due to Thin Cut

It may be seen that as the thickness of the plane of sharpness is reduced the contrast will also be reduced, until a point is reached when the selected layer will be infinitely thin, at which point the contrast will be infinitely low.

A further loss of apparent definition will be caused by the constantly changing angle at which the beam meets structures at right angles to the plane.

When linear tomography is used the tube is at one point vertical. The full thickness of the structure contributes to give an accentuated edge effect.

This gives an artificially thick layer for structures at right angles to the plane.

Using the hypocycloidal movement the beam is never absolutely vertical and so a really sharp edge will not be seen. This is shown in 17 Fig. 13.

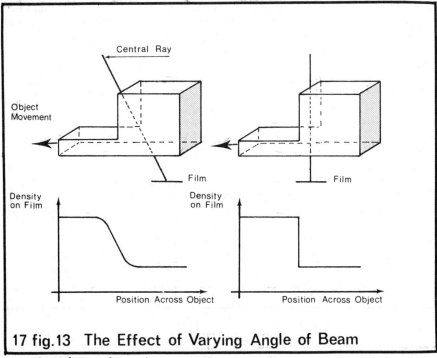

17 fig.13   The Effect of Varying Angle of Beam

In order to obtain the maximum amount of contrast all available measures should be adopted. This means low kV and high mA, small films, well coned down to reduce scatter, etc. For some types of work it will be found advantageous to remove the grid, since this will permit a further reduction in kV. For most complex movement tomography, noticeably better results are obtained using a fine focus tube (0.6 mm^2) and standard films and screens. This usually introduces problems with tube loading so that high speed tubes have to be used.

Since the length of exposure time will be determined by the mechanical arrangement of the tomographic unit, it is advisable to have stepless control of the tube current for tomography. This will be limited to a maximum of 50 to 100 mA because of the problem of tube loading, but since tomographic exposures are comparatively long, the required mAs product can be easily achieved. Having selected the speed of tube movement and the angle during which X-rays are emitted, the tube current is adjusted to give the required mAs.

With such a flexible piece of equipment it is vital to select the correct

282

combination of conditions for each exposure. For example, the thickness of cut should be sufficient to include the complete structure under examination, at least during the initial stages. This means that for some types of examination the complex movements should be avoided.

17.8 Multi-section Tomography

It should be noted that there is little point in using a conventional multi-section cassette when the hypocycloidal movement is used. One could take a set of films with such a device without gaining any useful information since the plane of sharpness is only about 1·0mm thick, whereas the films usually show layers about 1 cm apart. However, if a multi-section cassette is required for use with complex movements then one can be made by removing the usual felt from a standard cassette so that it will now take three films and three sets of screens. A certain amount of experimentation is needed to get good screen to film contact on all three films but, once this is achieved, one has the facility to obtain three films spaced just under 1 mm apart with only one exposure. Even so this system is far from perfect since all multi-section cassettes suffer from certain disadvantages :-

A multi-section cassette is made up of a certain number of sets (usually five) of graded intensifying screens. Three types of screen are commonly available.

High definition
Standard
High speed (fast tungstate)

The pack is made up as shown in 17 Fig. 14. The screens are graded so that slow screens are used at the top of the pack and fast screens at the bottom. This is to compensate for the radiation absorbed by each film and screen set in succession. When a three-film cassette is made up for use with a complex movement tomograph the top three combinations should be used.

It will be found in practice that the saving in dose to the patient will be less than expected, but there will be a saving in examination time. There is also the advantage that all the films are taken at the same instant, so that the patient cannot move between exposures. It is interesting to note that the magnification is the same for all films so that the size of structures at various levels can be compared. This is especially useful when the tomographic unit does not have fixed magnification. This applies to all types of multi-section cassettes. The main disadvantage is that the films are only comparable over a limited range of kV's and this tends to be between 80 and 100 kV, which is really too high for complex tomography. This is due to two factors, first of all the different types of screen tend to give differing results over a range of kV's and secondly the upper screens act as a filter - preventing a certain proportion of the softer radiation from reaching the films below. This effect is also kV dependent.

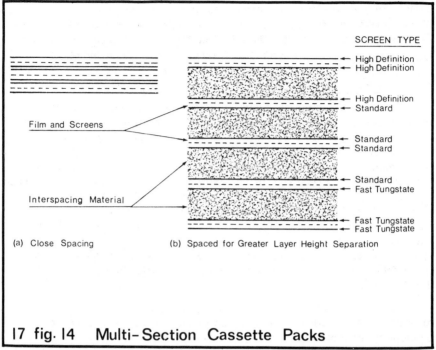

SCREEN TYPE

High Definition
High Definition

High Definition
Standard

Standard
Standard

Standard
Fast Tungstate

Fast Tungstate
Fast Tungstate

Film and Screens

Interspacing Material

(a) Close Spacing

(b) Spaced for Greater Layer Height Separation

17 fig. 14   Multi-Section Cassette Packs

Using the standard type of multi-section cassette no great problem
should be encountered with the required kV since, when a cassette yielding
films showing planes 1 cm apart is used, for the best results, the thickness
of cut should be just about 1 cm. Under these conditions there is sufficient
contrast for high kV's to be used, although some degradation of the film
itself will result because of scatter within the casstte.

17.9 Zonography

For some subjects the best results are obtained when only a very
narrow angle of movement is used, so that a relatively thick section is
shown on the film. This technique is called Zonography, a name coined
by its originator for what was initially called "planigraphy with slight
blurring".

The technique is particularly useful for such things as renal studies
where it can eliminate obstructing shadows whilst still showing the entire
kidney. For the best results there must be a free zone above and below the
plane of sharpness. The more remote the extraneous detail is from the
required plane the more completely is it eliminated.

Reduced to its simplest form the only equipment required for
Zonography is a co-operative patient. This is the basis of the technique of
auto tomography which is sometimes used in such examinations as air
encephalography in which the patient gently shakes his head during the
exposure.

Where a specialised tomographic unit is used for Zonography the circular movement is the one most suitable since the remaining shadows are rather less distracting than when a linear movement is used.

17.10 Axial Tomography

A further application of the basic tomographic technique is axial tomography. The schematic layout of such a unit is shown in 17 Fig. 15.

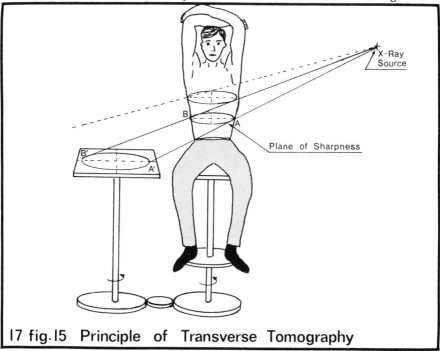

17 fig. 15 Principle of Transverse Tomography

The patient and film rotate together so that the shadow of an object on the plane of sharpness will always fall on the same point on the film. As in conventional tomography, shadows cast by structures above or below the plane will move over the film and so be blurred out.

It should be noted that this is an example of a tomographic unit in which the tube remains stationary while the patient and film are moved.

The illustration 17 Fig. 16a shows the unit in use with the film horizontal, whereas the second photograph 17 Fig. 16b shows the film tilted at an angle. As with other types of tomographic units, the plane of sharpness is determined by the plane of the film. Under normal conditions the film is horizontal so that an axial layer is recorded. If the film is tilted then the plane of sharpness will also be tilted, enabling radiographs to be produced at a wide variety of angles on an upright patient.

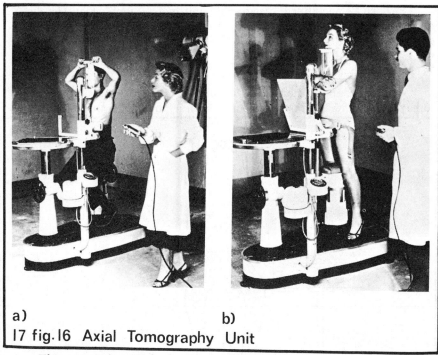

a)   b)

17 fig. 16 Axial Tomography Unit

This principle may be further exploited by mounting the film in a curved cassette so that the plane of sharpness follows a curve. This is particularly useful in showing up the entire jaw without the other structures of the skull being shown. The principle is shown in 17 Fig. 17.

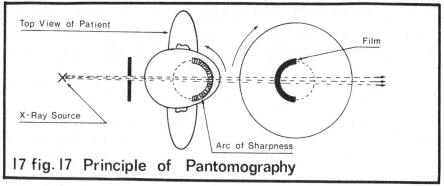

Top View of Patient

Film

X-Ray Source

Arc of Sharpness

17 fig. 17 Principle of Pantomography

17.11 Test Procedures

The simplest test involves the use of a ruler and a pin and is simply a check of the accuracy of the height scale. Various commercially available tomographic test blocks may be used, but if one is not available it is a simple matter to make one. (See Section 20.1.6).

When a comprehensive test is to be carried out on a tomographic unit, the largest film that can be fitted in the cassette tray should be used and the

286

film masked with lead so that five exposures can be made at the same height; one in the centre and one at each corner. This will show if the plane of sharpness is flat and also whether it is parallel to the table top.

When carrying out tests which involve the use of the bucky tray (for example measuring the height or the thickness of cut) it is essential that a cassette of the same type as will be used during an actual examination is selected, since variation in the vertical position of the film in the cassette tray will cause a variation in layer height. Other tests, in which the film is placed on the table top, can be done using double wrapped films as in this case the height of the film is not critical.

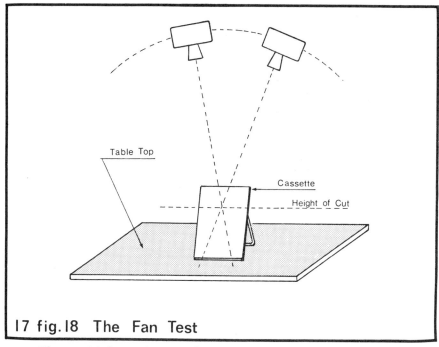

Table Top

Cassette

Height of Cut

17 fig. 18   The   Fan   Test

The most informative test that can be carried out on a linear tomographic unit is the fan exposure. For this a film is placed on the table top at a slight angle. (See 17 Fig. 18). If possible, the height of the film should be adjusted so that the centre of the film coincides with the pivot point. The light beam diaphragm is adjusted to give a narrow beam of radiation. A tomographic exposure is made and the film processed. This should show a fan shaped pattern which should be evenly blackened throughout the arc. Any variation in blackening indicates a variation in the angular velocity of the tube. In addition to this the shape of the crossover gives an indication of the alignment of the system (See 17 Fig.19).

Where the performance of a non linear unit has to be checked this test cannot be used. There is, however, an alternative which will give useful information. For this a plate made of brass or steel with a very

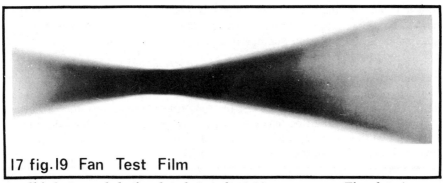

17 fig.19 Fan Test Film

small hole is needed, the plate being about 30 cm square. The plate is mounted on blocks at some distance above the table top. (See 17 Fig. 20). Ideally the plate should be at a distance above the table to equal twice the layer height selected. A film is placed on the table top, aligned with the hole in the plate and the light beam diaphragm closed down to give a narrow beam which should be centred on the hole. A tomographic exposure is now made. When the film is processed, a black line will have been traced out on the film showing the path of the tube during the exposure. Once again any variation in blackening during the exposure will indicate vibration of the tube. An example is shown in 17 Fig. 21. The final result is a pinhole picture of the tube focus, with the tube moving.

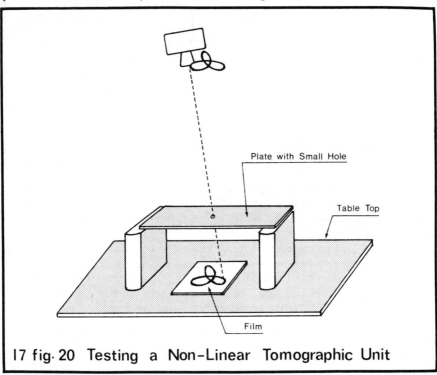

Plate with Small Hole

Table Top

Film

17 fig. 20 Testing a Non-Linear Tomographic Unit

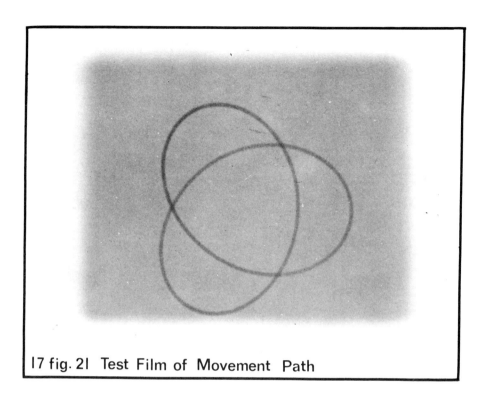

17 fig. 21 Test Film of Movement Path

Chapter 18

Skull Tables, Special Trolleys and Chairs

18.1 <u>Neuroradiography</u>

Radiological investigation of the skull and brain may be divided into four sections:-

    a) "Routine Skull" films.

    b) Special named views.

    c) Contrast examinations.

    d) Stereotactic procedures.

Routine skull films are the most frequent radiological examination of the skull and brain. These views usually comprise : an Antero-Posterior (AP), or a Postero-Anterior (PA), film, one or both lateral projections and a Townes view, as depicted in 18 Fig. 1 where the arrows indicate the direction of the normal ray. Routine skull films may be taken on a bucky table or vertical bucky combined with a head clamp and a tube column, floor or ceiling suspended. However, any view of the skull, be it routine or "special named view" is greatly facilitated by use of apparatus designed to acquire accuracy in the positioning of the patient and of the X-ray tube and film. Skull stands are produced for this purpose.

With a skull stand it is also possible to carry out many of the specialised examinations required in neuroradiology, for example carotid and vertebral arteriography or pneumo-encephalography.

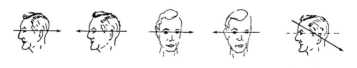

a - p   p - a   Left Lateral   Right Lateral   Townes

18 fig. 1 Positioning For 'Routine Skull Films'

Carotid and vertebral arteriography involve the rapid injection of a bolus of contrast medium which quickly flows along the arterial tree. This may be recorded by taking a rapid series of radiographs. As the contrast medium is more radiopaque than blood,its shadow appears lighter on the radiograph, and this is therefore referred to as a positive contrast procedure.

Pneumo-encephalography is an examination to show any structural abnormalities of ventricles of the brain and their connecting ducts. Gas, usually air or carbon dioxide,is injected by lumbar puncture, and passes up to the ventricles by displacing cerebro-spinal fluid (C.S.F.). As air is less radiopaque than the C.S.F., areas of gas appear darker on the resultant radiographs, and hence is termed a negative contrast medium.

Stereotaxy is the accurate insertion of an instrument into a selected area of the brain through a small opening or burr hole in the skull. This procedure obviously requires very accurate radiographic technique.

"Skull Stands" are designed to work by one of two basic principles; The Lysholm system and the Dulac system.

18.2　The Lysholm and Dulac Systems

The Lysholm system is the most commonly used. The distinguishing feature of this system is that the centre of rotation of the film holder and the X-ray tube support is in the centre of the film.

The other main feature of the Lysholm system is that the focus to film distance remains constant. The lateral view of the skull is taken in the prone position with the patient's head turned sideways. As can be seen from 18 Fig. 2 tomography is not possible with simple Lysholm equipment.

The Dulac system is often referred to as the isocentric method of skull radiography. The central X-ray beam remains perpendicular to the film. The X-ray tube and film combination rotate about a point in space. This point is chosen to be the centre of the area in the head under investigation. Since the centre of rotation is at a point in the patient's head, it is possible to increase or decrease the focus to film distance and, therefore, the patient to film distance, without altering the position of the patient.

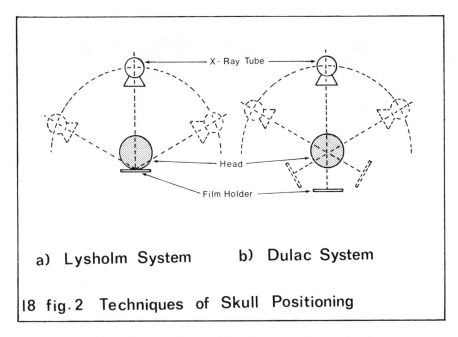

a) **Lysholm System**   b) **Dulac System**

18 fig. 2 Techniques of Skull Positioning

Macroradiography, direct radiographic enlargement, may be done routinely with the Dulac system.

If the film holder is placed in the axis of rotation of the X-ray tube and fixed whilst the tube support is still allowed to rotate, Lysholm techniques may be carried out.

The Lysholm system is the simplest to achieve mechanically. However, it has the following disadvantages : the patient's head must be placed on and secured to the film holder and bucky assembly; it is necessary to move the patient's head during examinations. Although it would be feasible to use an image intensifier and closed circuit television for fluoroscopy, a useful image could only be obtained when the normal ray is perpendicular to the film plane.

Equipment embodying the Dulac principle is necessarily more complicated and expensive. However, the advantages of the Dulac system are numerous. The patient's head can be supported by a headrest on a special chair or table and the X-ray tube and film combination rotated around the patient, thus obtaining any number of views without moving the patient. An image intensifier may be mounted beneath the film holder, allowing television fluoroscopy of any projection. With a little extra mechanical adaptation, it is also possible to make tomograms.

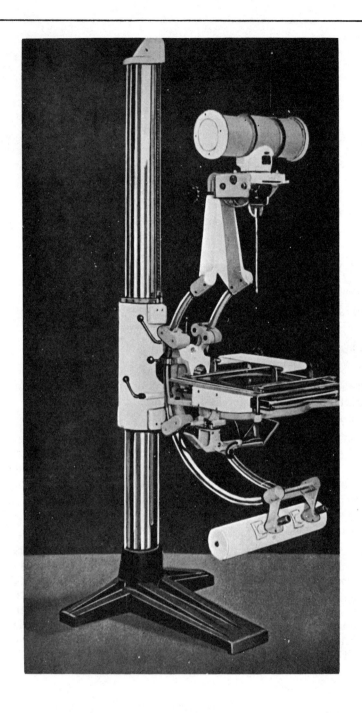

18 fig. 3 Skull Stand Designed to the Lysholm Technique

18.3 A Skull Stand Designed to the Lysholm Principle

The apparatus shown in 18 Fig. 3 consists of a rigid vertical column on which is mounted a freely sliding carriage, accurately counter-weighted. This carriage has a pivot about which a C-shaped arm supporting the X-ray tube may rotate. This pivot point is also the centre of rotation of an object table. The object table has a graduated transparent perspex top with two fixed and two moveable rails for a fixation device (18 Fig. 4) and a lateral cassette holder. Under the table is a rotatable support frame for the bucky, adjustable cassette holder and a mirror device used as an aid in positioning. The bucky and cassette holder take cassettes up to a maximum size of 24 x 30 cm which is large enough for a full view of the skull.

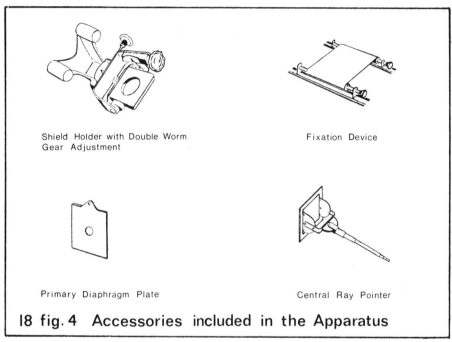

Shield Holder with Double Worm
Gear Adjustment

Fixation Device

Primary Diaphragm Plate

Central Ray Pointer

l8 fig. 4   Accessories included in the Apparatus

The X-ray tube is mounted at a fixed focus to film distance, and attached to the C-arm by two worm gear mechanisms, allowing angulation of the central beam to a point away from the centre of the film.

The comprehensive range of movements is shown in 18 Fig. 5. In neuroradiography, accuracy of positioning is vital and, as with other skull units, each movement has scales which are easy to read.

There are two devices which aid positioning. A telescopic pointer swivelled into position, indicates the direction of the central ray (18 Fig. 4); it shows the point of incidence of the beam on the patient. A mirror system (18 Fig. 6) indicates the point of exit of the central beam when the cassette holder is withdrawn (18 Fig. 7). Primary plate diaphragms allow accurate collimating to the area under examination.

With compound angulation, for example examination of the optic

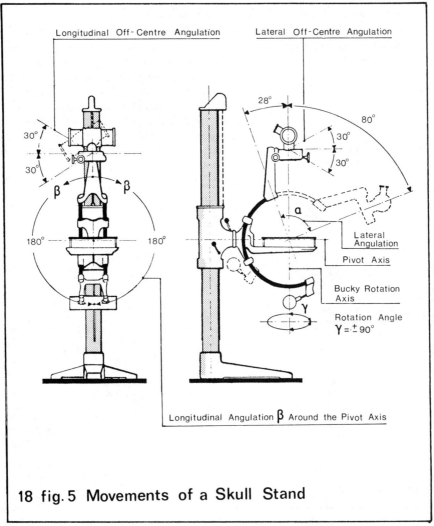

Longitudinal Off-Centre Angulation

Lateral Off-Centre Angulation

28°

80°

30°

30°

30°

30°

30°

β

β

180°

180°

α

Lateral Angulation

Pivot Axis

Bucky Rotation Axis

Rotation Angle
$\gamma = \pm 90°$

γ

Longitudinal Angulation β Around the Pivot Axis

18 fig. 5 Movements of a Skull Stand

foramina, it is necessary to rotate the bucky so that correct grid alignment is obtained. The following formula enables the bucky rotation angle to be calculated.

If the lateral angle is α , the longitudinal angle is β and the bucky rotation angle γ , the bucky rotation is given by the equation :-

$$\mathrm{Tan}\,\gamma = \mathrm{Cotan}\,\alpha\;\mathrm{Sin}\,\beta$$

The table shown in 18 Fig. 8 has been calculated in order to facilitate the determination of the necessary rotation angle for correct orientation of the bucky.

In pneumo-encephalography, when lateral radiographs are required

296

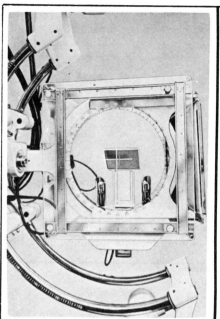

18 fig. 6
Mirror System

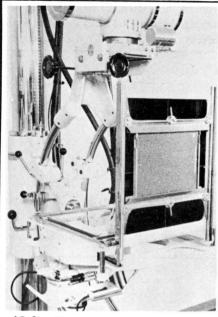

18 fig. 7
Cassette Holder Withdrawn

		Longitudinal Angulation ± β (Around Pivot Axis)																	
		1	2	3	4	6	8	10	12	14	16	18	20	22	24	26	28	30	35
Lateral Angulation α by Arc Adjustment	1	45	27	18	14	9	7	6	5	4	4	3	3	3	2	2	2	2	2
	2	63	45	33	26	18	14	11	10	8	7	7	6	5	5	5	4	4	3
	3	72	56	45	37	27	21	17	14	12	11	10	9	8	7	7	6	6	5
	4	76	63	53	45	34	27	22	19	16	14	13	12	11	10	9	8	8	7
	6	81	70	64	56	45	37	31	27	23	21	19	17	16	14	13	13	12	10
	8	83	76	70	64	53	45	39	34	30	27	24	22	20	19	18	17	16	14
	10	84	79	73	68	59	52	45	40	36	33	30	27	25	23	22	21	19	17
	12	85	81	76	72	64	57	51	46	41	38	35	32	30	28	26	24	23	20
	14	86	82	78	74	67	61	55	50	46	42	39	36	34	32	30	28	26	23
	16	86	83	80	76	70	64	59	54	50	46	43	40	38	35	33	31	30	28
	18	87	84	81	78	72	67	62	57	53	50	46	44	41	39	37	35	33	32
	20	87	85	82	79	74	69	65	60	56	53	50	47	44	42	40	38	36	35
	22	88	85	83	80	76	71	67	63	59	56	53	50	47	45	43	41	39	38
	24	88	86	83	81	77	73	69	65	62	58	55	52	50	48	45	43	42	41
	26	88	86	84	82	78	74	71	67	64	61	58	55	52	50	48	46	44	43
	28	88	86	84	83	79	75	72	69	66	63	60	57	55	53	51	49	47	45
	30	88	87	85	83	80	76	73	70	67	64	62	59	57	55	53	51	49	47
	35	89	87	86	84	82	79	76	73	71	68	66	64	62	60	58	56	54	51
		Bucky Rotation Angle ± γ																	

18 fig. 8   Table Relating α, β, γ

whilst the patient remains prone, it is necessary to use a lateral cassette holder (18 Fig. 9). This is because the examination is concerned with fluid levels and so it is not possible to turn the patient.

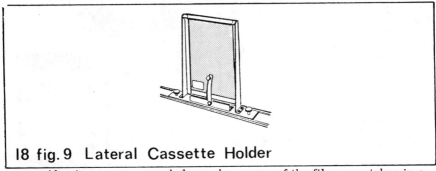

18 fig. 9 Lateral Cassette Holder

Also in pneumo-encephalography, some of the films are taken in a seated position. A head fixation device suitable for this technique is shown in 19 Fig. 10.

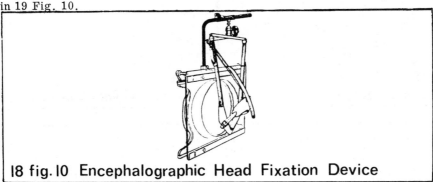

18 fig. 10 Encephalographic Head Fixation Device

18.4 An Apparatus Designed for Both Lysholm and Dulac Techniques

The unit shown in 18 Fig. 11, consists of a ceiling suspended column which can pivot about a vertical axis. Attached to the column is a sliding carriage which may be moved vertically. On this carriage is mounted an X-ray tube arm which may rotate in a vertical plane about a pivot on the carriage. The bucky and cassette carriage assembly may be moved along the rails on the X-ray tube arm, so that the focus to film distance may be varied. This assembly may also be tilted. Hence, with this apparatus both Lysholm and Dulac positioning techniques may be used. (18 Fig. 12 and 13).

The bucky and cassette holder assembly may be removed so that cerebral angiography with film changers may be carried out.

18.5 Equipment for Specialised Examinations

An example of apparatus designed especially for advanced neuro-radiological procedures is shown in 18 Fig. 14.

All skull projections, survey and detail, are possible with either Lysholm or Dulac positioning techniques; all positioning may be checked by

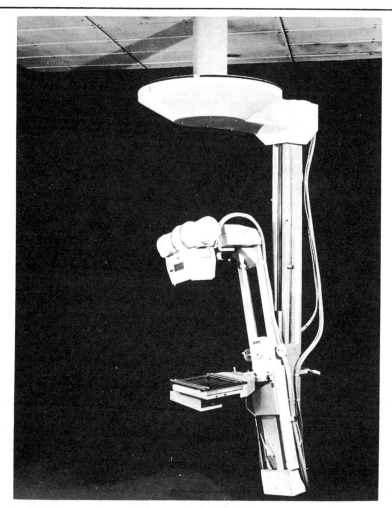

18 fig. II Apparatus for Lysholm and Dulac Techniques

T.V. fluoroscopy. Conventional radiography, 70 mm fluorography, cine fluorography, video recording and linear tomography are all possible with this apparatus. All movements are power driven and remotely controlled thus providing ease of operation and minimum radiation hazard (see 18 Fig. 15).

Routine cranial radiography, fractional pneumo-encephalography and ventriculography with positive or negative contrast medium, cerebral angiography, traumatology and stereotactic centring are all possible.

The component parts are shown in 18 Fig. 16 and the motorised movements available are shown in 18 Fig. 17. The apparatus may be used with a conventional skull table or with an isocentric chair, as described in the next section.

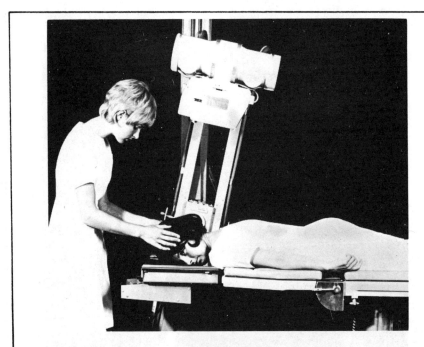

18 fig. 12   Stenvers   Positioning ~ Dulac

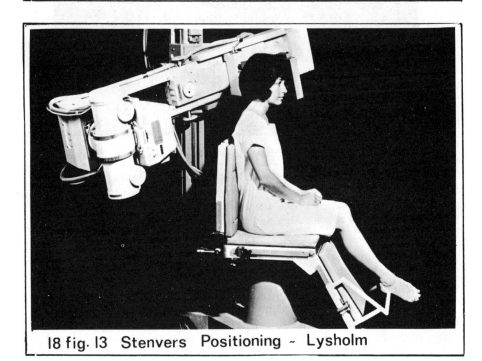

18 fig. 13   Stenvers   Positioning ~ Lysholm

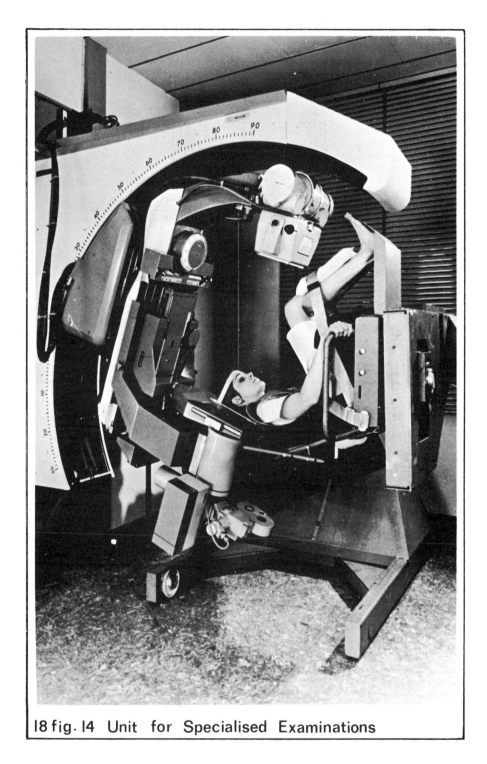

18 fig. 14 Unit for Specialised Examinations

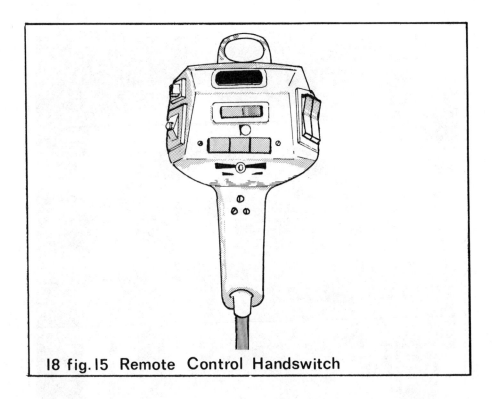

18 fig. 15 Remote Control Handswitch

18.6 Patient Tables

Two types of patient table or chair are used for neuroradiology; the conventional table/chair and the somersault chair.

The conventional patient table/chair (18 Fig. 18 + 19) is suitable for all routine views, cerebral angiography and stereotactic procedures. The somersault chair greatly facilitates positioning especially for procedures requiring movement of the patient to control fluid levels, as in pneumo-encephalography and cervical myelography. Patients under general anaesthetic can be easily handled.

There are two basic types of somersault chair. One system has its centre of rotation in the middle of the chair and the principle is shown in 18 Fig. 20.

With this type it is not possible to watch the movement of air in pneumo-encephalography by T.V. fluoroscopy during rotation of the chair, as the area of interest may move out of the field of view.

The isocentric chair, shown in 18 Fig. 21, has its centre of rotation in the patient's head. Thus the area of interest remains in the field of view throughout the examination regardless of the degree of rotation of the patient. This means that not only the moment of exposure can more

302

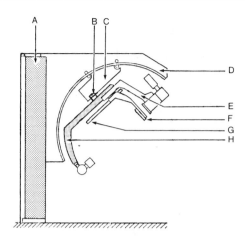

A = Column, attached to the wall for vertical travel of D

B = Pivot point about which X-Ray tube/image intensifier combination rotates

C = Motor-driven carriage, supporting X-Ray tube/image intensifier combination

D = Curved girder construction for travel of carriage C

E = Image intensifier holder; can slide along H to vary geometrical enlargement

F = Cassette holder; can slide along tomography arm G; for selecting technique and for setting layer height in tomography

G = Tomography arm

H = X-Ray tube/image intensifier combination; can rotate about pivot point B

18 fig. 16 Components of a Specialised Skull Unit

accurately be chosen, but also pathology, which otherwise might have been overlooked, may be detected.

The isocentric chair also offers the possibility of selective filling of the temporal horns. The isocentricity is particularly advantageous when general anaesthesia is used, because the head remains in the same area during the entire examination.

18.7   Image Intensifiers in Neuroradiology

Recent improvements made in image intensifiers have rendered them suitable for observation of the fine detail required in cranial neuroradiology In pneumo-encephalography, it is certainly very useful to observe intra-cranial movements of gas but this technique is restricted when an image

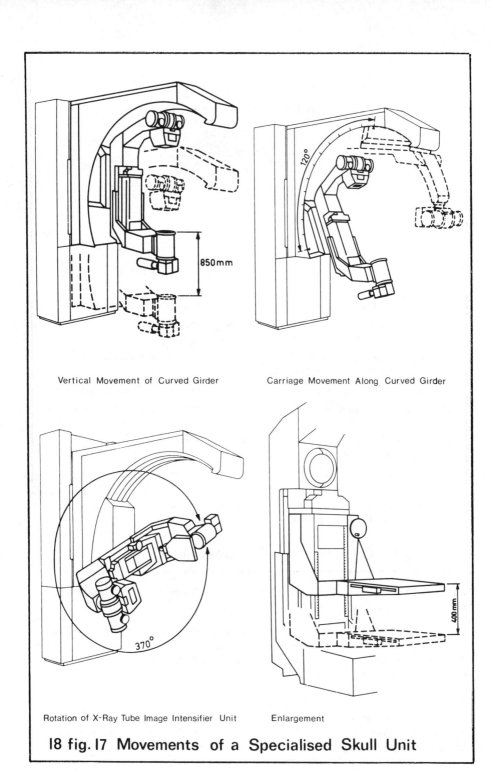

Vertical Movement of Curved Girder   Carriage Movement Along Curved Girder

850mm

120°

Rotation of X-Ray Tube Image Intensifier Unit   Enlargement

370°

400 mm

18 fig. 17 Movements of a Specialised Skull Unit

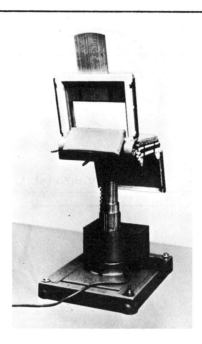

18 fig. 18   Conventional Table - Seated Position

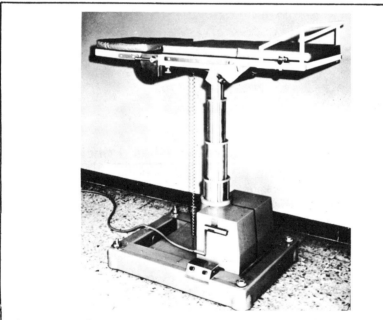

18 fig. 19 Conventional   Table - Lying   Position

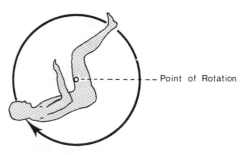

18 fig. 20 Principle of a Somersault Chair

Point of Rotation

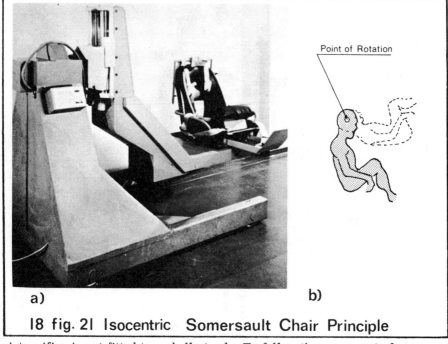

Point of Rotation

a)   b)

18 fig. 21 Isocentric   Somersault Chair Principle

intensifier is not fitted to a skull stand. To follow the movement of gas, without an image intensifier, requires a multiplicity of radiographs which is time consuming, expensive and entails a high radiation dose.

Great improvement in image quality of the intensifier, enabled the use of monoplane and even bi-plane techniques with closed circuit television for myelography on a conventional tilting fluoroscopic table.

The apparatus described in section 18.4 was specifically designed with a 6" image intensifier in mind. Not only may the course of gas filling be watched and therefore precisely controlled, but it may be filmed or recorded on video tape.

18.8   Cranial Angiography

The best equipment for cerebral angiography is a system solely designed for this technique. It should consist of bi-plane 24 x 30 cm automatic film changers, with a fixed lateral X-ray tube, and an AP X-ray tube on a pendulum system to allow for both AP and Townes views. Equipment for cerebral angiography must be simple to use as carotid angiograms are a common emergency technique which must be performed at any hour of the day, often by staff inexperienced in neuroradiology. However, for economic reasons, very few such systems have been made. Instead it is necessary to make equipment which can carry out routine radiography and contrast techniques - both negative and positive contrast being used.

Basic equipment for cerebral angiography in practice often consists of a simple skull stand with a manual bi-plane cassette changer fitted to the object table. Such a cassette changer is described in Chapter 19.

Although the specialised apparatus described in Section 18.5 is basically designed for pneumo-encephography it may also be used for cerebral angiography as in 19 Fig. 22 (a) and (b).

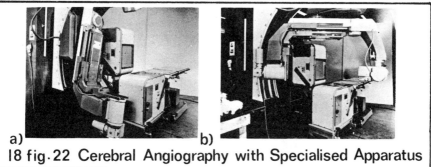

a)   b)
18 fig. 22 Cerebral Angiography with Specialised Apparatus

Both the simple skull stand and the specialised unit may only be used in one plane at a time. It is, therefore, possible to use a single film changer and a universal stand so that the one changer may be tilted to serve in examinations using horizontal or vertical X-ray beams.

With the ever increasing quality of fluorographic film and image detail of intensifiers, diagnostic cranial angiograms, using 70 mm fluorography or even 35 mm cine fluorography, are becoming a reasonable prospect. One would have the great advantage of being able to check whether the examination is a success by television fluoroscopy during filming. Cranial cine angiograms also offer the possibility of providing more evidence about cerebral blood flow.

Chapter 19

Serial Radiography

19.1 Introduction to Serial Radiography

In order to investigate lesions of the cardiovascular system which cannot be displayed by plain radiography, special techniques and equipment are required. A bolus of contrast medium is rapdily injected into a blood vessel and its progress along the vascular tree is followed by taking a rapid series of radiographs. As the rate of this series is impossible to attain with conventional equipment, special devices have been designed.

Equipment for rapid serial radiography using large film may be divided into two types, namely cassette changers which handle film in cassettes, and film changers which use film without cassettes. Cassette changers may be manually or automatically operated;whilst film changers, both cut film and roll film types, are power driven. Manual cassette changers may be operated at speeds of up to 1 exposure per second depending on the operator's dexterity. The automatic rapid cassette changers usually have a maximum exposure rate of 3 per second. Cut film changers have a maximum exposure rate of 6 per second and the roll film, 12 per second.

19.2 Manual Cassette Changers

Manual cassette changers are mainly used for cerebral angiography where the rate of blood flow is low. A typical unit shown is in 19 Fig. 1.

The diagram 19 Fig. 2 shows the basic construction of manual cassette changers. Each cassette is stoutly made with a handle or strap attached to one end. A thick lead sheet is fixed to the back so that no

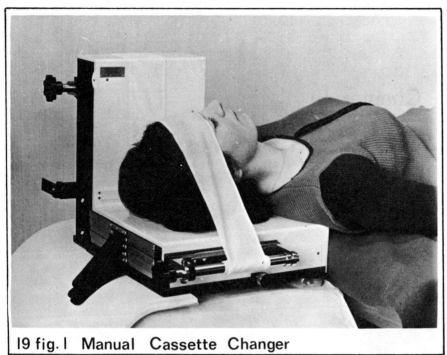

19 fig. I Manual Cassette Changer

radiation can pass through the cassette being exposed to fog subsequent cassettes in the pack. Three or five of these cassettes are held together in a holder by a large spring. After the first cassette has been exposed it is rapidly withdrawn, by pulling on the strap, and the spring presses the next cassette up against the grid ready for the second exposure. This sequence is continued for the rest of the cassettes.

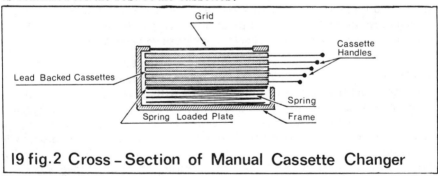

19 fig.2 Cross – Section of Manual Cassette Changer

19.3 Automatic Cassette Changers

Several types of automatic cassette changers are made for cassette sizes 24 x 30 cm, 35 x 70 cm, and 35 x 43 cm.

An example of an automatic cassette changer is shown in 19 Fig. 3.

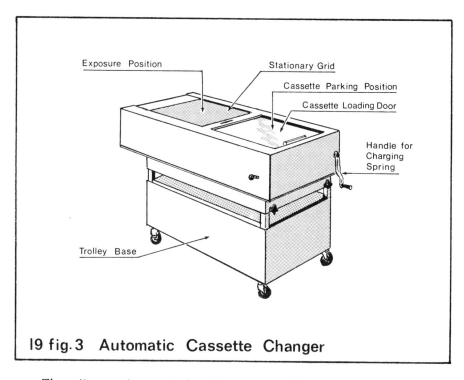

Exposure Position

Stationary Grid

Cassette Parking Position

Cassette Loading Door

Handle for
Charging
Spring

Trolley Base

19 fig. 3   Automatic Cassette Changer

The unit comprises a steel casing with nine cassette trays each
mounted on rails and lined with lead. The cassette trays each hold a
35 x 43 cm cassette. Prior to the exposure sequence the cassette trays are
all in the exposure position, one above the other under a stationary grid.
Each tray when loaded compresses a spring and is held in the exposure
position by a release catch and solenoid. After the first exposure, the top
catch is released and allows the spring to propel the uppermost tray to the
parking position where it is retained. The second exposure can then be
recorded on the next cassette. This sequence is controlled by a programme
selector and continues for up to nine cassettes. The programme selector
allows rates of one, two or three exposures per second or a single exposure.
Correct loading and the number of unexposed cassettes are indicated by
illuminated selector buttons.

This type is especially suited for abdominal and femoral arteriograms
where the increasing magnification with each film in the series is of little
consequence. This allows a higher exposure rate than is normal in a
manually operated cassette changer.

Cassette changers for 35 x 70 cm cassettes have been specially built
for use in aortography and arteriography of the lower limbs. They
can be placed under and coupled to a special bucky table with a fully floating
top. The table can be used separately for bucky examinations as a bucky
carriage and cassette tray are incorporated. When not in use the cassette
changer can be parked out of the way. For large differences in object

311

thickness a certain correction of radiation quality is required over the exposure area. This is effected with a wedge filter which is shaped to compensate for the reduction in thickness of, for example, the lower leg.

19.4 Automatic Film Changers

In angiocardiography (the examination of cardiac anatomy by means of contrast media injection) the rate of blood flow is too great for cassette changers to be of value. Automatic film changers have exposure rates of up to 12 exposures per second and are therefore designed for these examinations.

19.4.1 Cut Film Changer

The AOT cut film changer is the most common rapid film unit. They are available for two film sizes, namely 35 x 35 cm and 24 x 30 cm and are capable of exposure rates between 1 every 5 seconds and 6 per second. It is also possible to operate the film changer in a single exposure mode. A maximum of 30 films may be exposed in one run.

The photograph 19 Fig. 4 shows a pair of 35 x 35 cm AOT's on stand suitable for bi-plane operation. A single changer in the AP position with the loading magazine and take-up cassette partly inserted is shown in 19 Fig. 5.

When the film changer is operated the magazine is automatically opened, thus allowing the film to be advanced by two transport levers, protruding through holes in the magazine (19 Fig. 6). The film changer contains two sets of transport wheels, used for conveying the films. The first set of wheels advances the film from the open magazine to the exposure position, where it is compressed between two intensifying screens and pressure plates ready for exposure. After the film has been exposed it is advanced, by the second set of transport wheels, until it finally drops into a take-up magazine. When all exposures have been completed the take-up magazine is closed, by depressing a knob, then removed in daylight from the film changer, and taken to a normal darkroom to process the films. Before the loading magazine can be removed for reloading,the mechanism must be driven in reverse until the loading magazine is again adjacent to the door.

There are two types of control unit suitable for this film changer.

The velocity selector allows a series at one speed or a series of single exposures. The programme selector allows series of exposures at different rates with pause facilities. The programme selector shown in 19 Fig. 7 may control a pair of these film changers in bi-plane configuration.

The programmes may be varied by leaving gaps in the loading of films into the magazine. If films are missing the changer operates normally but an exposure is only initiated if there is a film between the intensifying screens actuating the exposure interlock micro-switch.

A device which automatically marks and numbers each film in a series of exposures, may be fitted. By inserting a patient data card, each film is automatically marked with the patients' name and number. A time marker

312

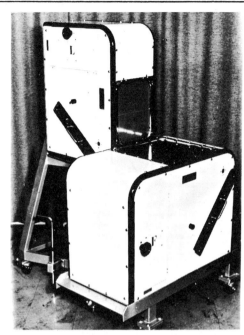

I9 fig.4 Bi~Plane Automatic Cut Film Changer

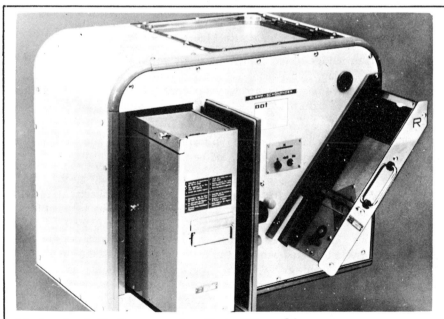

I9 fig.5 A.P. Automatic Cut Film Changer

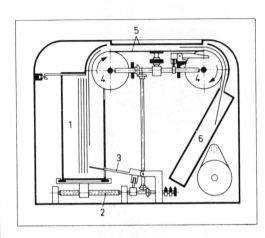

19 fig. 6 Principle of AOT Film Transport

is also incorporated which may be utilised, if required, instead of the numbering device.

19.4.2 Cut Film Changers with Fluoroscopic Facilities

The disadvantage of the cut film changer so far described is that it is impossible to conduct fluoroscopy without some inconvenience. Cut film changers have since been designed which permit fluoroscopy, although the maximum exposure rate may not be so high. Examples of such equipment are shown in 19 Fig. 8.

The Puck film changer is made in two types, type L and type U. The letter L or U indicates the path followed by the film.

The L type film changer has the take-up cassette at 90° to the exposure plane, whereas the type U film changer has its take-up cassette parallel to the exposure plane. With the U type, T.V. fluoroscopy may be used for positioning the patient and for control of catheterisation only whilst the take-up cassette is empty. Prior to taking a film series with the Puck U, a protective plate is inserted between the film plane and the take-up cassette. The L type may be used for TV fluoroscopy at any time during the programme and to check each exposure as it takes place, because the exposed films are not stored in the X-ray beam. The advantage of the U type is that it is more compact.

Both types will accept up to 20 films 35 x 35 cm in size. Each film is

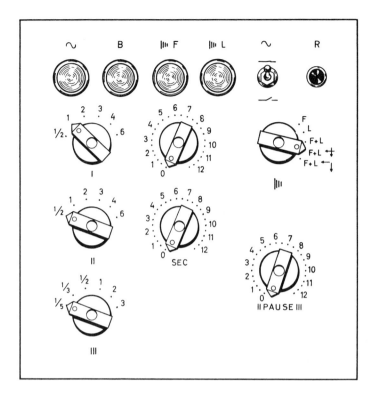

a) Programme Selector

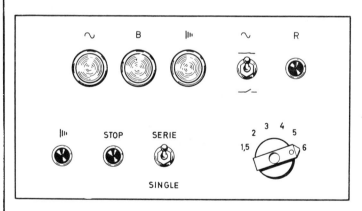

b) Velocity Selector

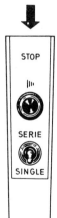

c) Handswitch

19 fig. 7   AOT   Control   Units

315

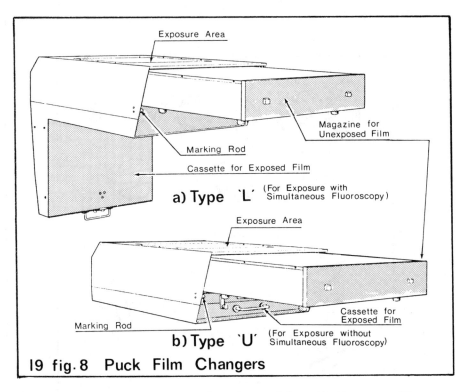

Exposure Area

Magazine for Unexposed Film

Marking Rod

Cassette for Exposed Film

a) Type `L´ (For Exposure with Simultaneous Fluoroscopy)

Exposure Area

Cassette for Exposed Film

Marking Rod

b) Type `U´ (For Exposure without Simultaneous Fluoroscopy)

19 fig. 8 Puck Film Changers

automatically marked with a serial number and the patient's name. The serial number changes with each film; the patient's name is inserted with a marking rod.

The principle of the film transport is as follows. On a command from the control unit a film is pushed by the film feeder on the loading magazine, through the feed rollers (See 19 Fig. 9). These feed the film into the exposure position, where the film is halted. The film is then compressed between a stationary intensifying screen and the moving pressure plate carrying another screen. The exposure then takes place, after which the film is released as the pressure plate is lowered, and the exit rollers drive the film into the take-up cassette. The marking rod holds the patient data strip and the patients' name is thus photographed onto the film in the exposure position.

This film changer is controlled by a programme selector and hand-switch as shown in 19 Fig. 10.

The programme selector controls the changer during both single exposures and programmed examinations. Programmed examinations are controlled by a computer punch card. The required programme is punched out by hand as shown in 19 Fig. 11 and then inserted into the cardholder in the programme selector. Punch card programme selectors are now becoming common with conventional cut film changers.

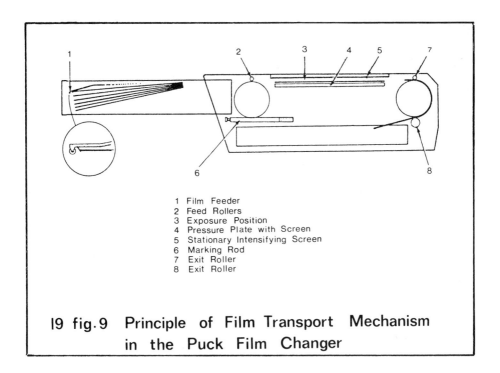

1 Film Feeder
2 Feed Rollers
3 Exposure Position
4 Pressure Plate with Screen
5 Stationary Intensifying Screen
6 Marking Rod
7 Exit Roller
8 Exit Roller

19 fig. 9 Principle of Film Transport Mechanism
in the Puck Film Changer

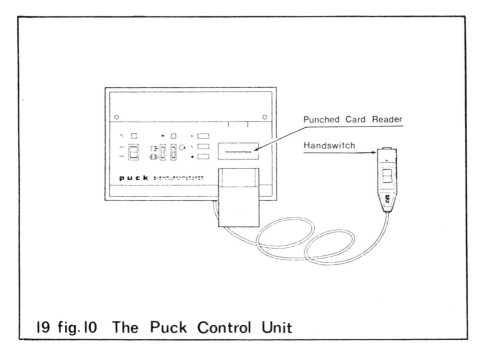

19 fig. 10 The Puck Control Unit

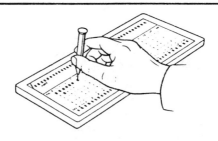

19 fig.11 Punching of Programme Card

19.4.3 Automatic Bi-plane Roll Film Changer

This unit, illustrated in 19 Fig. 12 may be used to make rapid serial radiographs in two perpendicular projections, on roll film 30 cm wide with a maximum length of 25 metres. The exposure rate is adjustable between one film in 10 seconds and 12 films per second. The exposure area of the lateral plane is 30 x 30 cm. and that of the frontal plane 35 x 30 cm. The unit was designed for angiocardiography and abdominal arteriography of children and adults.

The roll film changer is mounted on a mobile stand which can be raised and lowered. It is also possible to rotate the roll film changer about a horizontal axis which passes through the lateral exposure plane.

The film changer housing is a light-tight metal cabinet. The method of film transport is shown in 19 Fig. 13.

The rolls of films must be inserted into the changer under safelight conditions. The film is fed from the supply spools, between the intensifying screens, and the transport rollers, to the take-up spools. During film transport the rear screen, attached to the pressure plate is separated from the front screen which is stationary, thus allowing movement of the film. When the required amount of film has passed, it is braked and re-compressed between the screens. A single motor drives the entire mechanism for both planes. This motor has two speeds, one twice the other, corresponding to two of the possible exposure rates. Other rates are achieved by pulsing the electrical supply to the motor on and off.

A programme selector similar to that used for AOT film changers controls the rate and sequence of radiographs.

19.5 Processing and Viewing Angiograms

Radiographs from cassette changers and cut film changers may be processed and viewed in the normal way. However, in view of the large number of films produced in an angio examination, especially in bi-plane work, it is desirable to provide special viewing facilities. Automatic film display units have been designed which enable a large number of cut films to be presented simultaneously (See 19 Fig. 14).

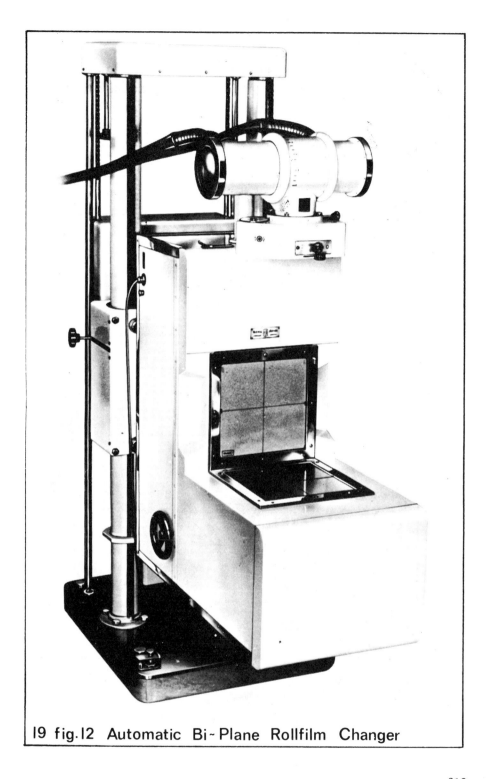

19 fig.12 Automatic Bi-Plane Rollfilm Changer

Groups of radiographs can be selected at will from a storage magazine.

Roll film presents special difficulties with regard to conventional processing and viewing as the film may be up to 25 metres in length. Processing of roll film is less of a problem with roller type automatic film processors except for the excessive processing time required because of its length. However, for manual processing of roll film a giant spiral film tank is available, similar in principle to that used for processing 70 mm or 35 mm film. Large film dryers are also available, again similar to those used for manually processed 70 mm film. In order to view roll film angiograms it is possible to cut the roll into a series of single radiographs, but this

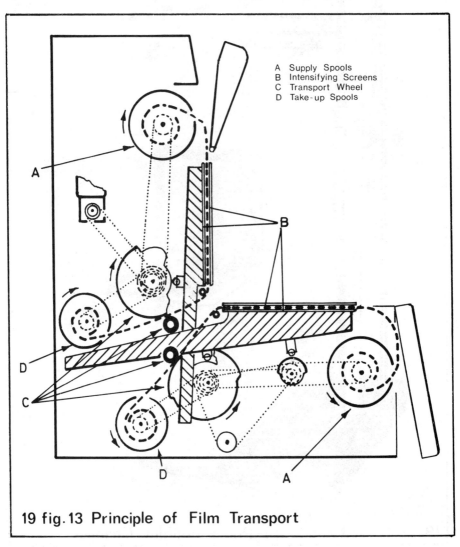

A Supply Spools
B Intensifying Screens
C Transport Wheel
D Take-up Spools

19 fig. 13 Principle of Film Transport

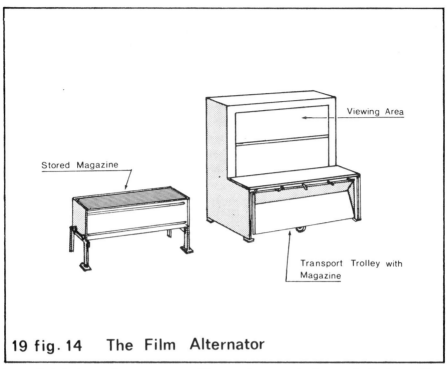

19 fig. 14   The Film Alternator

immediately loses the sequence. The most convenient way of viewing roll film is to use two three channel viewing boxes one above the other for the frontal and lateral views. At both ends of each box a roller mechanism with handles is fitted, so that the films may be rolled backwards and forwards as desired. It is then also possible to keep the lateral and frontal films in register with each other.

19.6 Injectors

In peripheral and cerebral arteriography it is usually possible to inject the required amount of contrast medium manually with a conventional syringe. However, intra-cardiac and great vessel blood flow is so fast that it is necessary to inject a bolus of contrast medium with great rapidity. This is difficult to do manually as catheters have narrow lumens and contrast medium has a high viscosity.

The above requirement led to the design of automatic injectors. There are two main types, pneumatically and motor operated. The former type consists of a pneumatic ram which bears upon the piston of the loaded syringe. The latter consists of a motor driven lead-screw coupled to the syringe piston.

Due to the high rate of blood flow it is usual to initiate the radiographic series by adjustable contacts on the injector, so that the series may begin as soon as the contrast medium has been injected. The injection itself may be initiated by a heart phase triggering device as described in Section 21.11.1.

The most advanced injectors may also make fractional injections in synchronism with cardiac function.

19.7 Event Marking

In angiocardiography it is of great advantage to know exactly in which phase of the heart each film was taken and also how much dye had been injected at any stage. It is possible to record these events in conjunction with the physiological recording apparatus. The tracing in 19 Fig. 15 shows a typical example of such a recording.

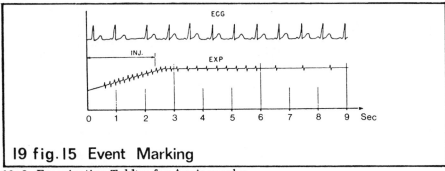

19 fig. 15   Event Marking

19.8 Examination Tables for Angiography

In smaller departments where arteriograms are not often carried out it is necessary to use existing equipment such as a tilting diagnostic table (See 19 Fig. 16). This may be adapted for angiography by the addition of a sliding table top.

It can be used in conjunction with cut film changers or cassette changers and still allows the possibility of TV fluoroscopy with the image intensifier. This offers optimum facilities for insertion of the catheter under fluoroscopic control. Two versions are available, one with a serial shift device which is motor driven and one for manual operation. The serial shift device allows stepwise movement of the table top between exposures during femoral arteriography of the lower limb. Each step takes one second and the X-ray tube voltage is automatically reduced from step to step, to allow for the decreasing thickness down the limb. When not in use the angio sliding table top is removed from the diagnostic table.

In departments where many vascular examinations are carried out a table as shown in 19 Fig. 17 is a great advantage.

The floating table top is fitted with electromagnetic brakes. Automatic serial shift is programmed by selector buttons. Again the X-ray tube voltage is automatically reduced from step to step.

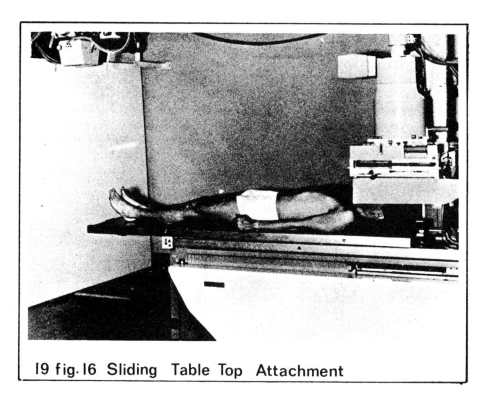

19 fig. 16 Sliding Table Top Attachment

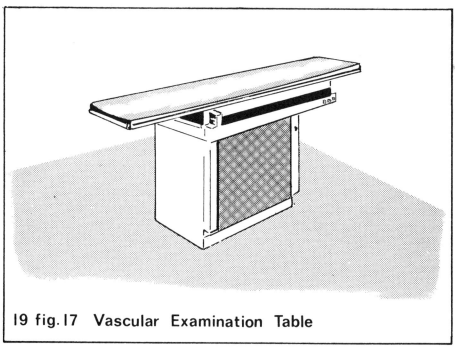

19 fig. 17 Vascular Examination Table

The size of an image on a direct radiograph is always larger than the object under examination due to the magnification which is dependent on the ratio of object-film and focus-object distances. This results in the need for films which may be as large as 43 x 35 cm for a chest examination. Film of this size is expensive and bulky to store. This has led to the development of photo-fluorographic cameras which will record the radiographic image, reduced in size, on small film.

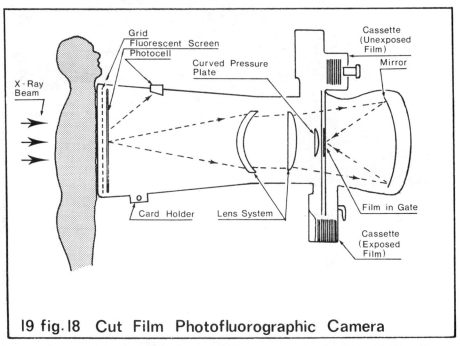

19 fig. 18   Cut Film Photofluorographic Camera

An example of a photo fluorographic camera is shown in 19 Fig. 18. A light image, formed on the fluorescent screen, is reduced in size and focussed onto film by a mirror-lens system. The entire assembly is light-tight. This system improves the light gathering ability. In the model illustrated, cut film (100 x 100 mm) is automatically fed from the feeder cassette into the gate where it is held for the exposure. The light from one point on the fluorescent screen can take many paths to one point on the film, therefore the film transport mechanism can be placed in the beam of light without producing problems. In a similar way the diaphragm in a normal camera lens system controls the light gathering capacity without affecting the angle of view. Once an exposure is completed, the film automatically feeds into the reception cassette. This cassette can be removed periodically for processing of the films. Alternatively the camera can be coupled to an automatic processor into which the exposed films are fed directly and which produces a miniature radiograph within minutes of the exposure.

A few more refinements make the camera ideal for mass surveys. The patients' data can be written onto a card which is inserted into a holder. During the exposure, the information on the card is automatically recorded on the film with the radiographic image of the patient. An interlock prevents another exposure until the card is exchanged, in order to minimise the risk of incorrect film identification.

A further refinement is the addition of photo-timing facilities. A photocell (usually the photo-multiplier type described in Chapter 10) views a section of the fluorescent screen and automatically cuts off the exposure at the correct density level.

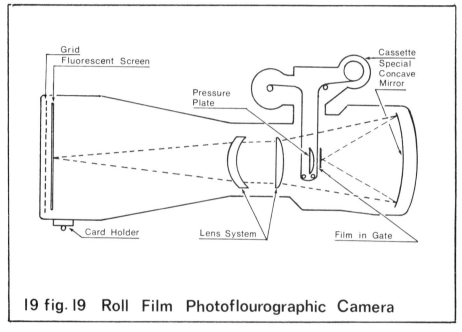

19 fig. 19   Roll   Film   Photoflourographic   Camera

A photo-fluorographic camera employing roll film (70 mm wide) is shown in 19 Fig. 19. The film is wound on automatically between exposures by the motorized cassette. Alternatively a hand wound cassette can be inserted.

Due to the high contrast and detail, photo-fluorographs are comparable to large-size radiographs. A grid is fitted in the camera to improve contrast by reducing the effect of scattered radiation. The 100 mm cut film camera offers greater flexibility in viewing and filing by producing individual photo-fluorographs. However the cost of film per exposure is less for the 70 mm version. Part of the saving in film cost for both cameras is due to the fact that the film used, unlike standard X-ray film, has emulsion only on one side of the base.

The miniature film is normally viewed magnified by a lens or projection system. Special processing and viewing equipment is available for 70 mm and 100 mm roll and cut film.

Photo fluorographic cameras are mainly used in routine chest surveys. Angled versions are available for undertable use which can be fitted with a rapid sequence cassette for up to 6 exposures per second and therefore may be used for arteriography.

One important disadvantage of this type of photofluorography is the increased radiation dose to the patient, over full size film radiography.

Chapter 20

Test Equipment and Fault Diagnosis

20.1 Test Equipment

20.1.1 The Spinning Top

The accuracy of an exposure timer, especially where exposures of under one second are involved, is very important. A simple way of testing this accuracy is with the spinning top. This consists of a metal disc in which one small hole is drilled near the circumference, and which is mounted on a pointed stem upon which it can be made to spin like a top (See 20 Fig. 1).

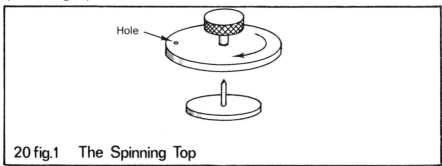

Hole

20 fig.1   The Spinning Top

To test the timer, the spinning top is placed on a loaded cassette (or double wrapped film) and the disc is spun while a radiograph is made with the tube positioned vertically over the spinning top. Each succeeding X-ray

pulse finds the hole of the spinning top in a different position on the circle
and irradiates the film over a very small area. When the film is developed
a series of dots will appear forming an arc of a circle (See 20 Fig. 2). The
speed of rotation of the top determines the spacing of these dots.   It is
obvious that if the speed is too slow, the dots will be very close together and
if the speed is too high, more than 1 revolution will be completed and the
dots will overlap.

Suppose now we have a fully-rectified, single phase unit and set the
timer for 0.10 sec. A 50 Hz supply, when fully rectified, produces 100 pulses
per second and hence 10 peaks in 0.10 sec. Therefore, if the timer is
accurate there should be 10 dots on our test film (20 Fig. 2).

With self-rectification (or half-wave rectification) only five dots will
be produced during 0.10 sec on 50 Hz. On three phase, 6 valve rectification,
due to the proximity of the dots and possibly the smoothing effect in the
circuit, a continuous band is produced with a series of denser zones. There
will be 30 of these denser zones in a 0.10 sec exposure

For a 60 Hz supply, the H.T. waveform will have a different pulse
frequency, producing a proportionately higher number of dots for the same
exposure time.

Generator type	H.T. Waveform	Appearance of test film
HALF - WAVE RECTIFIED (single pulse)	∩ ∩ ∩ ∩ ∩ 0·1 sec	5 dots
FULL - WAVE RECTIFIED (two pulse)	∿∿∿∿∿∿∿∿ 0·1 sec	10 dots
RECTIFIED THREE PHASE (six pulse)	‿‿‿‿‿‿‿‿‿‿‿ 0·1 sec	30 Dense Zones

20 fig. 2   Spinning Top Results (50 Hz Supply)

When a generator employs 12 pulse rectification or a smoothed H.T.
supply, the spinning top film will show a continuous black band. The
exposure time can then only be checked if the top is rotated at a known

constant speed and the length of arc measured.

The spinning top is of great value as a piece of test equipment, but care must be exercised in assessing the results. Suppose, for instance, a spinning top test is being conducted on a unit employing full-wave rectification at 0.10 sec and only 5 dots appear. This would indicate that the timer is operating for only 0.05 sec; but the timer could be working correctly while a rectifier failure in the H.T. generator is causing the unit to "half-wave".

20.1.2 The Timing Pencil

This consists of a solenoid coil with a metal core which is free to move. A short piece of pencil lead is fitted into the end of this core (20 Fig. 3). The leads from the coil are connected to the H.T. primary leads at a point in the circuit after the timer H.T. contactor. During an exposure the coil will be supplied with the H.T. primary voltage and the core will vibrate at the same frequency as the mains supply. Therefore if the pencil is moved over a piece of paper during the exposure period, dots will be produced.

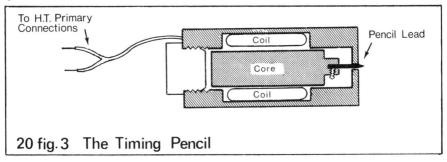

To H.T. Primary Connections

Pencil Lead

Coil

Core

Coil

20 fig. 3 The Timing Pencil

For single phase, full-wave rectification, the same number of dots will be produced as with the spinning top. However, used on a self rectified unit for an exposure of 0.10 sec, a timing pencil will produce 10 dots compared with the 5 produced by a spinning top. The pencil cannot be conveniently used in a three phase circuit as there are three primary H.T. coils to consider.

The timing pencil is a quicker method of checking than the spinning top, as it does not involve a developing procedure. However the spinning top does have the added advantage of proving that the H.T. rectifying circuit is functioning correctly.

20.1.3 The Step Wedge

X-radiation will penetrate a substance to varying degrees depending upon the thickness, the atomic number of the substance and the wavelength of the radiation. It has been shown in earlier chapters that the wavelength of radiation is proportional to the kV across the X-ray tube. If a wedge is made up in equal steps of a material of a certain atomic number (See 20

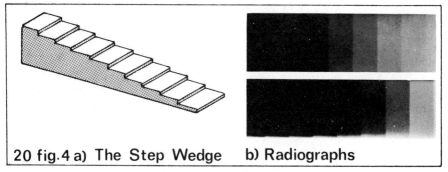

Fig. 4a), the penetration of each step will depend upon the applied kV.

If this wedge is placed on a cassette or double wrapped film and an exposure made, the resulting film will show, after development, a graduated pattern of film blackening corresponding to the steps (See 20 Fig. 4b). For X-ray units which have a kV range of 40 - 150 kV, the wedge is usually made of 3 mm steps of aluminium, but for low kV units, a more suitable material is perspex which has a lower absorption coefficient.

Although the step wedge cannot be used for direct measurement of kV, it can be used to compare the kV calibration on different mA ranges, for one tube. This test is usually only carried out at the time of manufacture and installation to verify that the kV compensation voltages (see Chapter 9) have been correctly set. The kV control is set to a certain value and step wedge films taken at each available mA setting, such that the mAs product is constant throughout the test. For example, if the check is being carried out on a 150 kV generator, the chosen tension may be 70 kV and the series of exposures in the order of 50 mA x 0.8 s, 100 mA x 0.4 s, 200 mA x 0.2s, and 400 mA x 0.1 s; each exposure giving 40 mAs. The resultant films should, after development, be of comparable density.

It is important to check, before each exposure, that the desired kV value and mains adaption adjustment are correctly set, otherwise the results of the test will be misleading. To avoid errors in developing, it is usual for all exposures to be made on one film, using a lead mask which allows only one strip of film to be exposed at a time.

20.1.4 The Pinhole Camera

We do not normally need to measure the size of the focal spot of an X-ray tube after manufacture. The accurate determination of actual focus size requires specialised equipment and a detailed definition of the criteria involved. It is sufficient here to describe the principle of the pinhole camera technique employed in this measurement.

Suppose we have an elongated source of light A - B (20 Fig. 5a) and a screen C - D. If there is no diaphragm between them, the screen C - D will be uniformly and diffusely illuminated by light from every point of A - B. If, however, we place between the source and screen a sheet of opaque

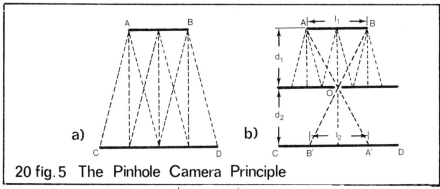

20 fig.5 The Pinhole Camera Principle

material having a pinhole at 0(20 Fig. 5b), then from each point along A - B, a very narrow pencil of rays will pass through 0 to a definite point on C - D.

There will then be produced on C - D an inverted image of A - B (B' - A'), and if the distances d_1 and d_2 are equal, we see (from similar triangles) that the image size will be exactly equal to the source. If the distances d_1 and d_2 are not equal, the source size can be obtained from the formula:-

$$I_1 \text{ (source size)} = \frac{I_2 \times d_1}{d_2}$$

This theory can be used to measure the size of an X-ray tube focal spot if the diaphragm is made out of a radio-opaque material (i.e. lead) and the screen replaced by a piece of double wrapped film.

Factors which cause a variation in the focal spot size are discussed in Chapter 8.

20.1.5 Kilovoltage Measurement

Until recently, the only way of checking the peak kilovoltage applied across an X-ray tube was that of connecting a spark gap in parallel with the tube.

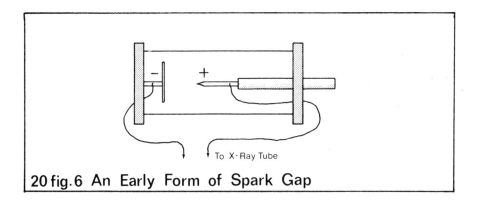

To X-Ray Tube

20 fig.6 An Early Form of Spark Gap

Originally, this consisted of a pointed rod and flat plate positioned in a glass housing, such that the point could be moved (20 Fig. 6). With high tension applied to the X-ray tube, the pointed stem was moved towards the plate until a spark jumped between the two electrodes. This gap was a measure of the kilvoltage across the tube. Unfortunately the instrument could not be accurately calibrated because the distance that the spark could jump also depended upon the humidity of the air and the corona discharge from the point.

It was found, however, that if the point and plate were replaced by polished copper spheres, the results were more consistent and a calibration table could be drawn up :-

Peak Kilovoltage	50	70	90	110	130	150
Spark gap in cm (for 10 cm spheres)	1.6	2.4	3.3	4.2	5.4	6.6

The copper sphere spark gap is only slightly affected by humidity (which can be allowed for in accurate measurement) and is still in use today. Such a unit is shown below (20 Fig. 7).

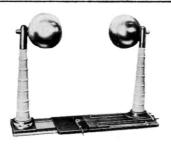

20 fig.7 The Sphere Spark Gap

The spheres are connected in parallel with the X-ray tube, via high value resistances to limit the spark current, and are mounted on insulating columns. One of these columns is fixed, while the other is movable but held back by a spring. With the aid of a cord it can be pulled towards the fixed column, against the action of the spring, and in moving forward it pushes a slider over a scale calibrated in kilovolts. With H.T. applied to the tube, the movable sphere is drawn towards the fixed one and, at the instant a spark jumps the gap, the peak kV is read off the scale.

Risks are involved in the use of this piece of test equipment, especially in hospitals, due to the danger of electric shock from the exposed high tension. A fairly recent innovation is the Philips electronic kV meter which has no exposed high tension and is not affected by humidity. This portable unit consists of two potential dividers and an electronic measuring unit. The potential divider is made up from high value resistors connected in series, between the H.T. cable receptacles and earth. The complete network is contained in a metal tank filled with oil

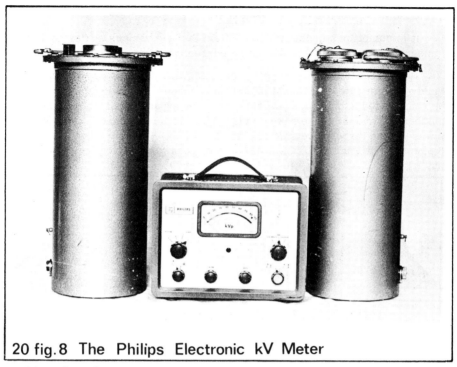

20 fig.8 The Philips Electronic kV Meter

and is referred to as a "pot".

The H.T. cables from the generator are plugged into the measuring "pots" which are then connected to the X-ray tube via short H.T. cables (See 20 Fig. 9). These "pots" scale down the H.T. voltage by a factor of 2000 and this signal voltage is fed to the electronic measuring unit, where it is used to charge a capacitor. The voltage developed across the capacitor is measured by an electronic circuit and displayed on a moving coil meter, whose deflection is then directly proportional to the kV across the X-ray tube. As the voltage across the capacitor does not disappear immediately the exposure finishes, the meter continues reading until it is reset, thus making it possible to measure the applied kV even though the exposure time may be very short. Once again the measurement recorded is the peak kV value.

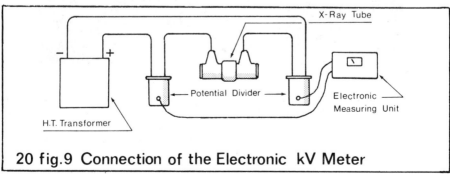

20 fig.9 Connection of the Electronic kV Meter

20.1.6 Tomography Test Equipment

It is sometimes necessary to confirm that the various scales on linear tomographic apparatus are indicating correctly.

Equipment to test the accuracy of tomographic planes need not be highly sophisticated, but must be carefully made. A simple phantom can be constructed using a block of balsa wood or expanded polystyrene and a number of straight dressmaking pins. With the block stood on its base, one pin is pushed through the side at a height of 1 cm , two pins at 2 cm , 3 pins at 3 cm and so in a similar progression to a vertical height of say 10 cm. (See 20 Fig. 10).

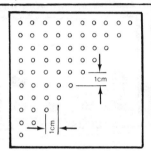

20 fig.10   A simple Tomographic Phantom for depth of cut.

The horizontal pins should also be spaced by 1 cm and all pins carefully placed so that they are parallel to the base of the block.

The assembly is placed on the tomographic table so that the axis of the pins is at right angles to the tube movement, and the fulcrum point of the machine aligned with any of the horizontal levels of pins. A radiograph is made, and when the film has been processed, the number of pins to be seen most clearly gives the height of the sectioned plane from the table top. (See 20 Fig. 11). This should, of course, coincide with the indication on the layer height scale.

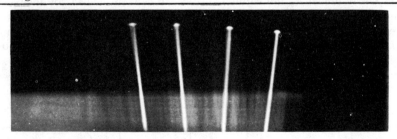

20 fig. 11 Layer Height Tomographic Test Film

Another interesting experiment that can be carried out on tomographic equipment is that of measuring the thickness of the defined layer obtained by using different angles of tube swing. The phantom for this test is similar to that described above, utilising the test block. A line is drawn

on the side of the block at 45° to the base and a number of pins pushed
through the side on this line at a spacing of 2 mm from each other   (See
20 Fig. 12). The fulcrum point of the apparatus is carefully aligned with
one of the pins (preferably one in the middle of the slope) and a tomograph
taken with a narrow angle of exposure set (say 25°). While this film is
being processed, another is taken with a wider angle of exposure set
(say 50°). A comparison of the two films will show that the wider angle of
exposure gives a thinner cut, and the actual thickness of cut can be
determined by the number of pins to be seen clearly (See 20 Fig. 13)

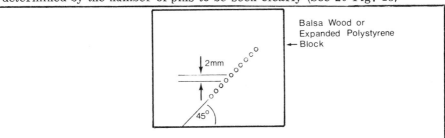

20 fig.12 Tomographic Test Phantom for thickness of cut.

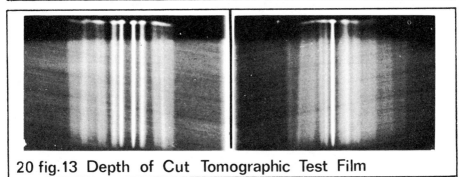

20 fig.13 Depth of Cut Tomographic Test Film

20.2 Measuring Instruments

Let us suppose that we have some instrument which will register a
change when a current flows through it. If we place this instrument M in a
circuit as shown in 20 Fig. 14 , it will indicate the current which is

20 fig.14 Current Indication   20 fig.15 Voltage Indication

flowing through the load P. The instrument M must have as low a resistance as possible, so that it will not add more than is absolutely necessary to the total resistance of the circuit.

If the same instrument M is placed in the position shown in 20 Fig. 15 , and the device still has a very low resistance, it will obviously allow all the current to flow through it and none will flow through the load P. It will, in fact, short circuit the supply. If, however, we make the resistance of the instrument very much higher, only a very small current flows through the instrument, whilst the bulk of the current from the supply will still flow through P. This small current must, however, obey Ohm's law of $V = IR$, and as the resistance of the instrument is constant, the current through it is directly proportional to the voltage. The instrument can therefore be calibrated directly in volts.

Thus the same type of instrument can read current, when it has low resistance, and voltage when its resistance is high. It is called an ammeter in the first case and a voltmeter in the second (See Section 20.2.4).

There are two main types of such instruments commonly employed in X-ray units. They are known as the moving-iron and moving-coil meters.

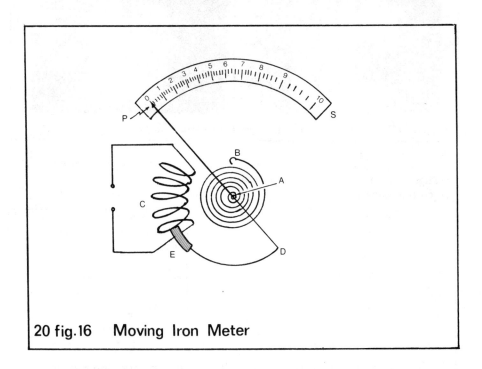

20 fig.16   Moving Iron Meter

20.2.1 The Moving-Iron Meter

A pointer 'P' moving over a scale 'S' (20 Fig. 16) is pivoted on an axle at 'A'. It is kept at rest on the zero line of the scale, when no current is flowing, by means of a spiral spring 'B'. Attached to the other end of the pointer is a short curved arm 'D' which carries a small block of iron 'E'. This can move into or out of a coil of wire 'C', the ends of which are connected into the circuit. When a current flows in 'C' it acts as a magnet and therefore pulls the iron block into the centre of the coil. The pull is resisted by the spiral spring 'B' and the pointer 'P' comes to rest at some point on the scale 'S'. The greater the current, the greater is the magnetism of 'C' and the greater therefore is the pull on 'E'. This relationship unfortunately is not a linear one, so the scale requires careful calibration.

The moving iron meter does however, have one great advantage, in that it can be used on either direct current (D.C.) or alternating currents (A.C.) because the effect of the current in the coil 'C' and the attraction on the iron 'E' is the same in both cases. In fact it can be used to indicate the R.M.S. (root mean square) value of any alternating waveform.

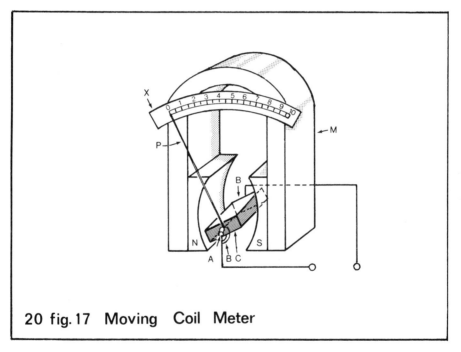

20 fig. 17 Moving Coil Meter

20.2.2 The Moving Coil Meter

Here a coil of wire 'C' is suspended on an axle 'A' between the poles of a permanent horseshoe magnet 'M' (See 20 Fig. 17) and a pointer 'P' is attached to it. Spiral springs 'B' keep the coil 'C' at rest when no current is flowing, in a position such that the pointer is then at rest on the zero line of the scale 'X'.

When a current flows through the coil, the latter acts as a magnet. Thus, remembering that unlike magnetic poles attract each other, the N pole formed in one face of the coil by the current flow will assume a position, against the restoring forces of the spiral springs, such that it is nearer the S pole of the permanent magnet. In doing this the pointer P moves over the scale 'X'.

The greater the current, the greater the force which pulls the coil around against the restoring force of the springs. With careful shaping of the permanent magnet pole faces, the relationship between pointer rotation and current flow through the coil can be made to be a linear one, simplifying the scale calibration.

The moving coil meter does have a disadvantage in that it can only be used with current which does not change its direction of flow (D.C. current). This is obvious when we remember that the magnetic polarity of the coil faces depends on the direction of flow of current. An alternating current (A.C. current) would therefore tend to make the coil and the pointer oscillate, which in effect would mean that neither would move.

20.2.3 The Milliampere-second (mAs) Meter

In order to obtain a radiograph which, after development, will have an optimum density, it is necessary to apply a certain tube tension (kV) and a certain tube current (mA) to the X-ray tube for a certain time. The product of the current and the time for which it flows is known as the milliampere-second (mAs) value.

A meter which will measure mAs is especially useful in the calibration of an X-ray unit, because exposures of less than 1 second do not give a milliampere (mA) meter sufficient time to give an accurate indication.

The construction of the mAs meter is essentially the same as that of a moving coil meter (See Section 20.2.2), except that the two spiral springs 'B' are replaced by a damping mechanism. The coil is thus free to rotate when current is passed through it and the distance the pointer moves across the scale depends upon the magnitude of the current and the time for which it flows. Since there is no spring to restore the pointer to zero after the exciting current has died down, the operator can read the mAs indication easily, even though the exposure time may be very short. Once the meter has been read, the pointer can be returned to zero either by a mechanical lever, or by passing a small current in the opposite direction, depending upon the meter type. As the pointer has a tendency to "creep" across the scale when it is not in use, it is important that the operator should zero the meter immediately prior to an exposure and read the indication as soon as the exposure has ended.

20.2.4 Meter Shunts and Multipliers.

On a high powered X-ray generator, the milliampere (mA) meter might be required to indicate a maximum of say, 1000 mA. If the meter had only one range, the tube current used for fluoroscopy (0.5 to 4 mA) would hardly register on the scale. It is obvious then, that the mA meter must have more than one scale and it is common to find desk mA meters with three ranges :- one for fluoroscopic currents (0 - 5 mA) and two for radiographic currents (0 - 100 mA and 0 - 1000 mA). (See 20 Fig. 18).

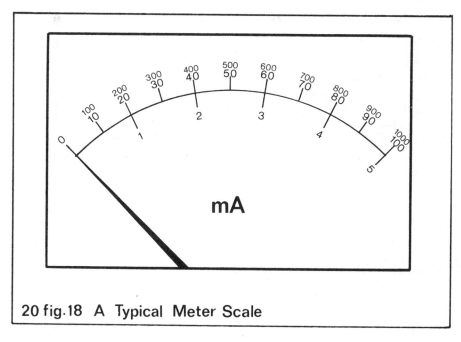

20 fig.18 A Typical Meter Scale

The basic meter movement commonly used for the mA meter is of the moving coil type because, having a linear scale, it is easy to read and is relatively robust. Suppose that a moving coil meter has a full scale deflection (f.s.d.) of 1 mA. This means that 1 mA passing through the coil moves the pointer as far across the scale as it can go. If this instrument is required to measure 5 mA it will be necessary to connect a resistor in parallel with it, so that only 1 mA goes through the meter and the other 4 mA goes through the resistor (known as a shunt). Thus for our 3 scale mA meter, there is a different shunt for each range of current, the shunts being lower in resistance as the range of current to be measured becomes higher.

In 20 Fig. 19 , switch S1 is shown in the 100 mA position. With 100 mA entering the circuit, R2 passes 99 mA leaving 1 mA to drive the meter to full deflection. The bridge rectifier D1 - D4 is necessary because a moving coil meter will only work on D.C. current (see Section

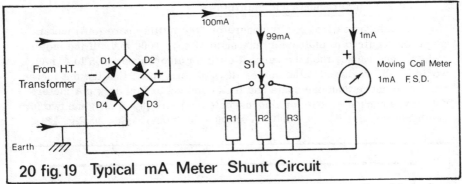

20 fig.19 Typical mA Meter Shunt Circuit

20.2.2). In a modern X-ray desk,the switch S1 would be replaced by relay contacts which automatically select the correct shunt for the meter. Thus, when fluoroscopy is selected, the tube current is read from the inner scale of 20 Fig. 18 . For radiographic currents of up to 100 mA, the lower of the two outer scales is used,and for radiographic currents greater than 100 mA the outermost scale is automatically selected.

A similar system of shunts would be fitted to the mAs meter (Section 20.2.3) to give suitable ranges, e.g. 10 mAs, 30 mAs, 100 mAs and 300 mAs full scale deflection.

At the beginning of this section (under 20.2) it was stated that the basic meter movement could be used to construct a voltmeter, providing that its resistance was high. With most meter coils this is not the case, so we have to connect a large value resistor (called a "multiplier") in series with the meter to increase its resistance (See 20 Fig. 20).

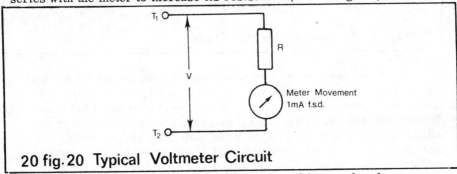

20 fig.20 Typical Voltmeter Circuit

In this circuit, the multiplier resistor R will have to be of a sufficiently high value to pass only 1 mA when the maximum voltage to be measured is applied to the terminals T_1 and T_2.

20.3 Radiographic Calibration

When a new X-ray control desk is delivered to a hospital it usually has been calibrated in the factory, using standard X-ray tubes and a nominal mains supply. The installing engineer has then to adjust the unit to suit the local mains supply and the X-ray tubes with which the room is to be equipped.

After connecting the X-ray desk to the mains supply and wiring in the ancilliary equipment, the engineer's first task is to switch on and check the operation of the Radiographic timer. This test is carried out with the H.T. transformer primary leads disconnected, and in the case of a 4 pulse unit, a timing pencil (See Section 20.1.2) is used to check the accuracy of the timer. If the unit is a 6 or 12 pulse generator, the engineer will have to use more sophisticated test equipment. The next step is to match the unit to the local mains resistance. Most X-ray generators are factory calibrated on a "worst case" mains resistance of about 0.5Ω and if the hospital mains supply is lower than this, extra resistance, called "padding resistance", will have to be added until the mains resistance plus the padding resistance equals 0.5Ω.

The unit is then ready to be adjusted for the X-ray tubes supplied. The following steps will also have to be carried out if an X-ray tube is replaced due to failure.

Each new X-ray tube is supplied with a radiographic rating chart, which is used by the engineer for setting the maximum kV limit and tube overload circuits. Most units can cope with a selection of different tubes so these limits will have to be set on each tube selection.

After certain other low tension checks have been made, the H.T. transformer primary leads are connected and each X-ray tube is "run in", using continuous fluoroscopy. This commences with settings of say 2.0 mA, 50 kV and the voltage is gradually increased in 5 kV steps during a period of 10 minutes, to 2.0 mA, 120 kV; after which the tube voltage is held at 120 kV for a further 10 minutes. During running in, some "disturbances" may occur, indicated by a sudden kick on the mA meter and sometimes accompanied by an audible "tick" from the shield. Under these circumstances, the kV must be immediately reduced by 10 - 15 kV and gradually increased again. A "disturbance" is a temporary breakdown of the vacuum insulation between the anode and cathode and, at this stage, is usually caused by the ionising of residual gas between the two electrodes. The object of running in is to try and make this gas settle in a safe part of the tube, such as the inside of the cathode structure.

Providing that the tube has "run in" satisfactorily, and been allowed to cool, a start can be made on setting up the radiographic tube currents. For a medium powered generator, a series of test exposures are made at say 90 kV, 0.1 second on the 300 mA range and the tube current adjusted until the mAs meter reads exactly 30 mAs.

With the same time and mA selected, the kV is set to a low value and another exposure made. If the mAs indication is now either too high or too low, compensation adjustments will have to be made for the "space charge effect" (See Chapter 7). It is extremely important that sufficient time is allowed between exposures for the tube to cool. Failure to do so will result in the tube overheating (See Chapter 8).

Once the unit has been calibrated so that the mA is consistent over the kV range, a test film is taken with the step wedge (Section 20.1.3), to check that the kV is constant throughout the mA range. Any discrepancies shown by the film can be corrected by adjusting the kV compensation (See Chapter 9).

20.4 Fault Diagnosis

In a continual effort to make X-ray equipment safer and more simple to operate, its design is becoming increasingly complex, both electrically and mechanically. It is important, therefore, that the radiographer should be able to analyse the symptoms of faulty equipment behaviour in order that the manufacturer's service department may be given an accurate fault diagnosis. This is becoming increasingly important as service engineers are having to carry specialised test equipment (for example oscilloscopes for closed circuit television). Thus, if a concise telephone report is given to the service department, an engineer, equipped with the relevant spare parts and tools can be sent, with an obvious saving in time and subsequent cost.

It would be impossible, within the scope of this book, to detail all the faults that could occur, but a logical check list for an X-ray control desk which fails to expose could be :-

(a) Can the generator H.T. switch be heard to change over when another tube selection is made?

(b) Does the preparation cycle sound normal?

(c) Is the tube overload warning light on?

(d) Can the tube anode rotation be heard?

(e) Does the mA meter register?

(f) Is the fault common to both focii of the faulty tube?

(g) Does the fault condition occur with other auxiliary apparatus associated with the same tube?

(h) It is possible to carry out fluoroscopy on the faulty tube using very low factors?

(i) Does this fault occur on another tube?

A similar procedure could be adopted for an X-ray table which refuses to tilt :-

(a) Have the horizontal or vertical position stop switches been selected?

(b) Are all the other table movements normal? (If not, ask the hospital engineer to check the main fuses).

(c) Is the fault common to both directions of table tilt?

(d) Are the safety stop bars on the moving table top free to move and operating correctly?

(e) Are there any obstructions such as foot stools, patient's chairs or footswitches causing other safety stops to operate?

Simple tests such as these can often isolate the fault and may even show that the malfunction is simply due to operator's error. In either case an accurate diagnosis may save valuable time in restoring the equipment to full working order.

20.5 Equipment Care and Maintenance

In any hospital the X-ray department is one of the most expensive to equip and maintain. A large number of breakdowns could be avoided by considerate use and simple routine maintenance.

20.5.1 Diagnostic Tables

Any liquid is a potential hazard to X-ray equipment. Examination tables are not usually equipped with water-tight covers, so liquids used in their vicinity should be handled carefully as a spill could provide an electrical short-circuit within the equipment.

In the course of a barium session, it is not unknown for drinks to be spilled and enemas to go out of control. The table should be "mopped up" at once if possible, but it should be ensured that the table and serial changer are thoroughly clean at the end of the session. This routine procedure will save staff the time consuming task of removing barium sulphate which has dried and hardened. Remnant opaque media on the table may produce artefacts.

The catheterization table in its turn is susceptible to jets of contrast media being sprayed from the needle of a syringe during the process of eliminating air from the injector prior to injection.

20.5.2 Tubestands and Tracks

X-ray equipment designers always try to provide easy movement of the tube column, whether it is ceiling mounted or runs on floor tracks. It is important, therefore, that this careful design is not abused by letting any of the movements hit their end stops violently, as this could result in permanent damage to the tube as well as the column. An X-ray tube subjected to this sort of mechanical shock may suffer a fractured filament or even a shattered insert.

With floor mounted tube columns, a common problem is the failure of a motorised column to move during tomography. This is often due to the accumulation of dust and grit in the floor track which is not removed by normal floor cleaning. This dirt may build up to such a level that it becomes very difficult to move the column manually without straining the cross-arm (or the radiographer). If the floor track is cleaned regularly with a stiff narrow brush, both the radiographer and column will benefit.

20.5.3 Brakes and Locks

Properly used, a friction type brake or lock should be just sufficiently tightened to keep the equipment under control in its desired position. This type of lock is never intended to lock the bearing surfaces solid and should not be over-tightened. This does mean, of course, that the equipment can, and often is; moved against the hold of a friction lock, which much reduces its life, eventually reaching a situation where the lock does not hold at all and has to be replaced. The brakes fitted to bucky trays and tube rotational movements are the ones most susceptible.

20.5.4 Electrical Cables

On many mobile units and ceiling suspended tube columns, the horizontal tube arm can be rotated 360° around the vertical support. This does give the tube great mobility, but can lead to major problems with misuse. The H.T cables become badly entangled and can lead to cable fracture, especially if they are bent into a loop of less than 50 cm (18 ins.) diameter.

Electrical equipment should never be moved or pulled by its cable as the fracture of a wire, especially an earth wire, could result in accidents. It is also important that earthing connections are regularly checked in an X-ray room, particularly where E.C.G. machines, patient monitoring systems and cardiac syringes are used.

20.5.5 Accessory Equipment

In an X-ray department, accessory equipment such as cones, grids and cassettes often have to be carried from one place to another. All these items can sustain quite considerable damage if accidentaly dropped. Any such accident should be reported immediately, as continued use of the item, even though it shows only moderate damage, could cause serious problems. For example, a cassette which is only slightly distorted or has a broken catch, could quite easily become jammed in a serial changer, putting the whole examination room out of operation.

Secondary radiation grids are inherently delicate and complex in structure, despite their simple appearance. If a grid is dropped and is damaged, it may become inefficient radiographically or even dangerous; for cracks in a grid can simulate fracture lines in bone or non-existent fluid levels in the abdomen on the film. A damaged grid cannot be economically repaired.

20.5.6 Mobile Units

Very often mobile X-ray units are moved from one department to another by hospital porters. As they may not be aware of the rather fragile nature of the X-ray tube and various other components, it is essential that the last radiographer to use the apparatus ensures that all movements and cables are safely secured. If, for instance, the tube column rotational movement is not locked, the tube may swing out and hit a wall or door frame whilst the unit is in motion. This could easily result in the fracture of the tube insert.

Many mobile units are fitted with an electric motor drive, normally utilising a battery similar to that used in a car. The battery should be topped up regularly such that the electrolyte level is just above the plates. It should be kept fully charged so that the unit is ready for use.

Chapter 21

Electromedical Equipment in the X-Ray Department

21.0 Medical Electronic Apparatus in the X-ray Department

The introduction during recent years of routine open heart surgery and the upsurge of interest in organ transplants has introduced a whole new range of electronic equipment into the hospital. Much of this equipment is to be seen in the X-ray department. Thus medical electronic equipment is encountered being used in conjunction with X-ray equipment for two distinct reasons. Frequently it is employed to achieve a diagnostic result, for example, the electrocardiograph, direct blood pressure monitor and oximeter are used during cardiac catheterization procedures. Electronic equipment may also be included just to monitor or support the patient during long and hazardous investigations, for example, pulse monitors and automatic lung ventilators.

A study of the basic principles of this equipment will enable its operation in the X-ray department to be readily understood and will prevent the "special procedures room" from becoming a jungle of mysterious electronic apparatus.

21.1 Monitoring Equipment

By employing the term monitoring we imply those items of equipment which have no direct part in the diagnostic procedures, but are used solely to check the condition of the patient. Occasionally, it will be difficult to differentiate between monitoring and diagnostic equipment where their functions overlap. Generally, it may be said that the technical requirements of diagnostic equipment will be far greater than those for monitoring purposes alone, where an indication of the parameters is often sufficient.

21.2 Basic Monitors

The simplest form of monitoring is a pulse-rate meter. This consists of a small lamp placed against an extremity (usually the finger or ear lobe) together with a photocell (See Section 3.4 and 21 Fig. 1).

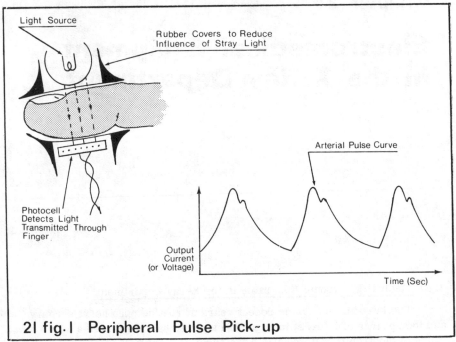

2l fig. l Peripheral Pulse Pick-up

The light is arranged to reach the cell after reflection under the skin or transmission through the periphery. Hence the light reaching the cell, and the electrical output from it, will vary according to the light absorbed by the volume of blood within the light path. The output will show the characteristic pulsations of the arterial pressure waveform and on some monitors will be displayed on an oscilloscope. The oscilloscope displays the amplitudes of the pulse waveform at any moment as a spot moves at a constant speed across the oscilloscope tube (called a cathode-ray tube or C.R.T). Several complete complexes may be shown if the C.R.T. screen is coated with a phosphor having a long persistence. (Note:- Here we are gainfully employing the principle of phosphorescence described in Section 3.5). By counting the peaks occurring over a few seconds, an average figure for the pulse-rate is obtained and displayed on a meter. Visual (and audible) high and low pulse-rate alarms are often added, either by using mechanical contacts on the pointer of the meter, or by way of electronic circuits set to compare reference voltages with a voltage produced by and proportional to the pulse-rate reading. The inclusion of a flashing light or audible bleep coincident with every pulse provides an indication of the heart rhythm.

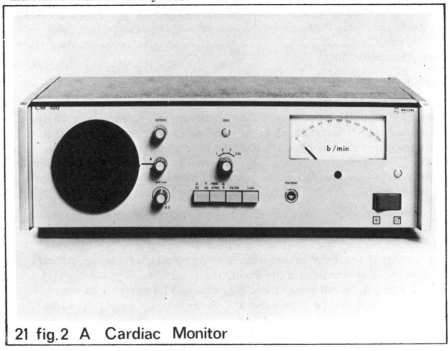

21 fig.2 A Cardiac Monitor

The concept of the basic monitor may be greatly extended by employing the patient's electrocardiogram (E.C.G.) as the input signal. Here the varying potentials produced by the heart during each cycle are detected by electrodes placed about the body and, after amplification, the waveform is displayed on the oscilloscope and used to derive a measurement of the heart rate. A more detailed account of the measurement of the E.C.G. is contained in the later section on diagnostic equipment (See Section 21.8). Equipment for detecting the occurrence of cardiac arrhythmia is also included in the section on E.C.G. measurements.

These two methods for detecting heart and pulse-rate differ in one important feature. The pulse-rate meter gives an indication of the blood circulation of the patient, while the E.C.G. is a measurement of the electrical activity of the heart. An E.C.G. waveform does not necessarily imply an effective circulation. Equipment is available to compare the E.C.G. with the pulse curve or arterial blood pressure waveform and indicate any deficit which may be present.

21.3 Temperature Measurement

The internal and skin temperatures may easily be measured by employing a thermistor probe. This simply comprises a piece of semi-conductor material (suitably encapsulated on the end of a cable) the electrical resistance of which is a simple function of its temperature. If, for example, a constant current is maintained through the thermistor, then an output voltage is obtained which is proportional to the resistance of the material (Ohm's Law). The output voltage obtained is therefore dependent on the temperature of the probe. For a small temperature range the relationship is almost linear and is amplified and corrected to give a truly linear meter reading.

21.4 Respiration Measurement

The respiration rate may be derived by a variety of techniques, but the simplest method also uses a thermistor probe. A thermistor having a short response time is placed in the air flow to and from the patient (i.e. the nasopharynx) to monitor the changes in temperature as cool air is inhaled and warm air expelled. By electrically counting the fluctuations over a period, the average respiration rate may be obtained and displayed on a meter, in a similar manner to the pulse-rate.

Other methods employed include :- switches attached to the thorax and operated by the expansion of the chest; the measurement of electrical impedence through the chest cavity where the resistance to the current varies with the pathway between the sensing electrodes; or the external impedence of a band across the chest, the resistance of which changes with its length. In all cases the signal obtained fluctuates with each respiration and may be processed to give the average respiration rate.

21.5 Electroencephalogram (E.E.G.)

The electroencephalogram is another measurement that may be encountered from time to time. The minute electrical signals originating in the various regions of the brain, up to about 200 μV ($\frac{1}{5000}$ Volt), are measured between pairs of electrodes attached to the scalp. Like the E.C.G., the signals are amplified and the waveform presented on an oscilloscope or paper chart. For full diagnostic procedures, 8 or even 16 different E.E.G. signals may be recorded simultaneously, but for monitoring purposes usually only 1 E.E.G. signal is taken together with the electrocardiogram (E.C.G.).

21.6 Indirect Blood Pressure Monitoring

Two basic methods exist for automated, indirect measurement of systolic and diastolic arterial blood pressures (these being the maximum and minimum pressures in the artery respectively). The first is an automation of the conventional cuff method and uses a microphone contained in the standard Riva - Rocci cuff to replace the doctors' stethoscope. The cuff is inflated to a pressure above systolic pressure and gradually leaked to atmosphere. The microphone detects the Korotkow sounds made as the blood passes down the brachial artery against the restraint of the cuff pressure. The first sound occurs as the cuff pressure nears the systolic arterial pressure, as blood just succeeds in pulsing under the cuff against the occluding pressure in the cuff. The sounds continue in rhythm with the heart beat until a characteristic change in tone occurs just before they fade away. The diastolic pressure is usually taken as the cuff pressure at the change of tone.

Automated systems based on the above principle frequently experience errors due to the microphone responding to ambient noise and to movement artefacts. It is also difficult to be certain of the diastolic tone change and one system is produced where the microphone output is printed out and the results visually interpreted.

The second important technique is based on the theory of pulse oscillometry, where pressure pulses in various segments of the human body are compared.

In the model shown in 21 Fig. 3 the measurement is made by a rheographic technique which is based on Ohm's Law. It will be remembered that in a conductor the Voltage (V) equals the product of the current (I) and the Resistance (R), (V = I x R). If the current is kept constant, the voltage across the conductor will be directly proportional to its resistance. As an example :-

1mA through a resistance of 1000 ohms = 1 volt across the resistance
1mA through a resistance of 3000 ohms = 3 volts across the resistance
(note 1mA = 0.001 Amps)

In this case, the constant current comes from a high frequency electric generator and travels through the arm between three electrodes fitted underneath a Riva-Rocci cuff (See 21 Fig. 3). The current is usually of the order of a few milliamps and a frequency of several hundred kHz. The blood flow in the artery causes variations in the conductivity of the arm under the cuff and consequently resistance changes occur between the electrodes. Since the electric current remains constant, voltage variations related to the heart beat appear at the outer electrodes, with respect to the centre, reference electrode.

The cuff is inflated automatically to a pressure at least 40 mm Hg above the expected systolic pressure and allowed to fall slowly by means of a leak to atmosphere. Voltage pulses will be obtained from the proximal (top) electrode while the cuff pressure is still above the systolic pressure, but no voltage pulses will be detected from the distal (lower) electrode until the cuff pressure has fallen to the systolic pressure. At this point, the arterial pressure will just overcome the occluding cuff pressure and blood will start to spurt through the occluded artery under the cuff, with each heart beat. Thus the first voltage pulse is detected from the distal electrode and a pointer, which falls with the cuff pressure, will then be held to indicate the systolic arterial pressure.

While the cuff pressure is intermediate between the systolic and diastolic pressures, the blood flow is restricted by the cuff. The voltage pulses from the distal electrode are consequently delayed by the occluding action of the cuff and occur fractionally after each pulse from the proximal electrode. As long as this "difference" signal is detected, a second pointer

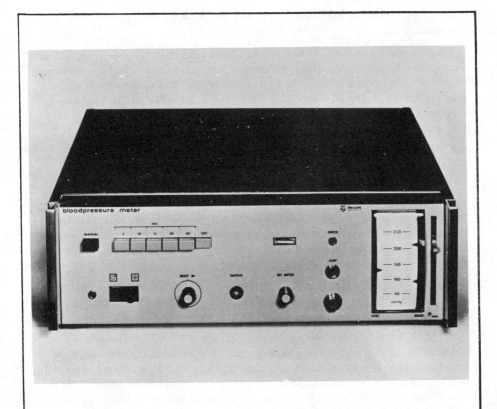

An indirect blood pressure meter operating on a rheographic principle

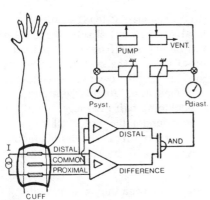

Principle of rheographic determination of systolic and diastolic blood pressure

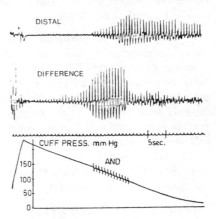

Electrode signals with AND–pulse series superimposed on pressure curve

21 fig.3 Indirect Blood Pressure Measurements

falls to the cuff pressure with each heart beat. When the cuff pressure equals the diastolic blood pressure, the arterial blood flow is no longer impeded by the cuff, and the voltage pulses from the proximal and distal electrodes become coincidental. Hence the difference signal rapidly disappears and the second pointer is stopped to indicate the diastolic blood pressure reading. After a lapse of about 3 seconds the cuff is completely deflated.

This method has several advantages in that :- it is more easily reproduced; the measurement is unaffected by ambient noise; and is less susceptible to motion artefacts or the patient being touched.

21.7 Direct Blood Pressure Monitoring

Here the pressure is recorded by directly connecting a measuring system with the blood in the arterial or venous system. This is usually achieved by inserting a fine bore catheter into the vessel and connecting it, either directly or via a connecting tube, to a pressure transducer and flushing system. A transducer is any device which converts an effect from one physical form to another, i.e. in this case, pressure into an electrical output. The hydraulic system so formed is completely filled with liquid, usually a saline solution to which Heparin has been added to avoid clotting, and this is infused into the patient through the catheter.

The transducer used comprises a diaphragm with the fluid system on one side; the other side, open to the atmosphere, has an electrical bridge network connected to it.

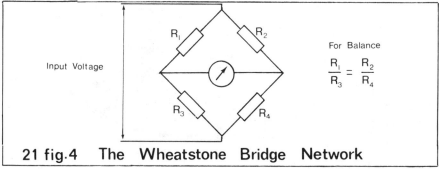

Input Voltage

For Balance

$$\frac{R_1}{R_3} = \frac{R_2}{R_4}$$

21 fig.4   The   Wheatstone   Bridge   Network

An electrical bridge network is shown in 21 Fig. 4 which consists of four resistive arms (Wheatstone Bridge). An A.C. or D.C. input voltage is connected across two opposite corners and the electrical output (or balance) of the bridge is measured across the other pair of corners. When all arms are of equal value no output reading will be obtained, but if the ratio of the arms is varied then the bridge is unbalanced and an output reading will be obtained. This arrangement is used for pressure transducers because it is a very sensitive measuring device. With equal pressures on both sides, the bridge is in balance and has zero output voltage. When a pressure difference is applied to the diaphragm, the resistance bridge attached to the diaphragm is unbalanced and an electrical voltage output, proportional to the pressure, is produced. An amplifier or electromanometer provides a meter reading and a signal for an oscilloscope display (or recording) of the pressure waveform.

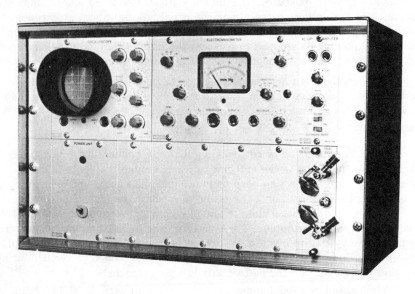

a)

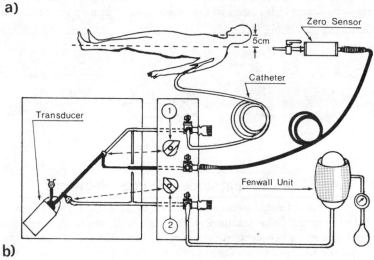

b)

The oscilloscope shown in (a) displays the blood pressure curve and
ECG simultaneously from the two modules on the right. The principle
of the transducer module (bottom right) is shown schematically in
(b). The top switch (1) enables either the catheter or the zero
reference sensor to be connected to the transducer. The lower switch
(2) enables 4ml/hr infusion rate through the catheter, from the
Fenwall pressure bag, to be increased after withdrawal of blood
samples.

21 fig. 5 Grandjean Microcatheter Apparatus

For arterial pressures the catheter used for monitoring purposes is normally about 10 cm. long and between 0.8 and 1.5 mm external diameter. It is usually inserted into the radial artery using the Seldinger's technique. The method is first to insert a needle into the artery and feed a guide wire (stilette) through the lumen of the needle. The needle is withdrawn over the stilette and replaced by the catheter. Lastly the stilette is removed and the catheter connected to the sterile manometer system.

For venous pressures the same system can be used but more frequently a long (90-130 cm.) "float" microcatheter is employed to give central venous pressure (CVP). The catheter is inserted through a needle and floats on the returning venous blood up and into the right side of the heart and may even be guided into the pulmonary artery (See 21 Fig. 6). The position of the catheter tip is monitored by observing the pressure waveform on the oscilloscope.

The purpose of these microcatheters is to enable the blood pressure to be monitored,but in addition blood samples may be removed for oxygen content determinations. It is not,however, possible to inject dyes through the fine bore of these catheters as is required in heart catheterization procedures for the detection of cardiac defects. Neither is it possible to monitor the pressures in the left side of the heart using microcatheters as these cannot float against the arterial pressure. See also Section (21.11).

21.8 Diagnostic Equipment - The Electrocardiograph

The electrocardiogram (E.C.G.) is a measurement of the electrical activity of the muscles forming the heart walls, as detected at convenient points on the body surface. It is necessary to give a brief description of the function of the heart if the E.C.G. is to be clearly understood.

21.8.1 The Heart

The heart can basically be described as a four chamber pump divided by the septum into two isolated parts, the right heart and the left heart. These form, with the arterial and venous systems, two distinct circuits around the body. (See 21 Fig. 6).

The left heart is the high pressure side, the left ventricle pumping freshly oxygenated blood around the body to all the organs and peripheries. The blood is returned from the organs to the right heart and pumped at much lower pressure to the lungs. The lungs exchange the carbon dioxide collected in the blood for oxygen and the blood passes on to the left heart for recirculation. The tricuspid valve between the chambers of the right heart and the mitral valve in the left heart ensure that blood does not flow in the wrong direction. There are also unidirectional valves at the entrances to the arteries to prevent blood returning to the ventricles.

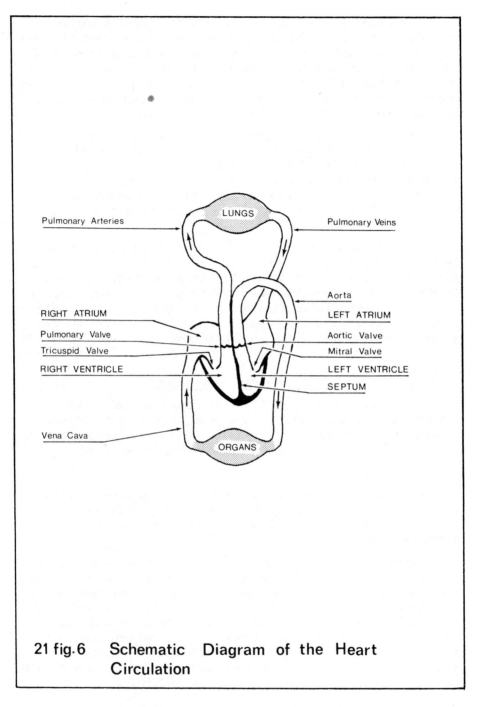

Pulmonary Arteries

LUNGS

Pulmonary Veins

Aorta

RIGHT ATRIUM

LEFT ATRIUM

Pulmonary Valve

Aortic Valve

Tricuspid Valve

Mitral Valve

RIGHT VENTRICLE

LEFT VENTRICLE

SEPTUM

Vena Cava

ORGANS

21 fig. 6   Schematic   Diagram   of   the   Heart
              Circulation

21.8.2 Generation of the E.C.G.

The electrical generation within the heart of the electrocardiogram will be briefly described with reference to the diagramatic representation of the E.C.G. shown in 21 Fig. 7.

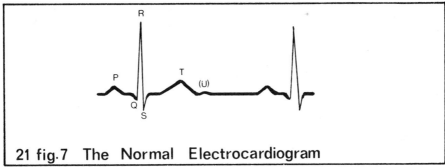

21 fig. 7   The   Normal   Electrocardiogram

The pumping action of the heart is normally started with a nerve impulse in the right atrium at a point called the Sinus Node. This impulse, electrical in nature, spreads out causing the activation of the muscles of both atria and gives rise to the P wave (duration 0.07 - 0.11 seconds) in the E.C.G. and the subsequent contraction of the atria. The contraction of the atria pumps blood into the ventricles.

The excitation wave passes from the atria through the Atrio-Ventricular Node and the "bundle of His" nerve pathway to the ventricles. This corresponds with a delay in the excitation of the ventricles and shows as a straight line close to the zero voltage (or isoelectric line) in the recording of the E.C.G. The normal delay (PR interval) is 0.10 - 0.20 seconds.

As soon as the excitation wave reaches the ventricles their activation, shown by the QRS complex, begins. This causes the ventricles to contract and force blood out into the aorta and pulmonary artery respectively. The duration of the QRS complex for a normal heart beat is between 0.05 and 0.10 seconds. It should be noted that either or both Q and S waves may be absent from the E.C.G.

The duration of QRS complex indicates the time required for activation of the ventricles and is followed in the normal heart by a return of the trace to the region of the isoelectric line. This is quickly followed by the T wave corresponding to the de-activation or repolarising of the ventricles.

The E.C.G. may also exhibit a low U wave following the T wave, the origin and significance of which is not clear.

21.8.3 Measurement of the E.C.G.

The patient is connected to the electrocardiograph via leads from electrodes attached to the body. The diagnosis of the electrocardiogram thus recorded is made by studying the shape of the waveform and time intervals observed in a series of standard "lead" configurations. Each "lead" is the voltage pattern measured between two active terminals with respect to a reference or "earth" terminal which is commonly attached to the right leg. The voltages measured at the extremities are nominally 1 mV ($\frac{1}{1000}$ Volt) and a differential amplifier is necessary to avoid interference, particularly that derived from the electrical supply (See Section 21.14).

The electrocardiograph (machine) may be encountered in many forms, each designed for its own particular application. The single channel battery unit is the most commonly encountered type and records one lead at a time. It can be seen in use in all parts of the hospital as well as in general practice. The E.C.G. voltage picked up from the patient is amplified over 1,000 times. The amplifier employed is called a differential amplifier, and is designed to cancel out interference signals (e.g. mains interference) to a large extent. Any signal which appears equally on both active electrodes is not amplified to any extent; only those signals where a difference voltage appears are amplified. Thus mains interference is reduced but not the assymmetrical interference due to muscle movement. The effects of different types of interference, likely to be encountered, are shown in 21 Fig. 8.

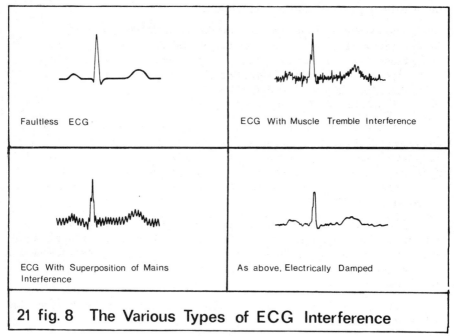

Faultless ECG

ECG With Muscle Tremble Interference

ECG With Superposition of Mains Interference

As above, Electrically Damped

21 fig. 8   The Various Types of ECG Interference

The amplified signal is next fed to a power amplifier which is used to drive the signal coil of the galvanometer, attached to which is the writing stylus. When a current flows in the coil, a magnetic field is produced which interacts with the field of a large permanent magnet. The force of

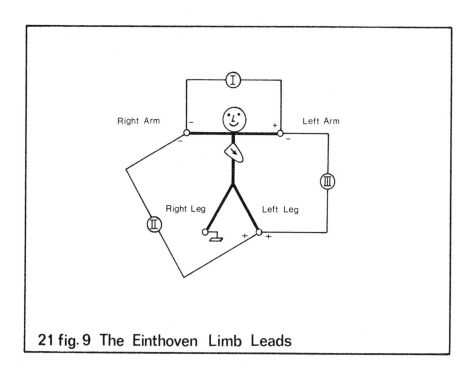

21 fig. 9 The Einthoven Limb Leads

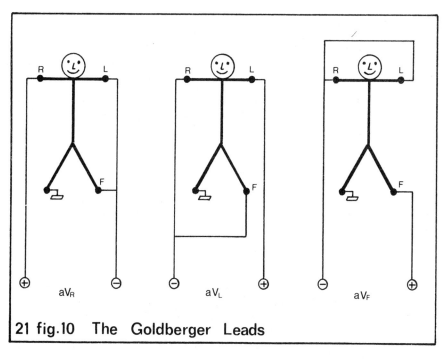

21 fig. 10 The Goldberger Leads

attraction (or repulsion) between these two fields results in the stylus being deflected. The permanent record is produced by heating the stylus to a faintly dull red heat and arranging for this to melt the white wax coating on a printed chart to reveal the black underlayer. The standard chart speed being 25 or sometimes 50 mm per second.

By careful design and the use of frequency correction it is possible to obtain a high standard of fidelity in the recording.

Multi-channel electrocardiographs are also popular in the larger hospitals. They are fundamentally similar in operation to the single channel instrument but enable two, three, or even six E.C.G. leads to be recorded simultaneously. They also offer the advantage of allowing several different parameters to be recorded together and time correlations to be made, for example, E.C.G., blood pressure curves, heart sound recordings. In the cardiac catheterization room the electrocardiograph may lose its identity and become a physiological monitor. This is a large monitoring console which contains all the electronic monitoring equipment together with large screen oscilloscopes and recorders. The recording may be made by a heated stylus, but other methods will also be seen, which include ultra-violet, photographic, ink and magnetic tape recording principles. The advantage of these latter types is their greatly extended high frequency response which ensures a more faithful representation of the original waveform. The great advantage of the heated stylus recorder is its technical simplicity and ease of use.

21.8.4 Einthoven Leads

These are the simplest lead configurations and the type most commonly encountered in monitoring situations. The Einthoven leads are defined as follows :-

Einthoven Lead I   Potential of Left Arm minus potential of Right Arm
Einthoven Lead II   Potential of Left Leg minus potential of Right Arm
Einthoven Lead III   Potential of Left Leg minus potential of Left Arm

Since the heart is usually in the direction shown in 21 Fig. 9, all the Einthoven leads normally show positive P, R and T complexes. This position of the heart generally causes Einthoven Lead II to exhibit the greatest amplitude and is normally used for routine monitoring applications. Clearly any deviation in the position of the main axis of the heart will be revealed by the Einthoven lead recordings.

21.8.5 Goldberger Leads

The Goldberger Leads, or augmented unipolar limb leads as they are also known, are derived as follows :- one of the three connections Right Arm (R), Left Arm (L) and Left Leg (F) is measured against the mean potential of the other two to give the three leads aVR, aVL and aVF respectively. Thus aVR is the potential of the Right Arm minus the potential of the Left Arm and Left Leg connected together. In the case of multi-channel electrocardiographs, the limbs are connected together by

100k ohms resistors to enable the three augmented leads to be recorded simultaneously without shorting one another out. Smaller resistors are usually retained in single channel units to cancel out the effects of imbalance in electrode impedances which would otherwise lead to errors in the tracings.

21.8.6 Wilson Leads

To record the Wilson precordial chest leads, the three active limb electrodes are connected together via resistors and used as a reference potential. An "Exploring" electrode is used to measure the potential at a series of well defined points around the heart on the chest wall, against the reference potential (See 21 Fig. 11) Six leads are normally recorded, V1 - V6, and with multi-channel machines these may also be recorded simultaneously.

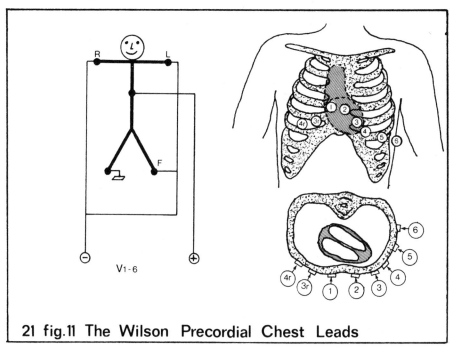

21 fig.11 The Wilson Precordial Chest Leads

In special examinations an electrode can be placed in the Oesophagus to obtain a reading very close to the left atrium, a point not accessible to the V leads. It is also possible to use catheters containing electrodes to record intracardiac leads from within the various heart chambers.

21.8.7 Cardiac Arrhythmias

This section on the detection of cardiac arrhythmias is strictly more appropriate to the sections on monitoring apparatus, but is included here for the sake of clarity. The normal E.C.G. waveform shown diagrammatically in 21 Fig. 7 is referred to as sinus rhythm, when the sinus node initiates the heart action. If however the heart muscle is damaged, say as the result of a recent coronary thrombosis, then all or some of the E.C.G. lead recordings will be distorted depending on the extent and position of the damage. Should the conducting pathways be affected, then the ventricles may cease to be triggered by the pulse originating at the sinus node, but may instead occasionally be precipitated by the AV node or another ventricular centre. This type of arrhythmia may indicate the onset of an important misfunction in the heart behaviour and consequently the principal forms of arrhythmia are constantly monitored on the "at risk" patient. The premature beat is clearly characterised by a reduction in the normal R to R interval. The ventricular premature beat or extrasystole is apparent by a gross widening of the QRS complex. Both types of arrhythmias can be monitored by comparing each complex with a series of stored reference heart beats and measuring the variation. It is also possible to indicate the occurrence of potentially dangerous runs of extrasystoles.

21.9 Phonocardiographs

Phonocardiography uses a microphone to record heart sounds and murmurs. Normal heart sounds are caused by the closing of the heart valves, the opening of the valves usually being inaudible. Two sounds are normally detected, the first heart sound corresponding with the closing of the valves between each atrium and ventricle as the latter contract. The second sound indicates the closing of the ventricle – artery valves when the arterial pressures exceed the ventricular pressures. In many heart conditions, for example valve stenosis (narrowing of the valve) and/or incompetence (a leaky valve), the heart sounds are modified and character-istic vibrations or murmurs are produced. Recording the heart sounds in relation to E.C.G. and blood pressure curves, etc., offers a powerful diagnostic tool, particularly in the case of defects of the heart valves.

To record the heart sounds a contact microphone containing a piezo-electric crystal element, which converts the mechanical sound vibrations into an electrical effect, is employed. It is held in contact with the chest wall (firmly but not too tight or the finer sounds and murmurs will be lost) using either a microphone stand or a rubber strap. The position of the microphone is generally between the apex and sternum, but good results are obtained directly on the sternum due to the efficient conduction of sound through the ribs, unless contra-indicated. The microphone output is amplified, filtered and then recorded on an electrocardiograph recorder. As an E.C.G. is normally required for comparison, and possibly a carotid or jugular pulse curve, a multi-channel machine having a high frequency response is used. For the high frequency sounds especially, the room must be very quiet (accoustically dead) as street noise and speech would also be recorded. The difficulty in recording the high frequencies is due to the low amplitude of these signals. Much useful information is contained in the high frequencies up to 350 Hz, detected by the microphone, but completely hidden by the very much greater amplitude of the lower frequencies. For example, the amplitude at 300 Hz is only 0.01% of the amplitude at 30 Hz. To enable this information to be observed a series of

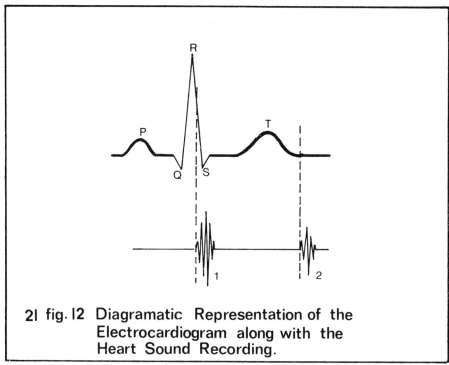

21 fig. 12 Diagramatic Representation of the Electrocardiogram along with the Heart Sound Recording.

high-pass filters are included, these cut-off the lower frequencies and leave only the high frequencies to be amplified.

The phonocardiograph is a very useful tool in diagnosing defects involving the heart valves, but is less effective in the case of septum defects, where it is normally necessary to resort to a radiographic procedure during cardiac catheterization. The two techniques are occasionally combined by the utilisation of special phonocatheters. These employ a special catheter having a rigid non-microphonic wall. A diaphragm at the end transmits the sound and conducts it through the air column to the microphone in the apparatus.

21.10 Pulse Wave Recording

Pulse curves are frequently recorded simultaneously with the phonocardiogram and electrocardiogram as a method of identifying the occurrence of events in the heart cycle. Thus the jugular venous pulse is used as a guide to events in the right side of the heart and the carotid arterial pulse when examining the left heart.

The technique of using a photo-electric pick-up to record peripheral arterial pulse curves for monitoring purposes was described in Section 21.2. The arterial pulse may also be detected by pick-ups employing a mechanical measuring technique, for example a compressible capacitor whose value is pressure dependent. To record a peripheral pulse a finger holder or strap is used to rigidly hold the capacitive pick-up in direct contact above the

363

artery. A constant polarising voltage is applied to the capacitor. Variations in the arterial pressure compress the capacitor and cause a change in the electrical output proportional to the pressure change. In recording arterial pulses closer to the heart, for example the carotid pulse, a bedstand is employed to position the pick-up, contact being made by an applicator.

The venous pulse in the jugular vein is frequently recorded by a photo-electric method so as not to damp the venous pressure changes. The pick-up is supported about 10 mm away from the skin. Light from its lamp is reflected from the area of skin superficial to the vein into the photocell.

The output of the venous or arterial pulse pick-up is fed to an A.C. amplifier prior to the recorder or display oscilloscope. The pulse curve obtained is representative of the pressure variations in the vessel (and heart chambers) but absolute measurements are not possible. To obtain the true blood pressure curves, catheterization is necessary.

21.11 Cardiovascular Catheterization

The technique of cardiac catheterization may be employed in conjunction with diagnostic X-ray equipment to investigate a wide range of heart and circulatory pathology. In most of these procedures, medical electronic equipment plays a major part in achieving the diagnosis.

Cardiac catheterization involves the insertion of catheters into the circulation and chambers of the heart. By employing radiopaque material in the construction of the catheters, these may be clearly visualised during fluoroscopy. The catheters, between 1 and 4 mm in diameter, are usually inserted into the artery by the Seldinger's technique   (see Section 21.7).

For catheterization of the right (venous) side of the heart, a vein in the arm is usually exposed and the catheter inserted. Heparin is added immediately to prevent clotting and the catheter is filled with saline or a similar solution to prevent the ingress of air. The saline also forms a convenient media for transmitting the blood pressure. The catheter is inserted in a vein and pushed via the superior vena cava into the right atrium under fluoroscopic control. It is possible to pass the catheter through the tricuspid valve into the right ventricle and on through the pulmonary valve to the pulmonary artery. If a septal defect exists the catheter can be passed through into the left heart. In the absence of a septal defect it is necessary to perform the more difficult left heart catheterization via a puncture of the femoral artery. Here the arterial pressures are much greater than those on the right side and since the direction of catheterization is against the blood flow, it is very easy to damage the heart valves if the passage through them is not correctly timed.

Having achieved a successful heart catheterization, a whole range of diagnostic procedures become possible. These are useful to confirm the results of the previously mentioned E.C.G. and phonocardiographic

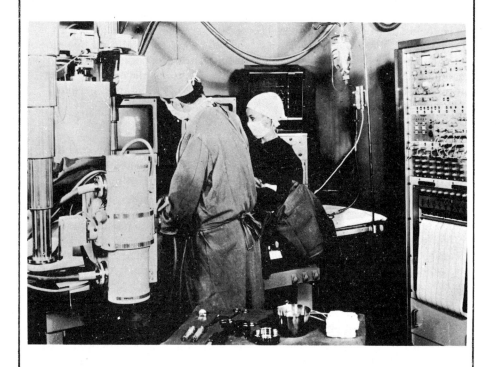

A cardiac examination room, containing a bi-plane installation with
image intensification, television and 35mm cine facilities.
On the right is the physiological monitoring console providing an
eight channel record of any of the following parameters; 2 direct
blood pressures, 6 ECG leads, 5 heart sounds, 2 EEG's a thermodilution
curve and the patients' temperature. In the rear is a remote multi-
channel oscilloscope display.

21 fig.13 A Cardiac Examination Room

examinations with which they may be combined. They are of particular value in investigating congenital abnormalities in children, holes between the heart chambers, valve defects and circulatory defects.

In Section 21.7 reference was made to the use of microcatheters for direct blood pressure measurements. Such catheters have a great value in monitoring central venous pressures, but cannot be used for investigations of the left heart. Cardiac catheters are much stiffer and can be positioned in the various heart chambers to enable the various blood pressure values and waveforms to be compared. The larger bore of the catheter allows a higher fidelity in the measurements, and offers the possibility of injection of dyes or the easy withdrawal of blood samples for analysis. Special catheters are also available to enable electrodes to be placed in the heart to record intra-cardiac E.C.G.'s or for the purpose of internal cardiac pacing (see Section 21.13.2).

21.11.1 Angiography

To determine the pattern of the blood flow around the heart and the condition of the heart valves a radiopaque dye can be injected into the heart via the catheter and its passage recorded by rapid serial films, cine fluorography, or video-tape recordings of the X-ray image. However, the injection of dye during the vunerable ascending T phase of the heart cycle can cause ventricular fibrillation, when the heart fails to pump blood effectively round the body. Consequently, the R wave of the E.C.G. is frequently used to trigger the injection after a pre-set delay, adjusted so as to avoid this vulnerable period. The special apparatus constructed for the purpose is the heart-phase trigger unit.

21.11.2 Cardiac Output

Cardiac catheterization permits a number of techniques for the determination of cardiac output by the Fick principle to be employed. All these measurements rely on the same basic principle. A known quantity of medium is injected into the right atrium and its concentration at a point downstream plotted on a graph against time. By calculating the area under the curve and applying the result to a formula, the cardiac output can be calculated, either by a tiresome manual calculation or more recently by employing a cardiac output computer. Three media are commonly available. The most frequent method involves the technique of dye-dilution. Cardio-Green or Evans-Blue dye is injected and the density measured downstream either via a second catheter or by employing an external photo pick-up if a further catheterization is not desirable.

The alternative methods are :- thermodilution, being the injection of saline at 4°C and measuring the blood temperature leaving the heart; or ascorbate dilution when vitamin C is injected and the hydrogen ion concentration measured downstream. Both these latter methods have the advantage that they avoid the recirculation characteristic of dye dilution. The cold saline and vitamin C are both rapidly absorbed and dissipated in the peripheral capillary blood vessels. Therefore it is possible to give a large number of injections (up to 50) in quick succession, which is not the case for dye techniques where recirculation and zero shifts, not to mention the colour of the patient, have to be allowed for.

In all these measurements it is also possible to confirm the existence of septal or circulatory defects, since the appearance of a premature recirculatory peak indicates the blood has taken a short cut in the circulation.

21.11.3 Oximetry

Cardiac catheterization permits the easy withdrawal of blood samples for analytical purposes, the most frequent of these in the X-ray department being oxygen content determinations.

The blood carries oxygen to all parts of the body, collecting on the way the carbon dioxide and other waste products of the body processes. In the alveolar sacs at the extremities of the two bronchial trees, the inspired gases in the lungs come into very close contact with the blood in the pulmonary capillaries. Consequently, it is possible for oxygen to be transferred across the dividing membrane from the air to the red blood cells and for carbon dioxide to be discharged to the air in the alveolar. The greater part of the oxygen in the blood is in loose chemical combination with a substance called haemoglobin (a part of the red blood cells) to form oxyhaemoglobin. A relatively small percentage of the oxygen is dissolved in the blood plasma.

The oxygen saturation of the blood is that percentage of the haemoglobin which has been converted to oxyhaemoglobin. The oxygen saturation of the blood returning to the left atrium from the lungs is commonly 95 - 98%,while that of blood going back to the lungs may typically be 60 - 80% (See 21 Fig. 14).

Oxygen saturation may be conveniently measured in the catheterization room by employing an oximeter. This method relies on the different absorption properties of haemoglobin and oxyhaemoglobin to light of different wavelengths.

The blood sample under test is brought into a cuvette and white light shone into the sample. This light, having passed through the blood, passes through monochromatic filters, each transmitting only one wavelength, and into photocells to measure the intensity transmitted at each wavelength. It is found that,at a wavelength of 805 nanometres (805 x 10^{-9} metres) the light absorption is independent of the quantity of oxygen in the blood. At this wavelength, which is in the infra-red region, haemoglobin and oxyhaemoglobin both have the same absorption factors. However,at other wavelengths,a difference in absorption occurs between these substances,this being a maximum at 650 nanometres (red light). Consequently, by taking a ratio of the output at 650 and 805 nanometres a reading is obtained which is dependent on the oxygen saturation of the blood. In many cases the instrument has to be calibrated for each patient as the output reading is also

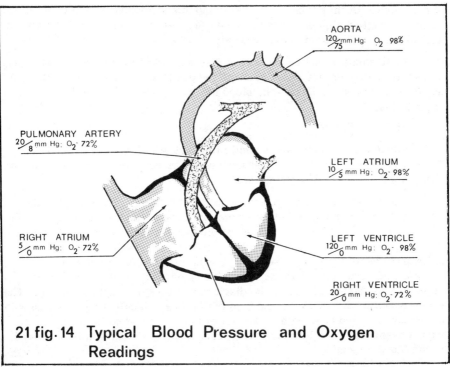

AORTA
$120/75$ mm Hg: O_2 98%

PULMONARY ARTERY
$20/8$ mm Hg: O_2^- 72%

LEFT ATRIUM
$10/5$ mm Hg: O_2 98%

RIGHT ATRIUM
$5/0$ mm Hg: O_2^- 72%

LEFT VENTRICLE
$120/0$ mm Hg: O_2^- 98%

RIGHT VENTRICLE
$20/0$ mm Hg: O_2^- 72%

21 fig. 14 Typical Blood Pressure and Oxygen Readings

dependent on other factors, such as haemoglobin concentration and the shape of the red blood cells. In one available model, the cuvette has been specially designed to eliminate the individual calibration for each patient, throughout the normal range of measurements, and thus provides a direct reading. A further feature is the incorporation of a second channel, also operating at 805 nanometres to obtain a measurement dependent on the concentration of haemoglobin and oxyhaemoglobin, but independent of oxygen saturation. This is used to provide an output reading for the total haemoglobin concentration expressed in grams per 100 millilitres. Both the oxygen saturation and the haemoglobin concentration may be measured with the cuvette connected to the catheter, the blood sample being returned to the patient (an in-vivo measurement). This instrument also has facilities for allowing dye dilution curves to be plotted.

Blood samples may be required for laboratory determinations of oxygen saturation, haemoglobin concentration and blood gas analysis, to obtain for example, the oxygen content (PO_2), carbon dioxide content (PCO_2), acidity (pH) and the concentration of potassium and sodium ions.

Note : The oxygen content PO_2 is a measurement based on the pressure exerted by a gas in solution as defined by Dalton's Law of partial pressures. This law states that the pressure of a gas in a mixture is identical with the pressure that gas would exert in isolation. When a gas is in contact with a liquid it will dissolve until the partial pressures reach a state of equilibrium. For example :- let us assume that the atmospheric pressure of dry air is 760 mm Hg. Atmospheric air contains about 21% oxygen but in the alveoli of the lungs this is down to around 14%. As PO_2 is always expressed in terms of dry air, we must compensate for the effect of water pressure,which is usually about 45 mm Hg.

Alveolar PO_2 $= \frac{14}{100}$ x (760 - 45) = 100 mm Hg.

The PO_2 of venous blood is typically 40 mm Hg and that of blood leaving the lungs 99 mm Hg.

21.12 Blood Flow Detectors

The presence of a blood flow may be detected in the X-ray department by subjecting the patient to an angiographic examination. It is also possible to use electronic monitoring equipment to confirm the existence of blood flow in a vessel. Two methods are commonly available and both allow a comparison of flow rates to be readily obtained.

One method involves the use of an electromagnetic detector, which consists of a magnet and an electric coil, encapsulated in an inert material to form a horseshoe-shaped probe. This is clipped over the exposed blood vessel so that the magnetic field cuts across the vessel, at right angles to the direction of blood flow. Now blood is an ionic fluid and the passage of these ions through the magnetic field causes a current, dependent on the flow rate, to be induced in the probes search coil. This current is amplified and used to provide an audible or visual output. This technique has the disadvantage that it is an invasive measurement.

The other technique is an ultrasonic application of the Doppler effect. Most readers will have heard the characteristic drop in frequency as a speeding train whistles past the observer. This effect is simply explained. Sound waves travel through any medium at a constant speed, the number of waves passing any one point being determined by the frequency of the sound. If however, the sound source has a motion relative to the medium,then there will either be an increase or a decrease in the number of waves passing the observer per second. Consequently the sound heard will have either a higher or lower frequency (pitch) dependent on the direction of the relative motion.

A similar effect occurs when the observer has a relative motion with respect to the medium, or when the sound waves are received after being reflected from a moving object; in this case a blood stream. The frequency of the reflected sound is dependent on the relative speed of the blood under the probe. Thus it is possible to check the blood flow through the skin, use being made of a gel to ensure a good acoustic coupling. The result is an indication of the blood flow, either as an amplified audible signal or as a graph.

21.13.0 Physical Therapy Equipment

We now come to those items of equipment which have a physical effect on the patient. When monitoring or measuring a phenomenon the intention is always to make the measurement with the least disturbance of the process being measured. For example,if a pretty nurse enters a room to record a reasonably healthy patient's pulse, then the reading may well be higher than it had been just a few moments before.

With therapy equipment the intention is just the opposite. Here, for example, a pacemaker may be used to control a patient's heart action and prevent the heart from beating too slowly. Conversely, the patient may be exercised to show a heart irregularity, enabling a firm diagnosis to be made The following sections describe various items of equipment of this type which may be found in the X-ray department.

21.13.1 Defibrillator

The defibrillator is a piece of equipment designed to give a large electric shock to the heart muscle, thus causing it to contract. There are two basic reasons for this action :- to restart the heart after a cardiac arrest, or to convert one heart rhythm to another.

Defibrillators encountered in the modern department will be of two types, depending on whether or not they are equipped with facilities for synchronising the time of application of the shock,with respect to the existing E.C.G. waveform. Those without this feature, the asynchronous defibrillators, are employed when no R-wave is present in the E.C.G. This would be the case for a patient in cardiac arrest or in ventricular fibrillation (a condition when the ventricles beat randomly and thus fail to pump blood effectively around the body). Since these conditions would both prove fatal,if the blood circulation to the brain and other essential organs is not restored within 3 to 4 minutes, a mains or battery operated asynchronous defibrillator is a vital part of the emergency "crash-cart" common to all large hospitals.

Frequently a patient develops an arrhythmia, perhaps following a coronary thrombosis, which although not directly life threatening may herald the onset of ventricular fibrillation. Hence, it is desirable to use drugs and/ or a defibrillator to convert the heart rhythm to a safer form, preferably normal sinus rhythm. In this case a recognisable ventricular contraction will exist and,therefore,a QRS and T wave pattern can be seen in the E.C.G. on the attached cardioscope. It has been shown by experience that a defibrillation shock applied to the heart during the "ascending T" period of the heart cycle, when the ventricles are repolarising, has a high probability of starting ventricular fibrillation. For this reason, cardio-version normally requires the use of a synchronous defibrillator. The application of the shock is then triggered by an R-wave, and applied to the patient either immediately, or after a delay, so as to avoid the critical period of the heart cycle shown by the "ascending - T"on the electrocardiogram. If no R-wave is detected, the shock may be arranged to be applied asynchronously as before. In more recent models, this can be arranged automatically, a feature that could be lifesaving in an emergency.

The shock can be administered by electrodes placed externally on the chest wall, or directly on the heart muscle during thoracic surgery. In a modern D.C. defibrillator a large capacitor is charged to a high potential, up to 7,000 volts for external defibrillation, and the energy stored (a maximum of 300 - 400 joules or watt seconds) discharged between electrodes applied to the chest wall. To prevent the patient receiving the added complication of burns, the electrodes must be in firm contact and electrode jelly is used to ensure a good conduction of the current. Usually the treatment is commenced with a lower energy value, this being increased for subsequent attempts if success is not achieved initially. When the chest wall is open then the shock may be given internally by electrode 'paddles' applied directly to the heart muscle, the energy required then being much less.

It should be added that defibrillators can be lethal weapons unless care is taken to ensure that attendant staff do not receive an accidental shock, through contact with the patient, during treatment. If, however, the instructions supplied are followed, no danger should arise.

21.13.2 Cardiac Pacemakers

Cardiac pacemakers are employed when a disruption of the normal conductive pathways, between the atria and the ventricles, causes an interruption of the normal heart rhythm. For example, in heart block, the ventricles beat at a lower rate than the atria. By applying a small, repetitive shock the ventricles can be made to contract and pump blood around the body at the desired rate.

Thus the simplest form of pacemaker is a device to deliver a current pulse, lasting a few milliseconds at a pre-set rate, between two electrodes. Both the number of pulses per minute and the current amplitude are adjustable, the maximum current available depending on whether external or internal electrodes are being employed. Pre-set, fixed-rate pacing (sometimes referred to as a manual or free-running mode of operation) has its main application for short term emergency use and for implantation in cases of irreversible complete heartblock. In the latter case, the impulse is applied to the muscles of the ventricles, either via catheter electrodes embedded inside the heart (intramural electrodes), or via electrodes stitched to the walls of the hearts' ventricles (epicardial electrodes). The pacemaker is inserted in the thorax or abdominal cavity and will of course be clearly visible on chest radiographs.

The external pacemaker is usually battery operated and employs an isolated output circuitry to ensure maximum patient safety. With internal electrodes making direct contact with the heart, a small patient leakage current could cause a serious cardiac arrhythmia (see Section 21.14).

An inherent disadvantage of the fixed rate pacemaker appears if heart conduction returns and the pacemaker pulses compete with the natural heart pulses. Here a pacemaker pulse may occur in the vulnerable "ascending T" period of the heart cycle and cause the heart to go into ventricular fibrillation. This is overcome by employing a variable rate, or 'on-demand', ventricular pacemaker for this class of patient. In the 'on demand' pacemaker, the natural R-wave inhibits the pacemaker and pulses are only generated when the time between successive R-waves exceeds the rate setting on the pacemaker. The pacemaker is inhibited by the presence of an R-wave, but may interpret a series of interference pulses as R-waves and fail to stimulate a heart which is not functioning. As patients may be encountered in the X-ray department with implanted, on-demand pacemakers, care should be exercised as high powered X-ray equipment may well interfere with the operation of the pacemaker and inhibit normal pacing of the patient.

A recent improvement which overcomes this problem is the QRS - synchronised pacemaker. In the case of normal heart action, this type is triggered by each R-wave and delivers a pulse just after the normal R-wave in the refractory phase of the heart cycle, when the heart is irresponsive to the additional electric current. In the event of a high frequency interference, the pacemaker is not inhibited by the interference pulses, but instead runs at a maximum rate of about two a second. In the absence of normal conduction, the pacemaker runs at a pre-set minimum heart rate.

21.13.3 Patient Ventilators

The prime purpose of artifical patient ventilation is to take over, or to assist,the natural respiratory effort of the patient when this either ceases or is insufficient. Basically, the Intermittent Positive Pressure Ventilator may be considered as an automated bag squeezer connected to the upper airway of the patient. Air, or another gas mixture, is forced into the lungs alveoli so that the oxygen may be collected by the blood and transported to the body cells to be exchanged for carbon dioxide waste. (see Sections 21.8.1 and 21.11.3). The connection to the patient can be made via an endotracheal tube or a tracheotomy tube directly into the trachea. The latter method is to be preferred for prolonged ventilation as the patient's mouth and vocal cords remain unobstructed, thus reducing the risk of ulceration of the throat.

The various types of ventilators may conveniently be characterised by specifying a number of their design features, although many of the more sophisticated models will cross these divisions.

The change from inspiratory to expiratory phase is initiated by one of three conditions depending on whether the ventilator is Time, Volume or Pressure cycled. In Time cycling, the inspiration and expiration times are set either independently or jointly adjusted in a fixed ratio (usually 1:2), the respiration rate consequently being determined at the same moment. In Volume cycling,the change from inspiration to expiration occurs when a pre-set volume has been delivered to the patient, and in Pressure cycled ventilators when the gas in the trachea reaches a pre-set pressure value.

Five main parameters are involved in the artificial ventilation of a patient. They are :-

Minute Volume   - the total gas supplied to the patient in one minute.
Tidal Volume   - the total gas supplied to the patient in each breath.
Inspiration Pressure - usually taken as the airway pressure at the end of inspiration.
Ventilation Rate   - the number of breaths per minute.
Compliance   - a measure of the elasticity of the lungs and chest wall.

These five parameters are related by the following equations :-

Minute Volume   = Tidal Volume x Respiration Rate.
Tidal Volume   = Inspiration Pressure x Compliance.

As the compliance is generally a quantity determined by the patient, only two independent variables need to be set. If for example, the minute volume and respiration rate (i.e. inspiratory and expiratory times) are set, then the tidal volume and inflation pressure are also determined for that patient, unless the compliance of the patient varies.

The ventilator may incorporate a trigger control. When this is switched on and the patient tries to breath spontaneously, then at a set suction pressure the machine automatically switches to inspiration. Ventilators designed specifically for this purpose are referred to as "Assistors". Another group of ventilators have a pre-set minute volume and are referred to as "Minute Volume Dividers". Once the minute volume has been set any change in respiration rate will effect the tidal volume,but not the total gas volume delivered to the lungs per minute. Lastly, the ventilator may include a negative phase control to assist the expiration of air from the lungs by applying a slight negative phase during expiration.

21.13.4 Exercise Equipment

Many patients present at the hospital with heart defects which are only apparent during stress. It is then necessary to carry out the examination during or immediately following a period of exercise. In the E.C.G. department, use may be made of a small set of stairs or a treadmill, but these methods are difficult to quantify and are not suitable for the catheterization room. Here it is possible to use an "Ergometer", this being a stationary bicycle which can even be mounted on the X-ray table. The patient pedals against the braking load of either a friction or an electromagnetic brake. The latter has the great advantage that it allows full control of the load applied to the patient and real quantitative measurements can be made.

21.13.5 Muscle Stimulators

Muscle stimulators may occasionally be encountered in the X-ray department. They are used to give a small electric shock to the muscle and thus to test the depth of anaesthesia and the effectiveness of muscle relaxant drugs. (Note. Electromyography is the measurement of muscle potentials).

21.14 Patient Safety

The need for regular maintenance of the equipment has been stressed in Chapter 20. This is particularly the case when medical electronic equipment is being used in direct contact with the heart, as even very small leakage currents (of the order of 50 microamps) through the heart muscle can cause dangerous fibrillation. Consequently, in the catheterization room, all metalwork within about 2 metres of the patient must be at the same earth potential. Any portable equipment must, likewise, be properly connected to a 3 pin mains socket. If special mains sockets have been provided for medical electronic equipment,they should always be employed.

Some of the latest types of equipment are provided with special circuits to isolate the patient,even during fault conditions, but nevertheless every precaution should be observed.

Closely associated with safety is the problem of interference. Interference, especially on the E.C.G., is likely if unshielded mains cables or high voltage cables are close to the patient or monitoring cables. Interference is also likely if the E.C.G. electrodes are not applied correctly. However, if the room and equipment are correctly maintained and due care taken with their use, good results should always be possible.

21.15 Equipment in the Operating Theatre

A wide range of diagnostic equipment has now been discussed. In the well equipped operating theatre and special radiological procedures room this equipment will play an important role in aiding the medical team to make a diagnosis,or to care for the patient.

Today, X-ray and medical electronic apparatus is specially designed for use in the operating theatre to ensure that the sterile conditions are maintained and that the limited space around the patient is used to maximum advantage. Sterilisable handles or covers for the controls are provided where necessary. Ceiling mounted apparatus is available so that the floor area around the operating table is free for the surgical team,or other equipment which has to be introduced.

Electrical leads, which have to be connected to electrodes or transducers on the patient, are often routed away from the surgical area via an underfloor duct or an overhead boom alongside the pipes carrying anaesthetic gases and suction facilities.

In modern suites, a monitoring room may be incorporated so that patients' physiological and radiological data from several operating rooms can be monitored or recorded centrally. This ensures efficient use of the wide range of apparatus which has to be employed. T.V. monitors or oscilloscopes in the individual theatres display information on the patient's condition.

21.16 Electronics in the Service of Medicine

We have now seen how it is possible to convert effects from one physical form into another. For example, it is possible to use an electrical stethoscope to listen to the amplified and filtered heart sounds. Why go to all this trouble? We could have listened to the patient's heart sound directly. The answer lies in the flexibility one gains by converting physical effects into an electrical signal. We can process the information for recording, transmission and remote display. Transducers are available which can convert mechanical displacement or stress, light, heat, pressure, sound, liquid level, humidity, weight or speed into an electrical output. Once such electrical signals have been obtained it is possible to process them in a variety of ways. Information or physiological data can be superimposed on the radiographic image displayed on a T.V. Monitor. Data can be transmitted to a neighbouring department or distant hospital for specialist advice or student instruction. It can be fed to a computer for overall assessment of the patient's condition based on a whole range of information.

In conclusion, it may be interesting, having discussed some of the problems which have been delegated to machines, to glance into the future. One problem which has not been solved and which presents major technological difficulties is pattern recognition.

To understand the problem it is necessary to draw attention to something we all do everyday and yet do not understand how it is achieved. Undoubtedly this morning you greeted one of your friends. It may have been by his face that you were able to recognise him. In general terms, you recognised a pattern. To read an electrocardiograph or a radiograph also requires pattern recognition and this is not an easy task for a machine. To release the medical specialist to deal with other medical problems, will require that in future these tasks are left to a machine to provide an automatic diagnosis. Already an E.C.G. machine has been constructed which can offer certain limited diagnostic suggestions. Document readers have been developed,but they have difficulty in reading ordinary, printed letters. Generally, the characters must be in magnetic ink and of a special shape. The machine cannot yet adapt itself to read handwriting of various styles. We can,however,read text in capital letters or gothic print, containing even major errors, and draw the correct conclusions.

Pattern recognition in reading a radiograph is a very complex process conducted by the brain. The radiograph may contain an error, such as a thumb print introduced during processing, which has to be ignored. To teach a machine this technique is a formidable task. All we can say at present is that research is being conducted on the problem and that one day the electronics industry may provide a solution,in the form of another machine in the service of the medical world.

Index

379